Atlas of Endoscopy with Narrow Band Imaging

Manabu Muto • Kenshi Yao • Yasushi Sano
Editors

Atlas of Endoscopy with Narrow Band Imaging

Springer

Editors
Manabu Muto
Department of Therapeutic Oncology
Kyoto University Graduate School
of Medicine
Kyoto
Japan

Yasushi Sano
Gastrointestinal Center, Sano Hospital
Kobe
Japan

Kenshi Yao
Department of Endoscopy
Fukuoka University Chikushi Hospital
Chikushino
Japan

This English translation is based on the Japanese original, M.Muto, K.Yao, Y.Sano
The Atlas of Endoscopy with Narrow Band Imaging
Published by Nankodo Co.,Ltd.

ISBN 978-4-431-54242-1 ISBN 978-4-431-54243-8 (eBook)
DOI 10.1007/978-4-431-54243-8

Library of Congress Control Number: 2015940409

Springer Tokyo Heidelberg New York Dordrecht London

Printed on acid-free paper

Springer Japan KK is part of Springer Science+Business Media (www.springer.com)

Foreword

It is my recollection that I dreamed of quantitative color analysis in the mid-1980s. At that time, we saw a rapid increase in flat nonulcerated early gastric cancers (gastritis-like early gastric cancers), and it became increasingly important to detect small changes in color or elevation. Our only available response was to "biopsy any suspicious lesions to confirm". In 1989, we received research funding for the First Comprehensive 10-year Strategy for Cancer Control and attempted to develop a colorimetry-capable dot sequential electronic endoscope at the National Cancer Center Hospital, in collaboration with Toshiba Medical Systems Corp. and the Oyama Research Department of the Tokyo Institute of Technology. This resulted in 1993 in a prototype capable of displaying the color of the target area as a coordinate on a color map using an algorithm. It was unable to identify cancer-specific colors, however, and we had to conclude that it had no clinical usefulness.

The reason for this was thought to be an insufficient quantity of information. Accordingly, as part of the Second Comprehensive 10-year Strategy for Cancer Control commencing in 1994, at the National Cancer Center Hospital East, in collaboration with Olympus Medical Systems Corp. and the Oyama Research Department of the Tokyo Institute of Technology, we first developed a spectrometer capable of endoscopic colorimetry, then collated spectrometric data concerning early cancers and noncancerous regions in the upper and lower gastrointestinal tract. Analysis of a large volume of textbook data from over 2,000 cases enabled differentiation between cancerous and noncancerous regions as groups, but it could not be applied at all to individual lesions, and this study reached an impasse after less than 5 years. It was Mr. Kazuhiro Gono, involved in this project on the Olympus side, who thought at that time, based on the fact that although the spectrometric pattern was different in each patient, the difference between the cancerous and noncancerous regions occurs within a narrow spectral range and that cancer screening might be possible using a narrow band filter. He photographed his own oral mucosa using a narrow band filter, finding that the surface microstructure was brought into particularly sharp relief when viewed through a short wavelength (blue light) filter. This was in December of 1999, as the end of the year drew close.

With patient consent, we promptly commenced clinical photography. At that time, however, we had no choice but to use monochromatic imaging, so at first we had no idea what we were seeing. Subsequently, we made rapid progress through basic studies and improvements in equipment (introduction of frame sequential pseudocolor imaging). Drs. Manabu Muto and Yasushi Sano, two of the editors of this atlas, worked on the clinical application of this method in examining pharyngeal and esophageal lesions, and colorectal lesions, respectively. They made steady progress in elucidating the mechanisms of observed phenomena and confirmed the usefulness of NBI through a number of clinical trials. Furthermore, for gastric lesions, where at first it was difficult to understand the NBI findings or discern any clinical benefits, the revolutionary approach by Dr. Kenshi Yao and his magnifying endoscopic methods made it possible to establish the diagnostic power of NBI.

In this way, with the publication of this atlas, edited by three pioneers involved in the development of NBI since the beginning, we can see that the contents are full of both a deep affection for this method and an understanding of its limitation. Reading this atlas, with its emphasis on actual cases, we are at first drawn to the beautiful images, but the structure is also practical, with thorough but concise explanations. This is an essential text for the endoscopist, of great interest to both the beginner just commencing NBI and to the experienced specialist. NBI can also be referred to as microangiography, as seen from the mucosal surface. Capillaries are found in every part of living organisms, so we anticipate clinical applications for NBI in many areas apart from gastroenterology, including examinations of the bronchi, bladder, uterine cervix, and also the retina. Accordingly, studies of the use of NBI in diagnosing disorders of the gastrointestinal tract have the potential to pave the way for a variety of future clinical applications, not confined to cancer detection alone. In anticipation of further deepening of these studies, it is my heartfelt wish that, with continual revisions, this atlas should become the “eternal textbook” in this field.

On a personal note, the resurrection of the experimental apparatus developed for the First Comprehensive 10-year Strategy for Cancer Control, as the Fuji Intelligent Chromo Endoscopy system in association with the discovery of NBI, was a great relief for me as one involved in the early stages. On reflection, it is somewhat ironic that our research, commenced with a vision of colorimetry (quantification of color tone), should abandon natural light and end up with endoscopic evaluation dependent on specific wavelengths. Nevertheless, reading this atlas will leave you in no doubt as to the great potential of examination using specific wavelengths.

I wish the authors all the best as they make further progress in their research in their respective areas, and I am pleased to recommend this atlas to anyone interested in the field of endoscopy with narrow band imaging.

Aomori, Japan Shigeaki Yoshida, MD

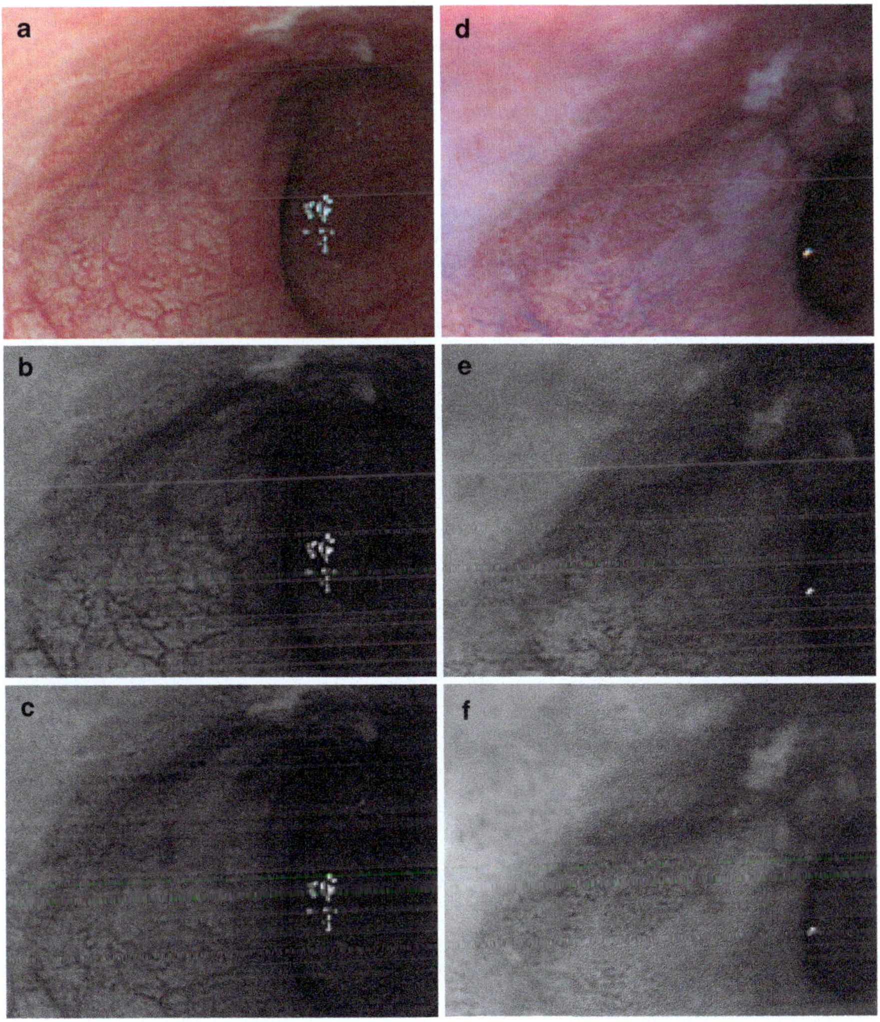

Prototype NBI photos (esophageal cancer: type 0-IIc): (**a**) standard filter, (**b**) green light filter, (**c**) blue light filter, (**d**) NBI filter, (**e**) green light filter, and (**f**) blue light filter

Preface

I believe that narrow band imaging (NBI) will soon become an essential modality of endoscopic examinations. During the planning discussions for this atlas, my fellow editors Dr. Kenshi Yao and Dr. Yasushi Sano and I were in agreement on the following three points: "The photos should be clear and easy to understand", "Diagnoses should be simple and reproducible", and "Explanations should be concise and easy to understand". You can also see from the layout design that this atlas was produced with these three principles in mind. Considering the size of this book, we aimed for something compact that could easily be taken into the endoscopy room. It is my recollection that it took less than 30 min to decide on these concepts.

In terms of content, we planned to present characteristic images of individual lesion types, based on the principles of NBI. The three authors are Dr. Sano, who has been involved in the development of NBI from the beginning and has studied the diagnosis of early colorectal cancer using magnifying endoscopy with narrow band imaging (M-NBI); Dr. Yao, who early on identified vascular abnormalities in early gastric cancers and has advanced the diagnosis of early gastric cancer using M-NBI; and I, working with Dr. Sano from the beginning in the development of NBI, and also studying risk factors for squamous cell carcinoma of the head and neck and esophagus, working towards methods of early detection.

NBI works best in combination with magnifying endoscopy, high-vision endoscopy, and high-vision monitors. Accordingly, wherever possible we have included photographs taken under these optimum conditions. We anticipate that the information in this volume, although it demonstrates that NBI is an advanced diagnostic modality, will be readily accessible to all new endoscopists, and not only to specialist gastroenterologists.

NBI can be said to have revolutionized the field of diagnostic endoscopy. One reason is that it enables a more objective assessment of a lesion. Along with improvements in the diagnostic ability of endoscopic examinations and training in endoscopic diagnosis, this provides considerable benefits for patients undergoing endoscopy. On the other hand, at the present time we still hear some endoscopists complain that they do not know how to use NBI or assess lesions. We have been very particular in presenting simple and easy-to-understand diagnoses with the aim of answering these complaints.

We cannot discuss the development of NBI without mentioning Dr. Shigeaki Yoshida (Medical Director Emeritus, National Cancer Center Hospital East, and

Aomori Prefectural Hospital Business Manager), Professor Hisao Tajiri (Jikei University School of Medicine), and Mr. Kazuhiro Gono (Olympus Medical Systems). NBI is unmistakably the successful product of industry–university joint research, from basic research to clinical application, with clear clinical significance. Following the development of NBI, we can expect more early gastric cancers to be detected. It can be considered a revolutionary technique that will save many people from suffering associated with cancer. The usefulness of NBI is now under wide scrutiny, not just in the field of gastroenterology, but also for the head and neck and bronchi, and in gynecology and urology. We anticipate that NBI will also prove useful in other fields in the future.

Kyoto, Japan Manabu Muto

Contents

Contributors

Takaya Aoki (Chaps. 16.6, 16.7), Department of Gastrointestinal Medicine, Makino Memorial Hospital, Kanagawa, Japan

Nobuo Aoyama (Chap. 15.4), GI Endoscopy and IBD Center, Aoyama Clinic, Kobe, Japan

Hideaki Arima (Chap. 3.5), Arima Surgical-Gastrointestinal Clinic, Chiba, Japan

Miwako Arima (Chap. 3.5), Department of Gastroenterology, Saitama Cancer Center, Saitama, Japan

Hisashi Doyama (Chaps. 9.7, 10.3, 10.9, 10.14, 12.1, 12.2, 12.3), Department of Gastroenterology, Ishikawa Prefectural Central Hospital, Kanazawa, Japan

Yasumasa Ezoe (Chaps. 5.1, 5.2, 5.3, 5.4), Department of Multidisciplinary Cancer Treatment, Kyoto University Graduate School of Medicine, Kyoto, Japan

Kougi Fu (Chap. 15.3), Kamma Memorial Hospital, Nasushiobara, Japan

Takahiro Fujii (Chap. 16.3), Department of Gastroenterology, Takahiro Fujii Clinic, Tokyo, Japan

Takahiro Fujimori (Chap. 16.15), Department of Pathology, Shinko Hospital, Kobe, Japan

Junko Fujiwara (Chap. 6.24), Department of Endoscopy, Tokyo Metropolitan Komagome Hospital, Tokyo, Japan

Kenichi Goda (Chaps. 3.3, 5.9, 5.10, 5.11, 6.21, 6.22, 6.23), Department of Endoscopy, The Jikei University School of Medicine, Tokyo, Japan

Santa Hattori (Chap. 16.15), Gastrointestinal Center, Sano Hospital, Kobe, Japan

Kazuhiro Gono (Chap. 1). R&D Planning Division, Olympus Medical Systems Corporation, Hachioji, Japan

Tomomasa Hayashi (Chap. 3.2), Department of Therapeutic Oncology, Kyoto University Graduate School of Medicine, Kyoto, Japan

Reiji Higashi (Chap. 16.1), Department of Internal Medicine, Hiroshima City Hospital, Hiroshima, Japan

Takahiro Horimatsu (Chaps. 16.4, 16.5), Department of Gastroenterology and Hepatology, Kyoto University Graduate School of Medicine, Kyoto, Japan

Masahiro Ikegami (Chaps. 5.9, 5.10), Department of Pathology, The Jikei University School of Medicine, Tokyo, Japan

Hiroaki Ikematsu (Chaps. 16.12, 16.16, 16.19), Division of Digestive Endoscopy and Gastrointestinal Oncology, National Cancer Center Hospital East, Kashiwa, Japan

Haruhiro Inoue (Chaps. 3.4, 6.2, 6.3), Digestive Disease Center, Showa University Koto Toyosu Hospital, Tokyo, Japan

Mineo Iwatate (Chap. 16.10), Gastrointestinal Center, Sano Hospital, Kobe, Japan

Chikatoshi Katada (Chaps. 16.3, 16.14), Department of Gastroenterology, Kitasato University School of Medicine, Sagamihara, Japan

Atsushi Katagiri (Chap. 16.11), Department of Gastroenterology, Showa University School of Medicine, Tokyo, Japan

Masahito Kotaka (Chap. 16.9), Gastrointestinal Center, Sano Hospital, Kobe, Japan

Shinei Kudo (Chap. 16.8), Digestive Disease Center, Showa University Northern Yokohama Hospital, Yokohama, Japan

Hirohisa Machida (Chaps. 9.10, 14.1, 14.2, 15.1, 15.2, 16.17), Machida Gastroenterical Hospital, Osaka, Japan

Takahisa Matsuda (Chap. 16.2), Endoscopy Division, National Cancer Center Central Hospital, Tokyo, Japan

Kumiko Monma (Chaps. 6.7, 6.8, 6.11, 6.18, 6.24), Department of Endoscopy, Tokyo Metropolitan Komagome Hospital, Tokyo, Japan

Shuko Morita (Chaps. 6.4, 6.5, 6.6, 6.10, 6.17), Department of Gastrointestinal Medicine, Kobe City Medical Center General Hospital, Kobe, Japan

Manabu Muto (Chaps. 2.1, 2.2, 3.1, 4, 5.5, 5.6, 5.7, 5.8, 6.1, 6.9, 6.19, 6.20), Department of Therapeutic Oncology, Kyoto University Graduate School of Medicine, Kyoto, Japan

Takashi Nagahama (Chaps. 10.16, 10.17), Department of Gastroenterology, Fukuoka University Chikushi Hospital, Chikushino, Japan

Takashi Narabayashi (Chap. 15.5), Department of Gastroenterology, Narabayashi Hospital, Kobe, Japan

Hogara Nishisaki (Chap. 16.18), Department of Gastroenterology, Hyogo Prefectural Kaibara Hospital, Hyogo, Japan

Masakazu Nishishita (Chap. 16.13), Department of Gastroenterology, Nishishita Gastrointestinal Hospital, Osaka, Japan

Shoko Ono (Chap. 10.18), Division of Endoscopy, Hokkaido University Hospital, Sapporo, Japan

Yasuhiro Ono (Chaps. 16.12, 16.16, 16.19), Division of Digestive Endoscopy and Gastrointestinal Oncology, National Cancer Center Hospital East, Kashiwa, Japan

Yutaka Saito (Chaps. 16.6, 16.7), Endoscopy Division, National Cancer Center Central Hospital, Tokyo, Japan

Taku Sakamoto (Chap. 16.2), Endoscopy Division, National Cancer Center Central Hospital, Tokyo, Japan

Yasushi Sano (Chaps. 2.5, 2.6, 13.1, 13.2, 14.3), Gastrointestinal Center, Sano Hospital, Kobe, Japan

Wataru Sano (Chap. 16.9), Gastrointestinal Center, Sano Hospital, Kobe, Japan

Masahiro Tada (Chap. 3.5), Cancer Treatment Center, Sainokuni Higashiomiya Medical Center, Saitama, Japan

Hisao Tajiri (Chaps. 3, 5.11, 6.21, 6.22, 6.23), Department of Gastroenterology and Hepatology, The Jikei University School of Medicine, Tokyo, Japan

Shinji Tanaka (Chaps. 3.5, 13.2), Department of Endoscopy, Hiroshima University Hospital, Hiroshima, Japan

Noriya Uedo (Chaps. 9.2, 9.6, 10.8, 10.13), Department of Gastrointestinal Oncology, Osaka Medical Center for Cancer and Cardiovascular Diseases, Osaka, Japan

Toshio Uraoka (Chap. 16.1), Department of Gastrointestinal Medicine, Tokyo Medical Center, Tokyo, Japan

Yoshiki Wada (Chap. 16.8), Department of Gastroenterology and Hepatology, The Tokyo Medical and Dental University School of Medicine, Tokyo, Japan

Kenji Watanabe (Chaps. 16.13, 16.14), Department of Gastroenterology, Osaka City University Graduate School of Medicine, Osaka, Japan

Hirokazu Yamagami (Chap. 16.14), Department of Gastroenterology, Osaka City University Graduate School of Medicine, Osaka, Japan

Yoshinobu Yamamoto (Chap. 16.18), Department of Gastrointestinal and Hepato Biliary Oncology, Hyogo Cancer Center, Akashi, Japan

Tomonori Yano (Chaps. 6.12, 6.15, 6.16), Division of Digestive Endoscopy and Gastrointestinal Oncology, National Cancer Center Hospital East, Kashiwa, Japan

Kenshi Yao (Chaps. 2.3, 2.4, 7, 8, 9.1, 9.3, 9.4, 9.5, 9.8, 9.9, 10.1, 10.2, 10.4, 10.5, 10.6, 10.7, 10.10, 11, 12.4), Department of Endoscopy, Fukuoka University Chikushi Hospital, Chikushino, Japan

Shigeaki Yoshida (Foreword), Aomori Prefectural Central Hospital, Aomori, Japan

Part I

Basics of NBI

Principles and History of NBI

1

Kazuhiro Gono

1.1 Introduction

Narrow band imaging (NBI) is a method of image enhancement [1, 2]. Although it is classified as an "optical digital method," it enhances images using optical technology, processing them in a different way to previous optical digital methods [3]. An understanding of the optical properties of living tissue was deeply involved in the development of NBI.

In this section, I will present the operating principles of NBI. To aid your understanding, I will also cover absorption and scattering and the interactions between living tissues and light. In addition, I will touch upon the two different imaging methods used with NBI, the simultaneous and frame sequential methods.

1.2 History of the Development of NBI

The development of NBI began with that of the endoscopic spectroscopy system (ESS). From the second half of the 1990s, as part of the "Comprehensive 10-year Strategy for Cancer Control," the National Cancer Center Hospital East, and the Oyama Research Department of the Tokyo Institute of Technology, in collaboration with Olympus Medical Systems Corp., we worked on quantitative colorimetry (spectrometry) of the gastrointestinal mucosa, with the aim of diagnostic application. As part of that study, we passed an optical fiber probe down an endoscope instrument channel, collected objective color data (spectral reflectance rates) from the stomach and colon, and developed an algorithm for their diagnostic application. Although we were able to show objective differences between tumor and nontumor

K. Gono
R&D Planning Division, Olympus Medical Systems Corporation,
2951 Ishikawa-machi, Hachioji 192-8507, Japan
e-mail: k_gono@ot.olympus.co.jp

M. Muto et al. (eds.), *Atlas of Endoscopy with Narrow Band Imaging*,
DOI 10.1007/978-4-431-54243-8_1

mucosa, there were a number of technical problems including a lack of functional stability, and our efforts failed to result in a diagnostic system.

Subsequently, further consideration of how we can observe the result of interactions between spectral reflectance rates and the living tissue led to the concept of NBI. In May 1999, we conducted an experiment to confirm the NBI concept using a multispectrum camera capable of taking spectroscopic images and a high radiant flux light source. This showed that the use of a narrow band of light with a central wavelength of 415 nm improved the contrast of images of capillaries difficult to discern using white light imaging (WLI), marking the start of the development of an NBI endoscopic system. In December 1999, Dr Yasushi Sano, then of the National Cancer Center Hospital East (now of Sano Hospital), started trials with an NBI prototype. The results were promising in both colonoscopy and esophagogastroduodenoscopy (EGD) areas. Subsequently, intensive effort by endoscopists not only in Japan, but also overseas, confirmed the clinical usefulness of NBI. In May 2006, Olympus announced the next generation NBI system, the EVIS LUCERA SPECTRUM.

1.3 Principles

1.3.1 Basic Knowledge Required to Understand the Principles of NBI (Optics and Bio-optics)

When white light is projected onto an apple, pigments in the skin of the apple absorb the green and blue wavelengths between 400 and 550 nm. The absorbed light is converted into heat. In other words, the wavelengths from blue to green from the white light are converted into heat. The wavelengths not absorbed, between 550 and 700 nm, are reflected. The reflected light reaches the eye, and the apple is perceived as red in color.

When light reaches the surface of a transparent material such as glass, part of the light energy is reflected and part is refracted to reach the interior of the material. In the case of milk, which contains fat globules 1–100 μm in diameter, light is dispersed randomly and three-dimensionally by the globules. This is scattering. When particles are present in large numbers, dispersed light encounters another particle to be dispersed again, causing multiple scattering. Accordingly, even if a narrow straight beam of light, such as a laser, is propagated, it is diffused by scattering in this way, becoming unrecognizable as a beam of light.

Based on this understanding of absorption and scattering, I have summarized the interactions between light and living tissue in Fig. 1.1. Light incident upon living tissue is in part reflected at the surface. Part of the light enters the tissue and impacts on small particles such as cell nuclei, intranuclear organelles, and nucleoli, causing multiple scattering. The degree of scattering and propagation depends on the wavelength of the incident light. Red light with a longer wavelength is propagated widely and deeply, whereas blue light with a shorter wavelength is propagated more narrowly and shallowly than red light. Part of the scattered light is absorbed by blood vessels. To be precise, blue (peak absorption at 415 nm) and green (peak absorption at 540 nm) wavelengths are absorbed by hemoglobin.

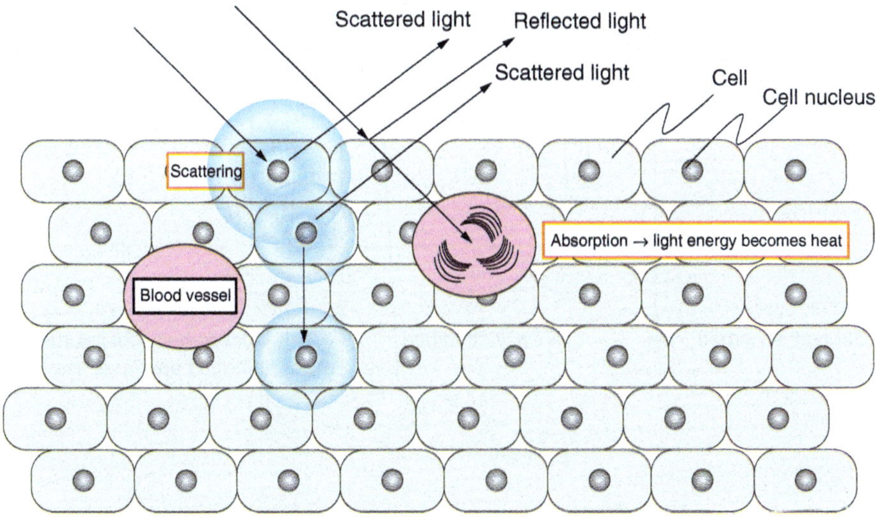

Fig. 1.1 Interaction between light and living tissue

1.3.2 Principles of NBI

Figure 1.2a shows the behavior of narrow band light with a central wavelength of 415 nm (light a) and narrow band light with a central wavelength of 540 nm (light b) projected onto a capillary in the superficial layer of the mucosa. The absorption peak of hemoglobin is in the vicinity of 415 nm, so light a is absorbed less by the blood vessel because it contains wavelengths longer than 415 nm, and it is also scattered less by the tissue and penetrates deeply. Light b is strongly absorbed by the blood vessel and returns from other areas through backward scattering. This results in strong contrast according to whether a blood vessel is present or not. On the other hand, with light b, part of the light energy is absorbed by the blood vessel, but some penetrates the blood vessel and is observed through backward scattering. Accordingly, even the position of the blood vessel does not become completely dark, showing it in low contrast.

Figure 1.2b shows the behavior of light projected onto a large blood vessel in the deep layer of the mucosa. Light with a central wavelength of 415 nm does not penetrate as far as the blood vessel due to strong scattering by the mucosa. On the other hand, light with a central wavelength of 540 nm is more weakly scattered by the mucosa than the 415 nm wavelength light and penetrates to the level of the blood vessel. Although less strongly absorbed than the shorter wavelength, the vessel itself is larger than a capillary, so the lower absorption is balanced by the greater size, and there is considerable light absorption by this deep vessel.

To summarize the above principles, NBI is a technique for observing living tissue taking the narrow band wavelengths that are strongly absorbed by blood and are not dispersed widely and deeply from conventional wide band white light. Images

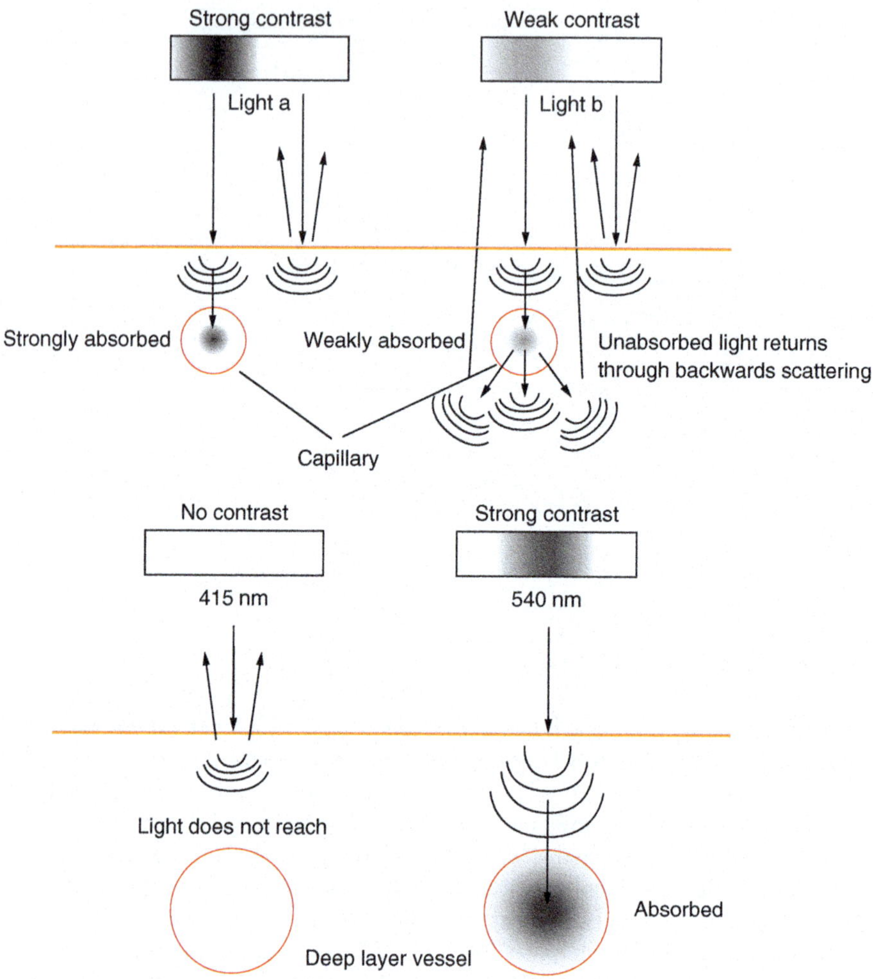

Fig. 1.2 Principles of NBI

taken with light with a central wavelength of 415 nm show capillaries in the superficial layers of the mucosa with high contrast, and images taken with light with a central wavelength of 540 nm show blood vessels in the deep layers with high contrast.

1.4 Two Imaging Methods

Electronic endoscopy systems use two different imaging systems. These are (1) frame sequential imaging, with sequential projection from a black and white charge-coupled device (CCD) and red-green-blue (RGB) light source and output color

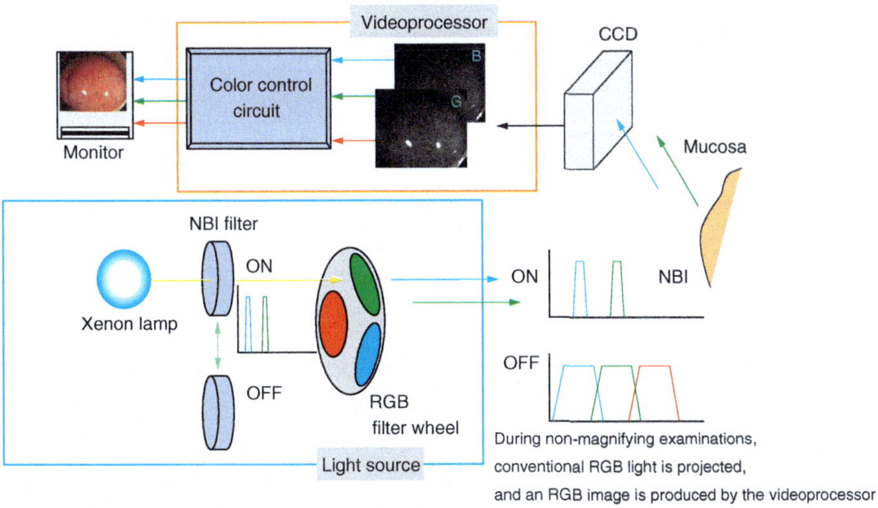

Fig. 1.3 NBI system diagram (EVIS LUCERA SPECTRUM)

images, and (2) simultaneous imaging projecting color CCD and white light. Olympus has product lines using both of these systems, respectively, the EVIS LUCERA SPECTRUM (Spectrum) and EVIS EXERA II (EXERA II).

1.4.1 EVIS LUCERA

1.4.1.1 NBI Using the LUCERA System

Figure 1.3 shows the Spectrum NBI system setup. An NBI optical filter is placed in front of the xenon lamp. This filter is two band specific to 415 and 540 nm (glass filter that only passes through light of the two narrowed bandwidths). During NBI examinations, the filter is inserted into the light path, and during conventional examinations, it is retracted from the light path. During NBI examinations, light with a central wavelength of 415 and 540 nm is projected onto the mucosa, yielding images with the two narrow bandwidths.

Variations are possible in the final color image according to which narrow bandwidth image from each wavelength is allocated to which color channel. However, from the viewpoint of making blood vessels highly visible, the image should be an enhanced reproduction with (1) a light and shade pattern showing the capillaries in the superficial layer of the mucosa and (2) a different coloration pattern to the capillaries for the blood vessels with a relatively large diameter in the deep layer of the mucosa. It is a characteristic of the visual sense in humans that fine patterns are easier to recognize when reproduced with a light and shade pattern rather than with a coloration pattern. On the other hand, thicker patterns can be clearly recognized when expressed with coloration. With these characteristics in mind, allocation of the 415 nm input to the B and G channels reproduces superficial vessels in a

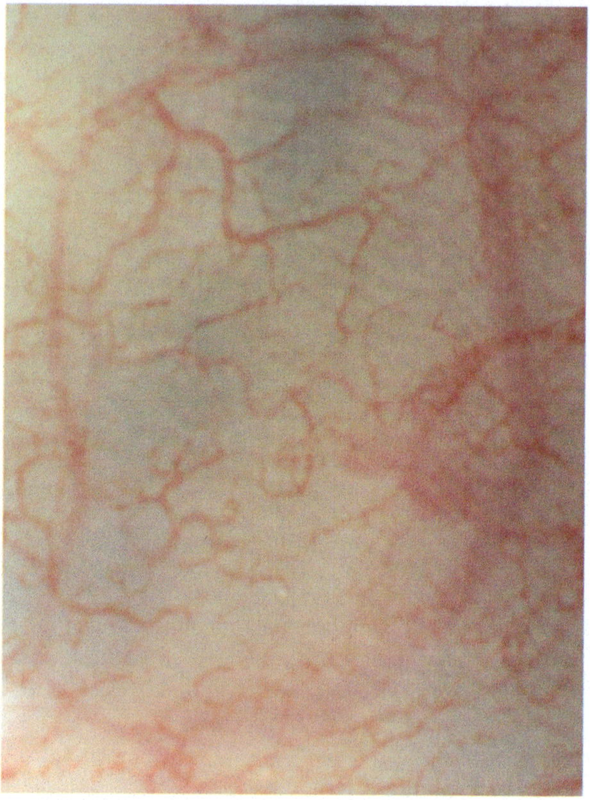

Fig. 1.4 White light image of the mucosa of the underside of the tongue

brownish pattern close to light and shade. Allocation of the 540 nm input to the R channel reproduces deep layer vessels as a cyan-colored pattern.

Figure 1.4 shows a white light image and Fig. 1.5 an NBI image of the mucosa of the underside of the tongue. As described above, in Fig. 1.5 the capillaries of the superficial layer of the mucosa appear brown and the deep layer vessels cyan, both reproduced in high contrast.

1.4.1.2 NBI Using the EXERA II System

NBI using the simultaneous output EXERA II system projects the same NBI light as the Spectrum and allocates the outputs to the same color channels, so it can be considered the same NBI as the Spectrum system. However, the endoscopes that can be used with the EXERA II and Spectrum systems are different, and they also yield different resolutions, magnifying ratios and brightnesses. Accordingly, when we compare NBI images obtained using the two systems, at the very least we should compare images taken with the same resolution and magnifying ratio.

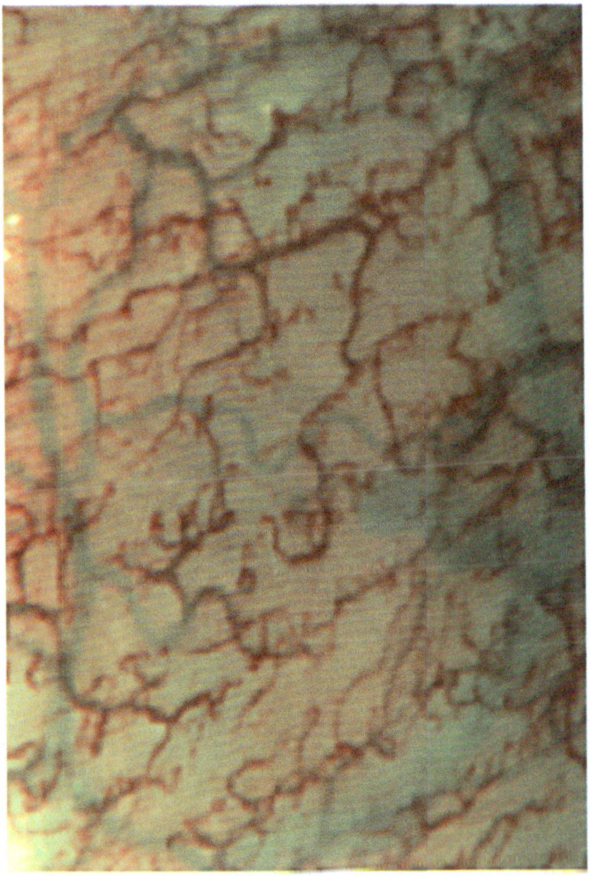

Fig. 1.5 NBI image of the mucosa of the underside of the tongue

Furthermore, the EXERA II and Spectrum systems do not give identical color reproduction even with white light. It follows that NBI color reproduction is also influenced by their basic configurations. However, this applies only to color reproduction, and the two systems provide similar results in the essential area of NBI, improving the contrast of images in comparison to those taken with white light.

Figure 1.6 shows a Spectrum NBI image and Fig. 1.7 an EXERA II NBI image of the mucosa of the underside of the tongue. The endoscopes used were the GIF-H260Z (Spectrum) and the GIF-H180 (EXERA II). We can see that, although there are differences in overall coloration and resolution, the basic NBI effect is the same. When comparing EXERA II and Spectrum NBI images, we should consider differences in endoscope characteristics and base color reproduction.

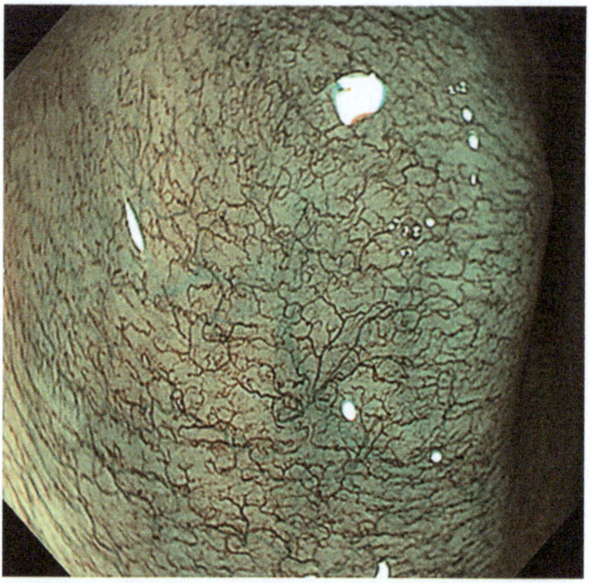

Fig. 1.6 Spectrum NBI image

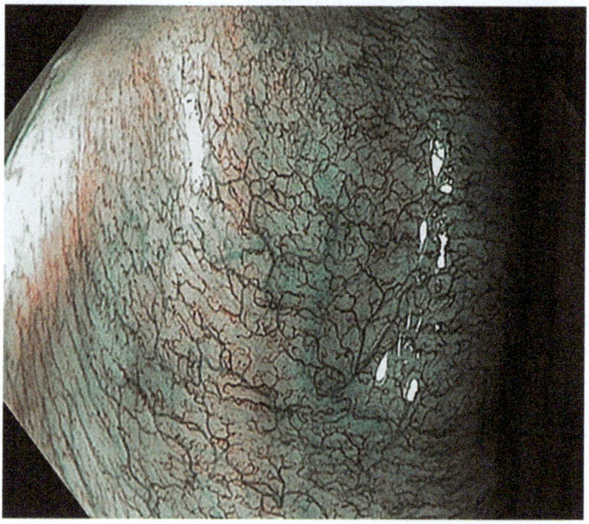

Fig. 1.7 EXERA II NBI image

References

1. Gono K, et al: J Biomed Opt 9:568–577, 2004
2. Gono K, et al: Optical Review 10 (4):211–215, 2003
3. Niwa H, et al: Clinical Gastroenterology 23:137–141, 2008

Tips for Obtaining Optimum Viewing Conditions Using NBI

2

Manabu Muto, Kenshi Yao, and Yasushi Sano

2.1 Pharynx

2.1.1 Prior Explanation

Before examining the pharynx and larynx, the procedure should be explained thoroughly to the patient. In particular, insertion of the endoscope into the pharynx triggers the gag reflex, so it is important to relieve the patient's anxiety to prevent or minimize the gag reflex.

2.1.2 Pretreatment

Secretions such as saliva often adhere to the mucosa of the oral cavity, pharynx, and larynx, interfering with examination. In these cases, before administering the pharyngeal anesthesia, we ask the patient to drink a glass of water, which may clear away some saliva. Lignocaine spray is used for the pharyngeal anesthesia. An antispasmodic agent such as butylscopolamine (Buscopan®) may also be administered to reduce salivary secretion.

M. Muto (✉)
Department of Therapeutic Oncology, Kyoto University Graduate
School of Medicine, 54 Kawahara-cho, Syogoin, Sakyo-ku, Kyoto 606-8507, Japan
e-mail: mmuto@kuhp.kyoto-u.ac.jp

K. Yao
Department of Endoscopy, Fukuoka University Chikushi Hospital, Chikushino, Japan

Y. Sano
Gastrointestinal Center, Sano Hospital, Kobe, Japan

M. Muto et al. (eds.), *Atlas of Endoscopy with Narrow Band Imaging*,
DOI 10.1007/978-4-431-54243-8_2

2.1.3 Premedication

Sedation may be administered to inhibit the gag reflex, but conversely the examination becomes more difficult if the patient goes to sleep after taking a hypnotic, so it is important to administer the appropriate sedation according to the situation.

At our endoscopy clinic, we use the following regimen:

A. Pethidine hydrochloride (Opystan®) 50 mg/1 mL + normal saline 4 mL to make up to 5 mL, 2–3 mL (20–30 mg) intravenously (IV)

or

B. Midazolam (Dormicum®) 10 mg/2 mL + normal saline 8 mL to make up to 10 mL, 2–3 mL (2–3 mg) intravenously (IV)

We almost always use A, as the examination is easier to perform if the patient is awake and can speak and alter their breathing for us. We use B if the patient is very nervous or has a strong gag reflex. Sometimes premedication is not needed for patients with a weak gag reflex.

2.1.4 Timing of NBI Examination

When we examine the pharyngeal and laryngeal regions, the best time to make our observations is during insertion of the endoscope, when the pharyngeal anesthesia is working well and there is little saliva collected. The pharynx can be examined following EGD, but an adequate examination is often difficult during withdrawal of the endoscope due to the patient's psychological state (feeling that the examination has been completed) and accumulation of saliva.

There may be a question of whether it is better to make an examination using NBI first or to use WLI. At present, considering the facts that there is little of clinical significance in the laryngopharyngeal region apart from detecting "cancer" and NBI is significantly better than WLI in terms of cancer detection rate [1], then examination using NBI should be the first choice. As melanosis cannot be diagnosed with NBI alone, the switch should be made to WLI.

2.1.5 Examination Sequence

When examining the pharynx and larynx, we should take great care in avoiding contact between the endoscope and the mucosa, in particular that of the pharynx. Care should also be taken to avoid contact between the tip of the endoscope and the base of the tongue, as this can induce the vomiting reflex.

If saliva or mucous is present in large quantities, it can be cleared by carefully placing the endoscope tip against the mucosa, pressing the water feed button to slightly irrigate the area with a small amount of water, then suctioning up the saliva/mucous with the water. A pointer for this situation is to continue the suction for a longish time.

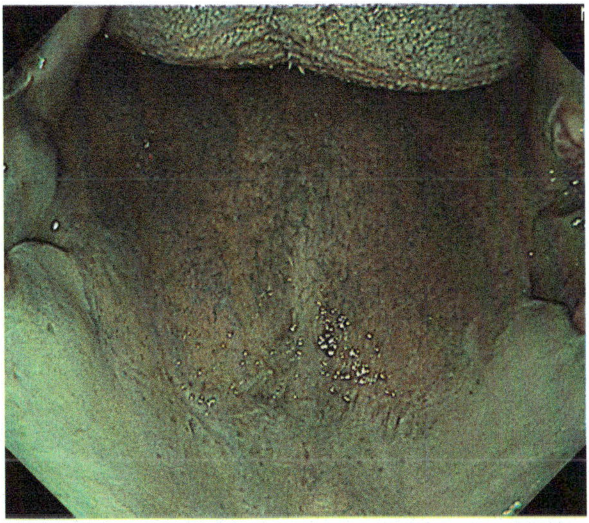

Fig. 2.1 NBI image of hard palate and soft palate

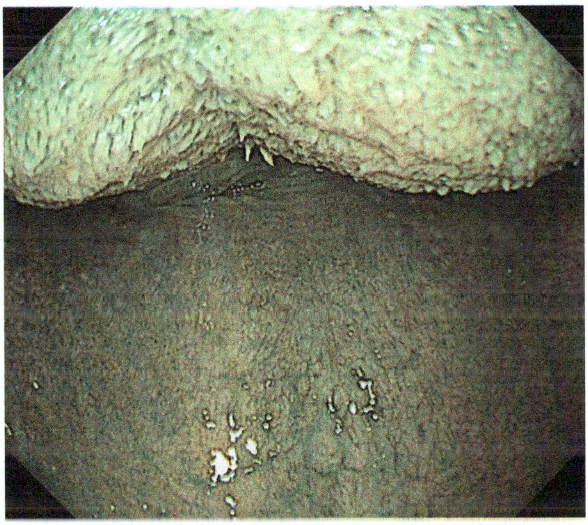

Fig. 2.2 NBI image of soft palate and tongue

2.1.5.1 Oral Cavity to Oropharynx (Fig. 2.1)

First, we examine the hard and soft palate. The retromolar areas on each side should also be examined in patients with a history of head and neck cancer, drinkers, and smokers. We examine the right anterior pillar of the fauces, tonsil, posterior pillar, and uvula, followed by the left anterior pillar of the fauces, tonsil, and posterior pillar. We then insert the endoscope into the oropharynx.

When the proximity of the soft palate to the tongue makes examination of the tonsillar region difficult (Fig. 2.2), ask the patient to say "Ah," thereby elevating the uvula and clearing the visual field (Fig. 2.3).

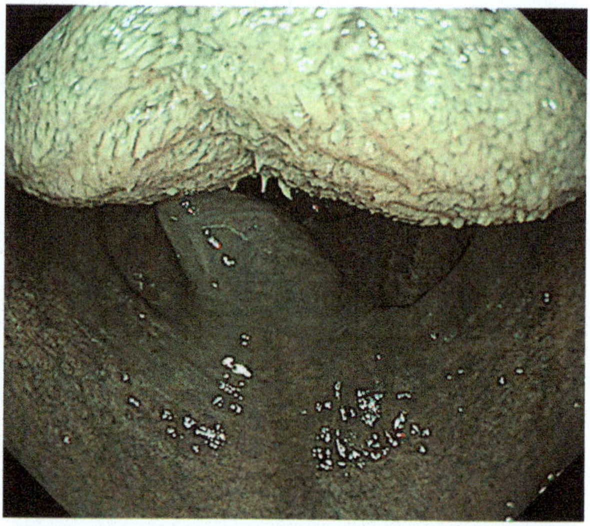

Fig. 2.3 NBI image of uvula when patient says "Ah"

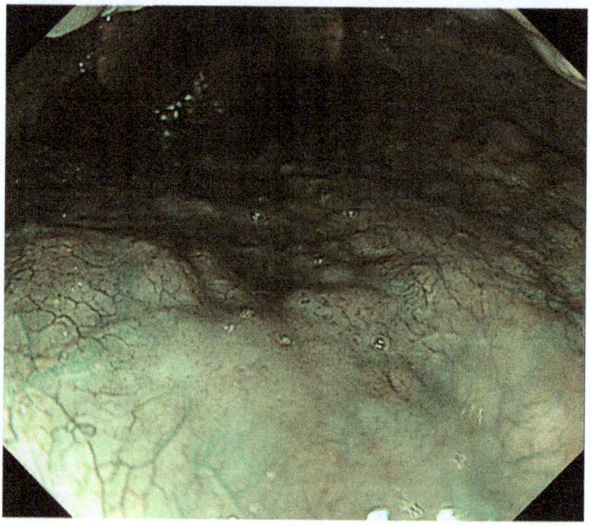

Fig. 2.4 NBI image of posterior wall of oropharynx

2.1.5.2 Oropharynx (Fig. 2.4)

In the oropharynx, we examine the posterior wall and then the right wall. Examination as far as the lower pole of the tonsil eliminates a blind spot. We then slowly advance the endoscope along the lateral wall, examining the epiglottic vallecula from right to left. We examine the left wall while slowly withdrawing the endoscope, up to the lower pole of left side of the tonsil.

We then advance the endoscope as far as the right piriform sinus. We can observe the larynx from a distance at this point. If the epiglottis interferes with advancing the endoscope, forcing the scope past may bring it into contact with the epiglottis, inducing the gag reflex. Instead, we ask the patient to breathe in, moving the epiglottis anteriorly to allow the intake of air and making space for the endoscope to pass distally.

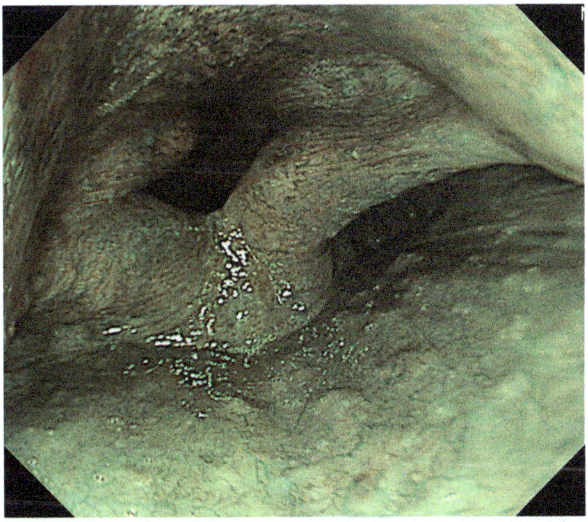

Fig. 2.5 NBI image of close position of posterior wall of hypopharynx and larynx

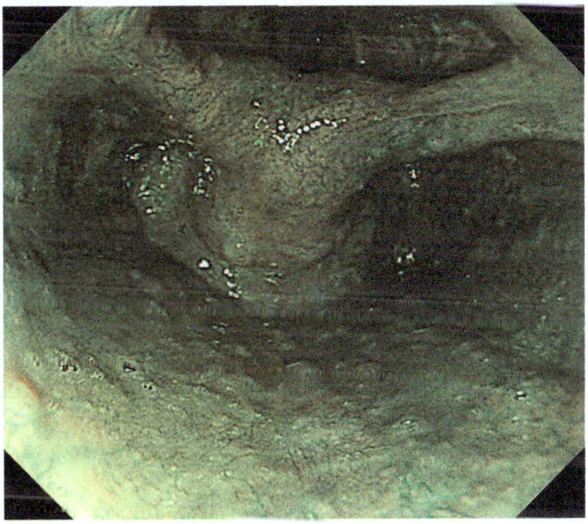

Fig. 2.6 NBI image of wider lumen between posterior wall of oropharynx and larynx when patient breaths out

2.1.5.3 Hypopharynx

After examining the left wall of the oropharynx, we advance the endoscope diagonally to examine the posterior wall of the oropharynx and hypopharynx, then the right piriform sinus. In general, the piriform sinus is a narrow recess and difficult to examine (Fig. 2.5). We first advance the endoscope as far as the apex of the right piriform sinus and ask the patient to breathe out or say "Air," as we withdraw the endoscope, thereby providing a view of the entire recess (Fig. 2.6).

At this time, we examine the arytenoid area, posterior wall, and left piriform sinus. As for the right side, we advance the endoscope as far as the apex of the left piriform sinus, get the patient to breathe out or say "Air," and withdraw the endoscope to obtain a view of the entire recess.

2.1.6 Magnifying Examination

When performing magnifying endoscopy with narrow band imaging (M-NBI), to avoid contact bleeding, it is best to always examine a lesion from the oral side. In the pharyngeal region, anatomical proliferation of abnormal blood vessels is common within lesions, so we must take care not to cause hemorrhage by rupturing any microvessels. Attaching a soft hood (MB 162 for the Q240Z, MB 46 for the H260Z, Olympus Medical Systems) to the endoscope tip helps maintain a clear field of view, but caution is required because it can cause unnecessary contact and bleeding.

2.1.7 Biopsy

Biopsies should be targeted and as few in number as possible (one per lesion). Small biopsy forceps f are sufficient for all lesions in the pharynx and larynx. Biopsies are often difficult to perform during withdrawal of the endoscope, due to the patient's psychological state and accumulation of saliva. Biopsy specimens should therefore be taken as the scope is inserted, when a lesion is first detected.

The patient should be informed when a biopsy is taken, as sometimes blood will come out of their mouth. No patients complain of pain from biopsies distal to the soft palate, as there is little feeling.

2.2 Esophagus

2.2.1 Pretreatment

Copious amounts of secretions such as saliva also interfere with endoscopic examinations of the esophagus, so we ask the patient to drink a glass of water before the procedure, clearing our field of vision. Lignocaine spray is used for the pharyngeal anesthesia. An antispasmodic agent such as Buscopan may also be administered to reduce salivary secretion.

2.2.2 Premedication

Sedation may be administered to inhibit the vomiting reflex, and we may perform iodine staining, so at our endoscopy clinic, we use the following regimen:

A. When iodine staining is planned: pethidine hydrochloride (Opystan®) 50 mg/1 mL + normal saline 4 mL to make up to 5 mL, 2–3 mL (20–30 mg) IV
B. When we anticipate a difficult examination due a strong gag reflex: midazolam (Dormicum®) 10 mg/2 mL + normal saline 8 mL to make up to 10 mL, 2–3 mL (2–3 mg) intravenously (IV)

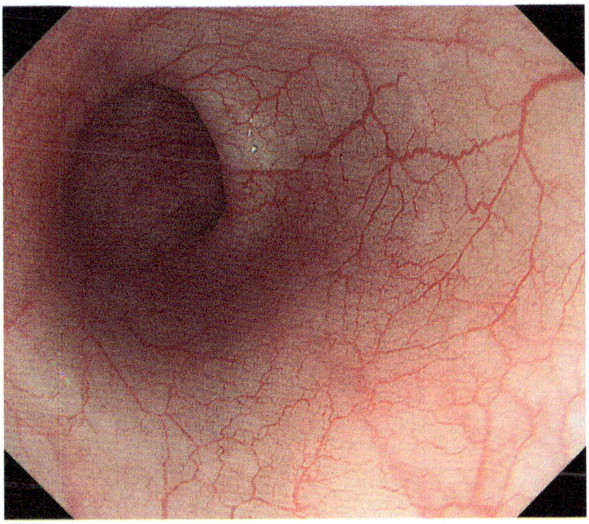

Fig. 2.7 WLI image of middle esophagus

2.2.3 Timing and Sequence of NBI Examination

Immediately after NBI examination of the pharyngeal and laryngeal regions, we insert the endoscope into the esophagus, so we can see that continued use of NBI allows for a smoother procedure. During scope insertion, examination for the cervical esophagus (approximately 16–18 cm from the incisors) is difficult, so this region must be examined at the time of scope withdrawal. Accordingly, during scope insertion, examination commences approximately 18 cm from the incisors in the upper esophagus. The examination proceeds with the esophageal lumen as widely dilated as possible, with irrigation and suction of saliva and other secretions as needed (Figs. 2.7 and 2.8). The esophagogastric junction is examined using both NBI and WLI (Fig. 2.9), to ascertain whether reflux esophagitis or Barrett's epithelium is present. We look for dysplasia within the Barrett's epithelium using M-NBI.

Since WLI examination is the standard method for the stomach at this moment due to limitations with lighting intensity, so examination of the esophagus during scope withdrawal is performed using WLI as for the stomach, enabling examination of inflammatory changes and other features difficult to identify using NBI during scope insertion. At 18–20 cm from the incisors, we switch over from WLI to NBI and examine the upper esophagus and cervical esophagus, not examined during insertion, as we withdraw the scope (Fig. 2.10). If the lumen cannot be maintained, we can either examine when peristaltic waves open the lumen or ask the patient to breathe out, thereby opening the cervical esophageal lumen. As we continue to withdraw the scope, we examine the esophageal introitus, completing the examination (Fig. 2.10).

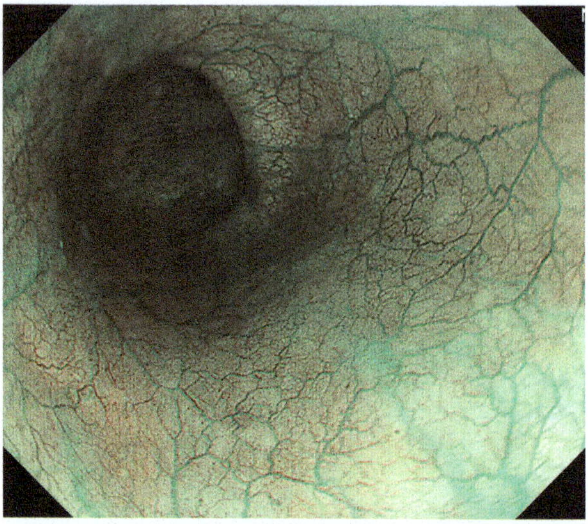

Fig. 2.8 NBI image of the same area as in Fig. 2.1

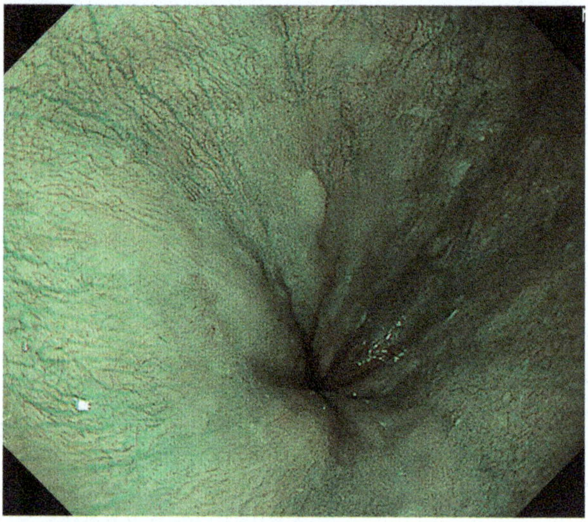

Fig. 2.9 NBI image of lower esophagus

2.2.4 Magnifying Examination

When performing M-NBI, to avoid contact bleeding, it is best to always examine a lesion from the oral side. In the pharyngeal region, anatomical proliferation of abnormal blood vessels is common within lesions, so we must take care not to cause hemorrhage by rupturing any microvessels. Attaching a soft hood (MB 162 for the Q240Z, MB 46 for the H260Z) to the endoscope tip helps maintain a clear field of view, but caution is required because it can cause unnecessary contact and bleeding.

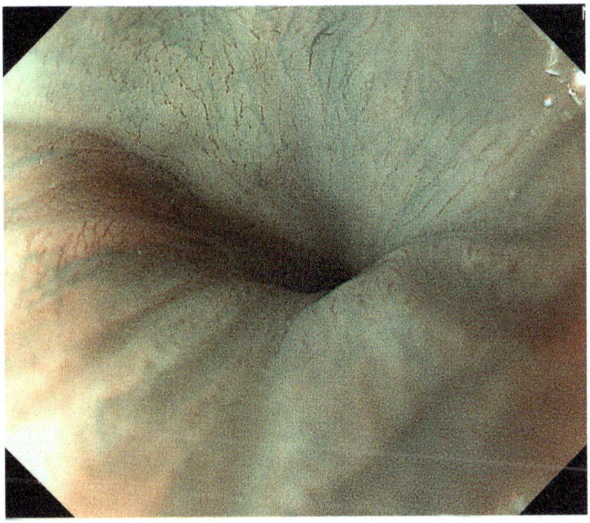

Fig. 2.10 NBI image of esophageal introitus (during scope withdrawal)

2.2.5 Iodine Staining

During an NBI examination, if features suggestive of cancer (brownish area with clear margins, proliferation of atypical blood vessels) are seen, we perform iodine staining as a next step. Since esophageal cancers are often multifocal, we recommend iodine staining the entire esophagus. However, if the possibility of iodine staining was not explained in advance or it is a screening endoscopy, then it is reasonable to only stain the area surrounding the suspect lesion and perform a detailed examination at a later date if necessary.

2.3 Stomach

2.3.1 Principles

The basis of a scientific approach to diagnostic imaging is analysis, using a reliable technique, of images obtained with a conventional observation method at the same resolution. Concerning clinical application of NBI in examinations of the gastric mucosa, the gastric lumen is considerably larger than those of the esophagus or colon, and images obtained by non-magnifying endoscopy with NBI are dark, noisy, and of no practical use. In this section, I will describe how to obtain the optimum conditions for M-NBI examination of the stomach [2].

2.3.2 Pretreatment and Irrigation (Removal of Mucous and Bile on the Mucosal Surface)

At my endoscopy clinic, we ask patients to fast from 9 p.m. the day before the procedure but allow them to drink water. On the day of the endoscopy, we prepare a solution of Pronase® 20,000 U, sodium bicarbonate ($NaHCO_3$) 1 g, and Baros® (dimethicone) antifoaming agent 10 mL in 100 mL of water and ask the patient to drink this solution 30 min before their procedure [3].

For detailed examinations, we administer a suppressor of gastric acid secretion (H2 blocker or proton pump inhibitor) for 1 week prior to the procedure to reduce nonspecific inflammation of the non-lesion background mucosa.

During the procedure, the presence of mucous overlying the lesion, or yellow bile visualized as red using NBI, interferes with the examination. In such cases, we vigorously rinse the mucosal surface with Gascon® (dimethicone) solution using a 20 mL syringe through the instrument port.

2.3.3 Video Processor Settings

The settings for the standard functions incorporated in the electronic endoscopy system video processor and switching between these functions during an examination are both important. Since this Atlas is aimed at NBI users, I will describe the structure enhancement function of the Olympus video system center CV 260LS and CV 180.

Pressing the user settings button on the keyboard brings up the Settings screen on the system monitor. On this screen, we adjust the various settings. The structure enhancement function has two modalities, an A mode and a B mode, for each of which there are 8 levels, from which 3 can be selected. Independent mode and level settings for the structure enhancement function can also be made for WLI and NBI. Because blood vessel diameters increase as the level is raised with the A mode, I use the B mode. I preset levels 4, 6, and 8, and for non-magnifying examinations, I use B mode level 4 or 6, and for magnified examinations, I use B mode level 8.

The NBI color mode is adjusted separately. After switching over to NBI, press the color button on the front of the video system center, not the keyboard, selecting one of mode 1, 2, or 3. Mode 1 is recommended for NBI examinations of the upper gastrointestinal tract.

2.3.4 Use of a Soft Black Hood for Magnifying Examinations

2.3.4.1 Fundamentals of Magnifying Examinations

Here I will present a standard technique for magnifying examinations that provides consistent images at the maximal magnifying ratio.

The stomach has the widest lumen in the gastrointestinal tract, making it difficult to draw close to the mucosa. Respiration and vascular pulsations made it difficult to focus the image at the maximal magnifying ratio during magnifying examinations. To resolve

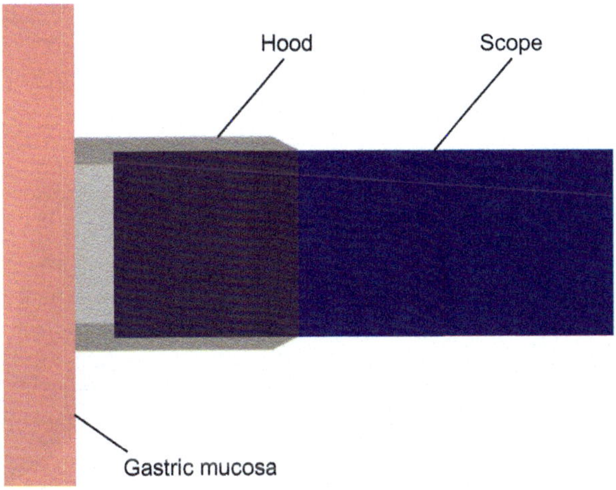

Fig. 2.11 Relationship between endoscope tip, hood for magnifying endoscopy, and gastric mucosa. The hood is attached to the tip of the endoscope, and the hood placed closely against the mucosa, maintaining a constant distance between the endoscope tip and the mucosa, consistently providing images at maximum magnification and in focus

these technical problems, I developed a simple but highly precise method of magnifying endoscopic examination of the stomach using a soft black hood [4]. In other words, we attach a soft hood to the tip of the magnifying endoscope. The depth of the hood is the same as the focal distance for the magnifying endoscope at its maximum optical magnifying ratio, so placing the hood right up against the mucosal surface enables us to consistently maintain a distance between the mucosal surface and the endoscope tip the same as the focal distance at the maximal magnifying ratio (Fig. 2.11).

For magnifying examinations down to the level of capillaries with a minimum diameter of approximately 8 μm, a hood must be attached. I attach a hood before commencing all examinations, whether routine or detailed examinations (the diameter of the endoscope tip varies with the upper gastrointestinal magnifying endoscope used, the MAJ-1989 for use with the GIF-Q240Z and GIF H290Z, the MAJ-1990 with the GIF-H260Z; both soft black hoods, Olympus).

2.3.4.2 Approach to Flat Lesions

Approaching the lesion, we place the tip of the hood lightly against the non-lesion mucosa and look for the lesion demarcation line (DL) under low magnification (Fig. 2.12). Once the DL has been identified, we increase the magnification, and with the tip of the hood in contact with the non-lesion mucosa, aspirate intragastric air to draw the mucosa up into close contact with the hood (Fig. 2.13). This is the best tip for obtaining images in focus at the maximal magnifying ratio.

When the mucosa is drawn in too close (Fig. 2.14a), we should move it away through insufflation of a small amount of air, and if the mucosa is too far away (Fig. 2.14b), we aspirate a small amount of air to bring the mucosa closer. An important point to grasp when examining flat lesions is that we do not press the scope tip onto the mucosa, closely applying the tip of the hood perpendicularly to the mucosal surface, but rather apply the hood tip to the mucosa through repeated insufflation and suction, adjusting the intragastric air volume to achieve close approximation of hood tip to mucosa.

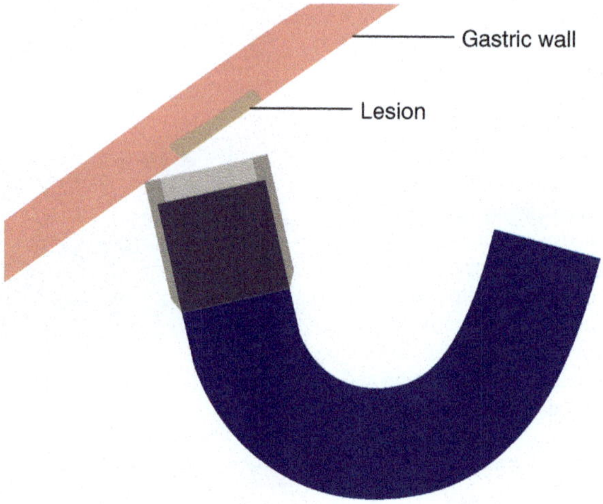

Fig. 2.12 Approaching the lesion, the tip of the hood is lightly placed against the non-lesion mucosa

2.3.5 Water Immersion Technique

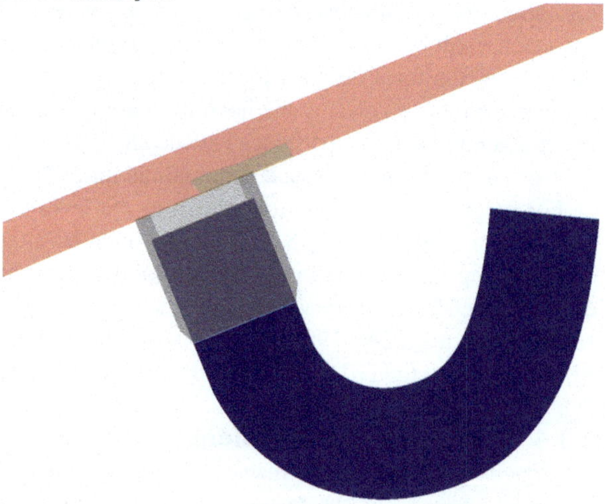

Fig. 2.13 Suction to aspirate intragastric air. From the situation shown in Fig. 2.12, we do not push the scope down but rather aspirate intragastric air to draw the mucosa up to the hood

Filling the narrow space bounded by the mucosa, hood lumen, and scope tip with water during magnifying examinations is known as the water immersion technique. This method has the following merits:

1. Elimination of halation (diffuse light reflection from the mucosal surface).
2. The depth of field increases, making it easier to focus even at the maximal magnifying ratio.
3. The resolution increases.
4. The hood slides more easily across the mucosal surface, reducing mucosal bleeding or mucous hypersecretion.
5. The problem of mucus obscuring the lens is reduced.
6. Gastric peristalsis is reduced if the stomach is filled with water.

Possible demerits include the following:

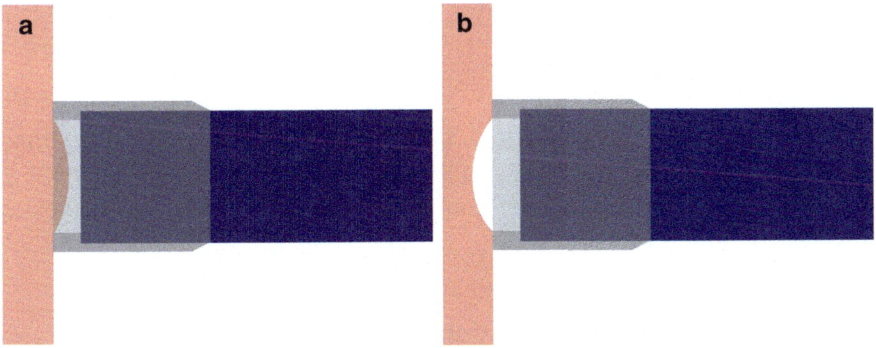

Fig. 2.14 Fine adjustments of the distance between mucosa and endoscope. (**a**) Adjustment by insufflation. When the mucosa is drawn in too close, insufflate a small amount of air, thereby moving the mucosa away from the scope tip to the position where it is in focus at the maximal magnifying ratio. (**b**) Adjustment by suction. If the mucosa is slightly far away and out of focus, aspirate a small amount of air to bring it into focus

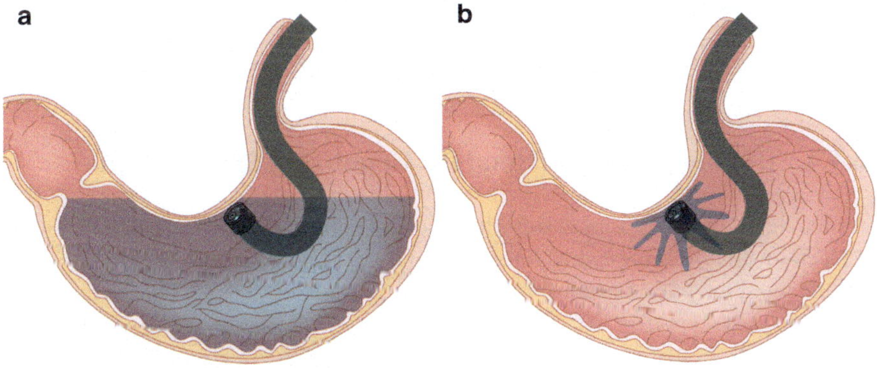

Fig. 2.15 Water immersion technique. (**a**) Water-filling method; (**b**) irrigation method

1. Perspective is somewhat distorted.
2. When the water is clouded, non-magnifying examination becomes difficult.

Although there are some demerits, use of the water immersion technique provides images in focus at the maximal magnifying ratio, enabling rapid image evaluation, tending to reduce procedure durations.

There are two variations of this technique: (1) the water-filling method, in which the gastric lumen is filled with water, as for endoscopic ultrasound (EUS) (Fig. 2.15a, b), and (2) the irrigation method, in which water is instilled through the instrument channel (Fig. 2.15b). Irrigation can be performed using a syringe (50 mL) or an EUS water supply pump unit (UWS-1, Olympus). With the GIF-H260Z and GIF-H290Z, we use the endoscope water jet function.

2.4 Duodenum

2.4.1 Principles

Although the duodenum has a narrow lumen, at present the usefulness of NBI in combination with non-magnifying endoscopy is uncertain. Accordingly, NBI is mainly used in combination with magnifying endoscopy following non-magnifying examination with WLI.

2.4.2 Preparation and Irrigation

Preparation is similar to examinations of the stomach. Large pools of bile in the duodenum, visualized as bright red using NBI, interfere with the examination, so we rinse the mucosa with Gascon® (dimethicone) solution before the examination.

2.4.3 Video Processor Settings

These are the same as for examinations of the stomach.

2.4.4 Use of a Soft Black Hood for Magnifying Examinations

As for the stomach, use of a soft black hood for magnifying examinations of the duodenum allows us to readily and consistently obtain magnified images in focus at the maximal magnifying ratio.

2.4.5 Water Immersion Technique

The merits of the water immersion technique in the duodenum are that, in addition to the merits of this technique in examinations of the stomach, we can examine the duodenum as we rinse bile mucosal surface, and irrigation with water allows us to see the normal duodenal villi swaying in the moving water, as well as the detailed structure of the mobile villi. Loss of villous motility is used as a diagnostic marker of conditions such as celiac disease [5].

2.5 Colon and Rectum

2.5.1 Non-magnifying NBI Examination

Clinical application of NBI in examinations of the colorectal mucosa requires a specific technique, as non-magnifying NBI images taken from the center of the lumen tend to be rather dark and noisy due to the large lumen in the colorectum.

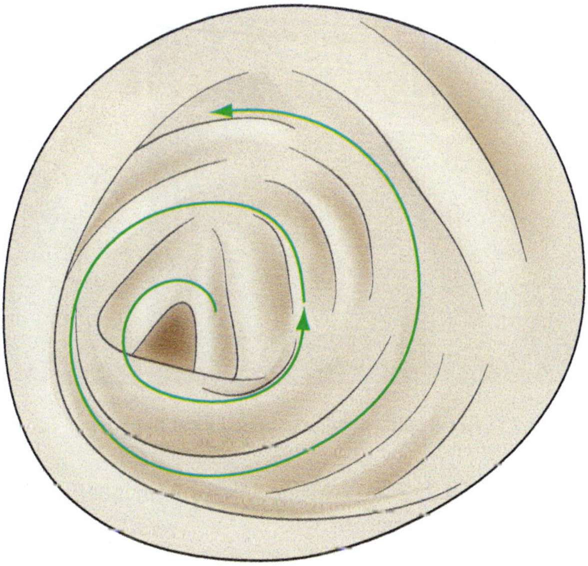

Fig. 2.16 Diagram of the withdrawal path for NBI examinations

To counter this, we maneuver the scope around the colorectal lumen as if drawing a spiral (Fig. 2.16).

2.5.2 Pretreatment and Irrigation (Removal of Fecal Fluid and Bile)

Fecal matter and fecal fluid adherent to the colorectal mucosa is shown as red using NBI, resembling a polyp or blood, interfering with the recognition of lesions (Fig. 2.17a, b). Adequate preparation is extremely important to avoid such interference with the identification of important pathology such as superficial flat lesions.

As preparation, the authors prescribe picosulfate sodium hydrate 7.5 g (Laxodate®, 1 bottle) the night before the procedure, then mosapride citrate 5 mg (Gasmotin®) the next day 3–4 hours before the procedure. The examination is commenced after bowel lavage with polyethylene glycol 2 L.

2.5.3 Video Processor Settings

The settings for the standard functions incorporated in the electronic endoscopy system video processor and switching between these functions during an examination are both important. Since this Atlas is aimed at NBI users, I will describe the structure enhancement function of the Olympus video system center CV 260LS and CV 180. I use the A mode. I preset the 3 levels, 4, 6, and 8, and I use A mode level 4 or 6 for non-magnifying examinations and level 8 for magnifying examinations.

The NBI color mode is adjusted separately. After switching over to NBI, press the color button on the front of the video system center, not the keyboard, selecting

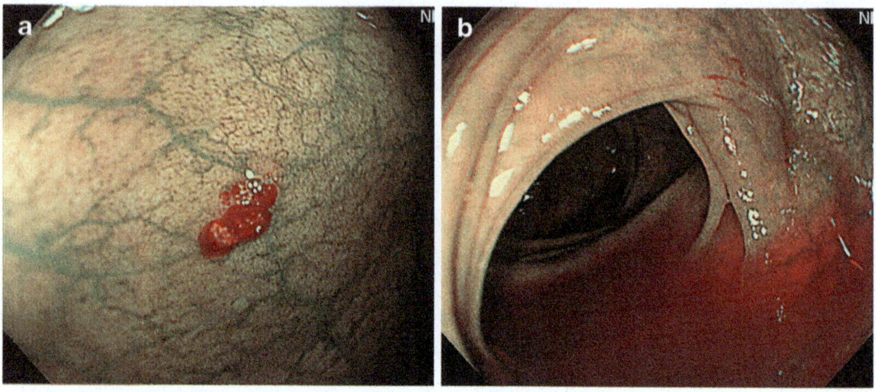

Fig. 2.17 Residual fecal matter (**a**) and fecal fluid (**b**)

one of modes 1, 2, or 3. Mode 3 is recommended for NBI examinations of the lower gastrointestinal tract [6].

2.5.4 How to Use the Optical Zoom Function with a Nontraumatic Catheter

In comparison with the esophagus and stomach, colonoscopy is characterized by (1) difficulty of insertion, (2) difficulty in maintaining the position of the scope tip in some regions, and (3) changes due to fecal fluid, peristalsis, and respiration. Magnifying colonoscopy therefore requires the acquisition of certain skills and techniques. Magnified examination of the pit pattern in the colorectal mucosa has been performed since the 1990s, and we now have available magnifying optical zoom colonoscopes. I usually use an Olympus H2607 ZI scope. In addition to moving the left knob on the control section, magnification can also be adjusted using a foot switch.

The following points are important in performing M-NBI examinations of the colorectal region:

1. Examine the lesion in its entirety, and determine from surface irregularities, redness, etc., which areas will be diagnostically important.
2. Through contact M-NBI examination of the mucosa, determine whether meshed capillaries are present. Determine the capillary pattern and conduct a qualitative analysis at low magnification. Increasing the magnification, look for areas suspicious for malignancy, e.g., CP type III (NICE type 2/3) (Fig. 2.18a, b).
3. For an irregular vascular network in a defined area, using the nontraumatic catheter, we adjust the focus to zoom in on the area of interest in the center of the field of view (Fig. 2.19a, b). In this situation, we must never use the maximal magnifying ratio (increasing the magnification too far makes comparison with the surrounding vascular structure difficult and accurate diagnosis impossible).

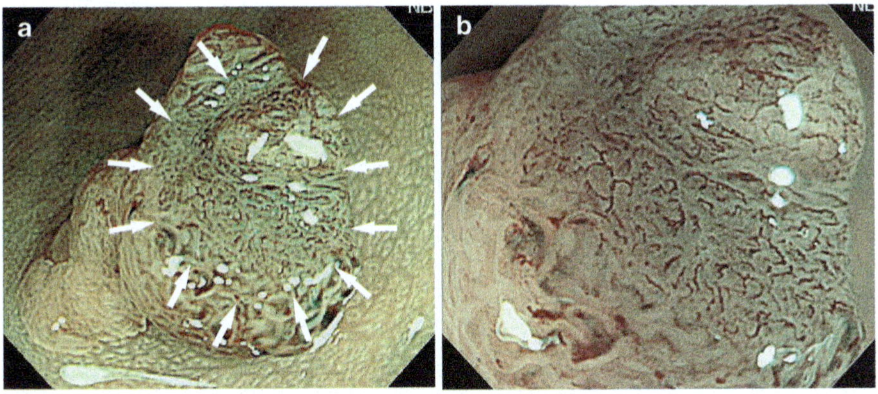

Fig. 2.18 Optical Zoom (**a**) Non magnifying NBI showed irregular vessels in the right side of the lesion (*arrow*). (**b**) When using optical magnification, adjusting focus as the area showing irregular vessels displayed in the full scale of screen. Irregular vessel was classified as CP type III A (NICE type 3)

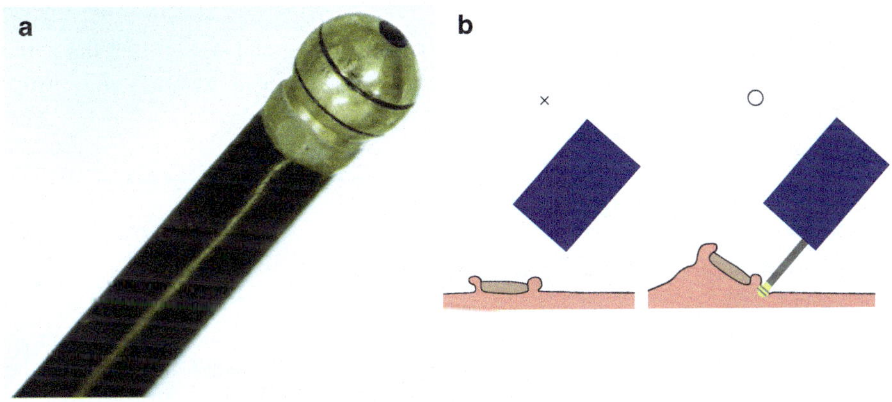

Fig. 2.19 How to use a nontraumatic catheter (Olympus 6233064). (**a**) Nontraumatic catheter. The diameter of the tip is 2.8 mm, and it is rounded to prevent mucosal surface damage and bleeding. (**b**) Even for lesions that cannot be directly visualized, using the nontraumatic catheter to adjust the amount of air makes direct visualization possible. It is also useful in quelling respiration-associated movement, such as in the transverse colon

4. Diagnose CP type III A (NICE type 2) and III B (NICE type 3) lesions, and determine the depth of invasion. At present, it is desirable to also determine the pit pattern using crystal violet staining.

I use a nontraumatic catheter when I perform magnified colorectal examinations. The rounded tip prevents damage to, and bleeding from, the mucosal surface. Furthermore, as shown in Fig. 2.19, even for lesions not amenable to direct examination, through adjustment of the amount of air within the lumen using the nontraumatic catheter, it is possible to examine the lesion directly. The nontraumatic catheter is also useful in quelling respiration-related movements, e.g., for lesions of

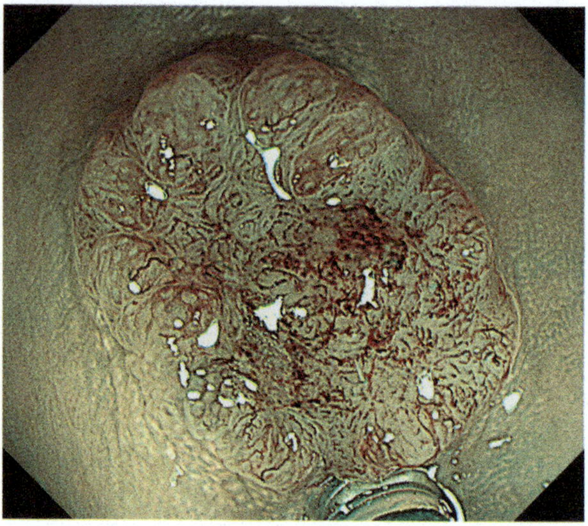

Fig. 2.20 IIa+IIc lesion and the nontraumatic catheter. The nontraumatic catheter has made direct visualization possible. We can clearly see irregular CP type III A blood vessels within the depressed area

the transverse colon. It also functions as a spray catheter and is useful for the elimination of mucous from the mucosal surface during NBI examinations and for dye spraying following NBI examination [7].

2.6 Lower Rectum and Anal Canal

2.6.1 Anatomy of the Anal Canal

The dentate line is the boundary between the ectodermal proctodeum (primitive anus) and endodermal hindgut (primitive rectum), above which the anal papillae and anal crypts extend as far as the anorectal ring (where these disappear is also called Herrmann's line). The oral side of the dentate line is covered in simple columnar epithelium and the anal side in stratified squamous epithelium (see Chapter 14.3 for anatomical diagram).

During defecation, cerebral suppression of defecation ceases and the internal and external anal sphincters relax, opening the anal canal.

2.6.2 Order of Examination

Endoscopic examination of the anal canal is mainly retroflexed. During the procedure, the patient is often tense and trying not to pass flatus, so the anal canal is more tightly closed than usual. Examination of the anal canal is impossible in this state. Telling the patient, "It's all right if you pass gas, please breathe out slowly and relax your bottom," we get the patient to slowly breathe in and out several times, after which the anal sphincters relax and examination is possible (Figs. 2.20, 2.21, 2.22, and 2.23). It is my belief that examination of the anal canal is not possible without

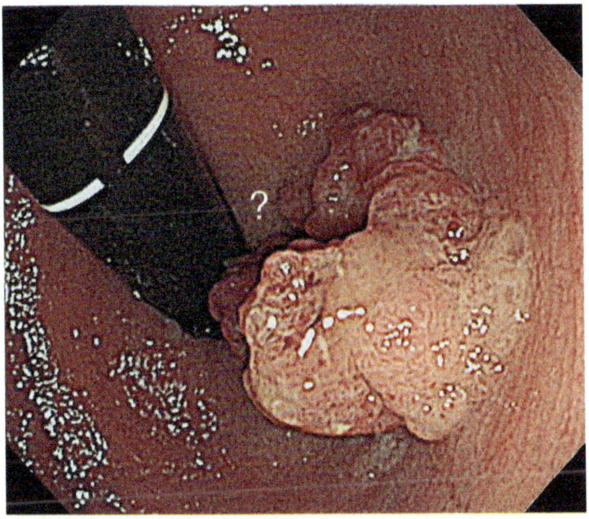

Fig. 2.21 Retroflexed view of the lower rectum (Rb), preoperative endoscopic examination of Rb rectal cancer. We can see a type 2 advanced cancer of the lower rectum (Rb), 3 cm in size. From this image, it is unclear whether it touches the anal canal (dentate line) or not

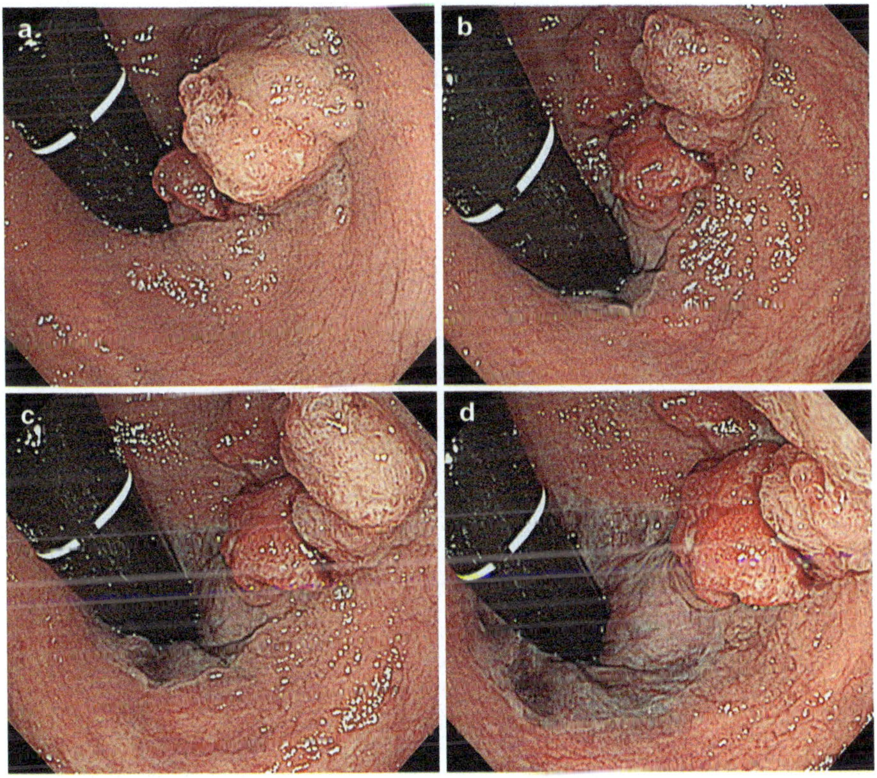

Fig. 2.22 (**a–d**) Examining the anal canal from the lower rectum. Asking the patient to slowly breathe in and out several times and relax, the oral portion of the anal canal can be clearly delineated

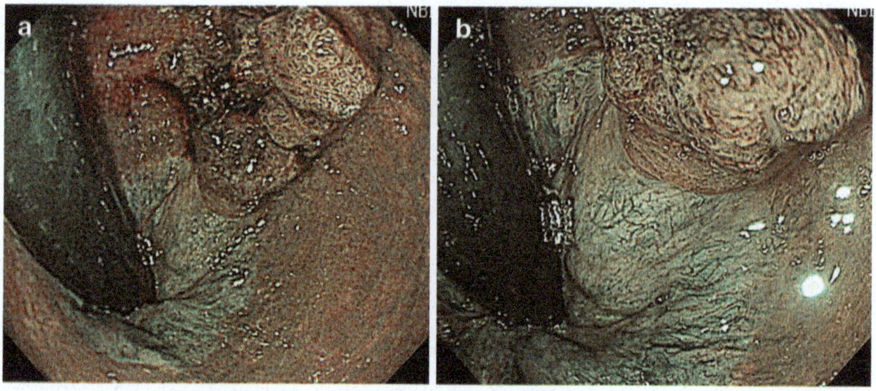

Fig. 2.23 (**a**, **b**) NBI findings of the same region shown in Fig. 2.22. NBI examination clearly shows the transitional zones of the simple columnar epithelium as brown and of the stratified squamous epithelium as greenish-white (**a**, **b**). This lower rectal lesion invades approximately 5 mm beyond the pectinate line at the 2 o'clock position

speaking to the patient in this way. It is important to develop a reliable system of examining this region, as accurate preoperative information, in terms of the distance from the anal verge (AV) and Hermann's ring is required before anorectal surgery.

From the anal verge, attachment of a hood to the endoscope tip is useful in performing detailed examinations of the anal canal.

References

1. Muto M, et al: J Clin Oncol 28:1566–1572, 2010
2. Yao, K (ed.) Zoom gastroscopy, Japan Medical Center, pp15–25, 2009
3. Yao K, et al: Endoscopy 41:462–467, 2009
4. Yao, K, et al: Gastroenterol Endosc 50:1145–1153, 2008
5. Badreldin R, et al: Endoscopy 37:994–998, 2005
6. Uraoka T, et al: GUT 58:604–605, 2009
7. Sano Y, et al: Dig Endosc 17: 105–116, 2005

Part II

Atlas of NBI: Pharynx to Esophagus

Overview

3

Manabu Muto, Tomomasa Hayashi, Kenichi Goda,
Hisao Tajiri, Haruhiro Inoue, Miwako Arima, Hideaki Arima,
and Masahiro Tada

3.1 Diagnostic System

During endoscopic examinations of the laryngopharyngeal region, insertion of the scope induces the gag reflex, and examinations have tended to be inadequate because of the desire to minimize patient discomfort. The laryngopharyngeal region is of course under the aegis of the ear, nose, and throat (ENT) specialty, but even in the ENT field, early detection of cancers in this region has been considered extremely difficult. Detection of superficial esophageal cancers is also far from easy, requiring considerable experience.

M. Muto (✉)
Department of Therapeutic Oncology,
Kyoto University Graduate School of Medicine,
54 Kawahara-cho, Syogoin, Sakyo-ku, Kyoto 606-8507, Japan
e-mail: mmuto@kuhp.kyoto-u.ac.jp

T. Hayashi
Department of Therapeutic Oncology, Kyoto University Graduate School of Medicine, Kyoto, Japan

K. Goda
Department of Endoscopy, The Jikei University School of Medicine, Tokyo, Japan

H. Tajiri
Department of Gastroenterology and Hepatology, The Jikei University School of Medicine, Tokyo, Japan

H. Inoue
Digestive Disease Center, Showa University Koto Toyosu Hospital, Tokyo, Japan

M. Arima
Department of Gastroenterology, Saitama Cancer Center, Saitama, Japan

H. Arima
Arima Surgical-Gastrointestinal Clinic, Chiba, Japan

M. Tada
Cancer Treatment Center, Sainokuni Higashiomiya Medical Center, Saitama, Japan

M. Muto et al. (eds.), *Atlas of Endoscopy with Narrow Band Imaging*,
DOI 10.1007/978-4-431-54243-8_3

3.1.1 Basics of Detection

The majority of laryngopharyngeal cancers are squamous cell carcinomas (SCCs), and in Japan 90 % of esophageal cancers are SCCs, making it essential in this area to master the diagnostic system for SCCs of the larynx, pharynx, and esophagus. Although iodine staining is useful for the early detection of SCCs, it is also highly irritating, causing pain and discomfort. Allergic reactions to iodine can sometimes cause hypotension or drug eruptions, making iodine staining difficult to perform as part of endoscopies at the health check or clinic level. In this respect, the addition of NBI enables detection of SCCs with a high degree of accuracy but no invasiveness and can be expected to contribute to the early detection of cancers in this region. A diagnostic flowchart using NBI is shown in Fig. 3.1.

3.1.2 High-Risk Group

For efficient early detection of cancers of the larynx, pharynx, and esophagus, we need to target the high-risk group. The high-risk groups comprise patients with a history of alcohol consumption and smoking, in particular those with decreased aldehyde dehydrogenase-2 (ALDH2) enzyme activity, associated with difficulty metabolizing acetaldehyde, the first metabolite of ethanol. Individuals with ALDH2 deficiency can be identified with about 90 % accuracy according to whether they experience facial flushing after ingestion of small amounts of alcohol.

3.1.3 Non-magnifying NBI Examination

For suspected SCCs, a useful marker for differentiating between cancer and non-cancer is whether a well-demarcated brownish area is present or not. Even if the brownish area cannot be delineated over its entire circumference, if the lesion is cancerous somewhere on its margin, a distinct demarcation line will be discernible. Lesions with a strong tendency to keratinization appear as low flat whitish protuberances.

3.1.4 Magnifying NBI Examination

For lesions presenting as a well-demarcated brownish area or a low flat whitish protuberance, identification of abnormal blood vessels (Inoue's classification ≥ type III or Arima's classification ≥ type 2; see the relevant sections) using M-NBI allows us to diagnose malignancy with an accuracy exceeding 90 %.

On the other hand, when magnified examination reveals no abnormal blood vessels within a well-demarcated brownish area, melanosis is likely, and switching over to WLI will make it easy to make the differential diagnosis. When a brownish area with unclear margins is detected, with no abnormal blood vessels within (only a ground glass appearance), this likely represents inflammatory changes.

Low flat whitish protuberances with a papillary surface structure are often papillomas.

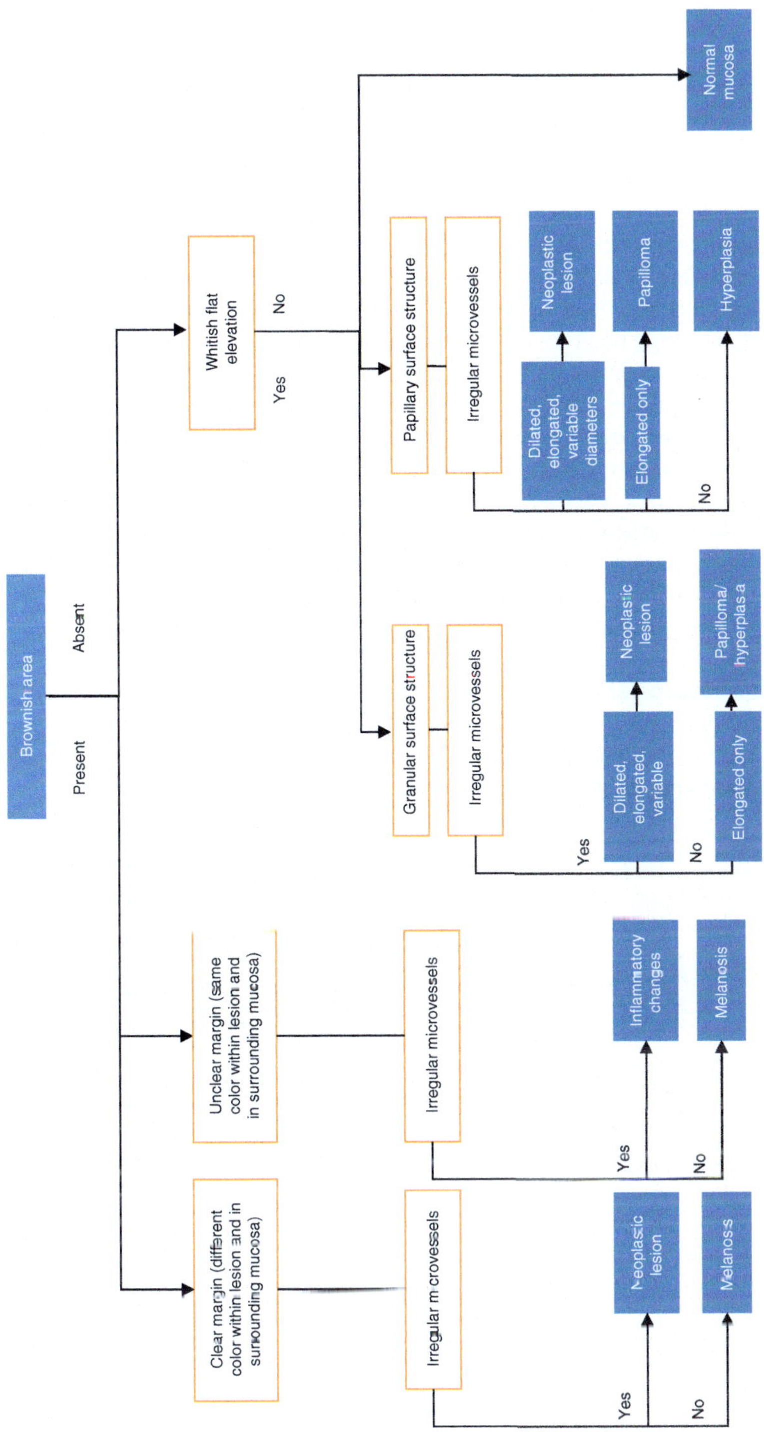

Fig. 3.1 NBI diagnostic flowchart

3.2 Anatomy of the Pharynx (1)

3.2.1 Correlation Between Endoscopic Images and Anatomical Subsites

In recent years with the development of NBI and improvements in endoscopes, we can now detect small and superficial lesions such as superficial cancers. This has been particularly beneficial in the laryngopharyngeal region, with important functions including swallowing and speech, as the patients can preserve these functions. This region is also dealt with by ENT and faciomaxillary surgeons, so careful consideration should be given to the anatomical subsite.

The "General Rules for Clinical Studies on Head and Neck Cancer" [1] discuss the anatomy of the laryngopharyngeal region but do not mention the endoscopic anatomy. In particular the larynx is located anterior to the hypopharynx, and definition of the boundaries of the hypopharyngeal subsites is complicated. The hypopharyngeal subsites are defined by their spatial relationship to the adjacent cartilages, making them difficult to identify during an endoscopic examination.

In this section, we will examine the correlation between endoscopic images and anatomical subsites, with the emphasis on the hypopharynx.

3.2.2 Regional Classification of the Pharynx

The pharynx is divided into the epipharynx (nasopharynx), mesopharynx (oropharynx), and hypopharynx (laryngopharynx), as shown in Fig. 3.2.

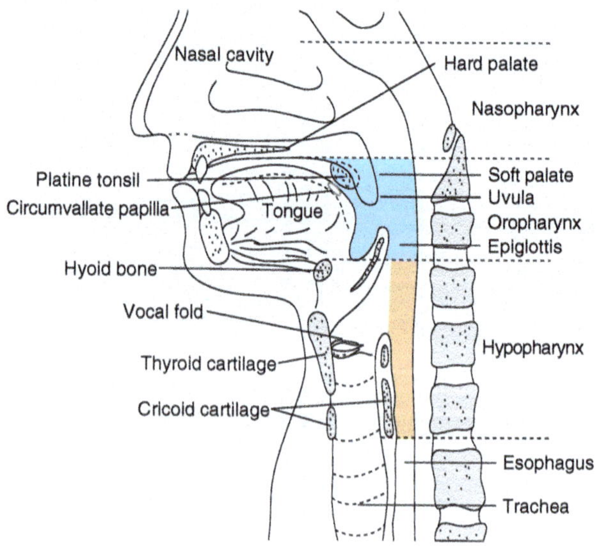

Fig. 3.2 Parts of the pharynx

There are also boundaries between the oropharynx and the oral cavity and between the hypopharynx and the larynx and cervical esophagus, making identification of the respective regions difficult (Fig. 3.3). The hypopharyngeal subsites are particularly complicated and difficult to understand.

Figure 3.4 shows the subsites of the hypopharynx, with the boundaries as determined by the positions of the cartilages drawn on the mucosal surface of a resected specimen of the laryngopharynx and cervical esophagus. The borders as seen at endoscopic examination are shown in Fig. 3.5.

3.2.3 Pointers for Endoscopic Identification of Boundaries Between Hypopharyngeal Subsites

The hypopharyngeal region is divided into: (1) the piriform sinus (PS), (2) the postcricoid area (PC), and (3) the posterior wall (PW). Comparison of the

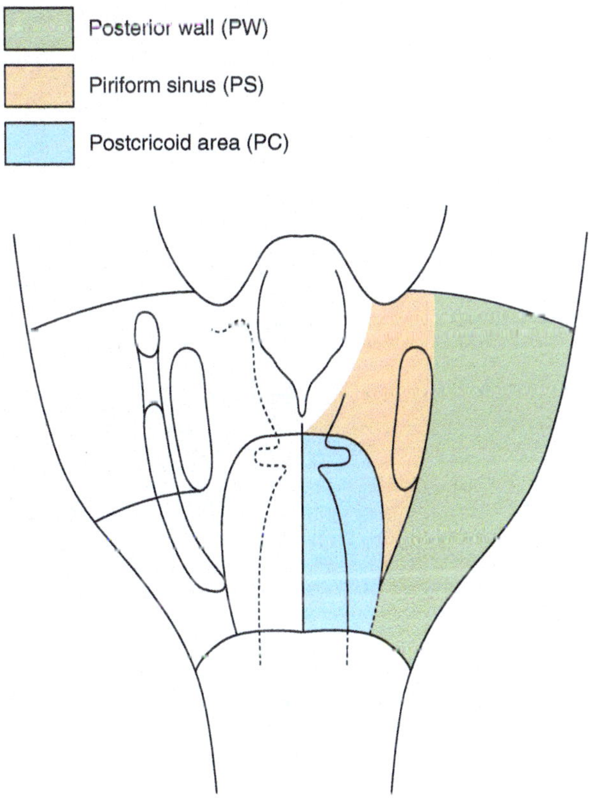

Fig. 3.3 Subsites of the hypopharynx

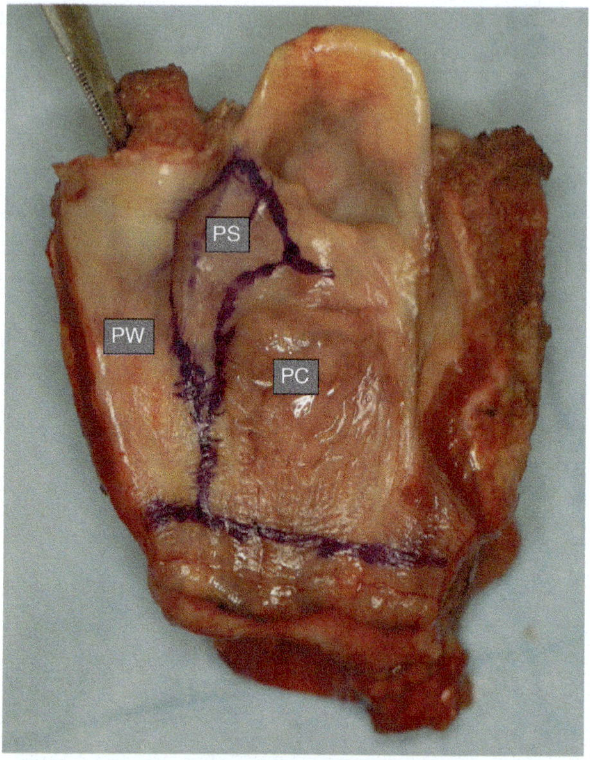

Fig. 3.4 Resected specimen of the laryngopharynx and cervical esophagus

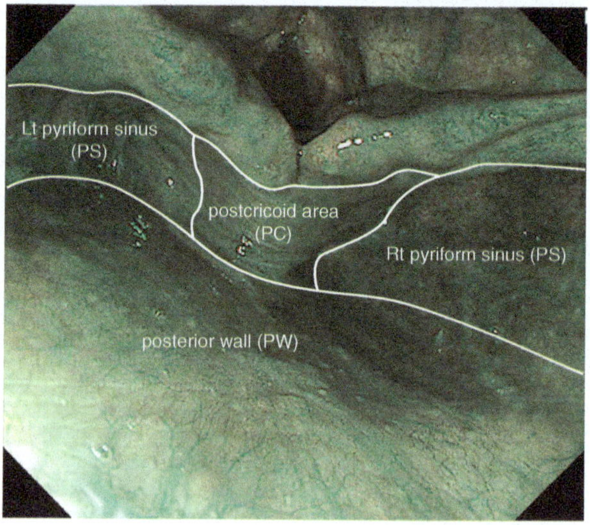

Fig. 3.5 Endoscopic boundaries between hypopharyngeal subsites

abovementioned spatial relationship to the cartilages and the endoscopic findings yields the following boundaries:

- Boundary between PS and PW = line along the fold between posterior and lateral walls
- Boundary between PS and PC = line from inferior tip of the arytenoid apex extended anally, at rest
- Boundary between hypopharynx and mesopharynx = line joining the left and right edges of the epiglottic valleculae

The boundaries between the PC and PW, and the boundaries between the hypopharynx (PC and PW) and cervical esophagus, are difficult to delineate endoscopically and will not be covered in this section.

3.3 Anatomy of the Pharynx (2): Anatomical Location of Subsites

The pharynx is a hollow organ located between the nasal cavity, oral cavity, and esophagus, and it is surrounded by muscle and connective tissue. The pharynx is vertically divided into the epipharynx (nasopharynx), mesopharynx (oropharynx), and hypopharynx (laryngopharynx) (Fig. 3.2). The oropharynx and oral cavity are separated by the circumvallate papillae of the tongue, the oropharyngeal isthmus, and the posterior margin of the hard palate. The boundary between the hypopharynx and the esophagus is the lower margin of the cricoid cartilage.

3.3.1 Oropharynx

According to the "General Rules for Clinical Studies on Head and Neck Cancer" [1], the oropharynx extends from the transition zone between the hard and soft palates to the level of the upper margin of the hyoid bone (or the base of the epiglottic valleculae) and is divided into the following subsites (Fig. 3.6):

1. Anterior wall (glossoepiglottic region): base of tongue (tongue posterior to the circumvallate papillae or posterior 1/3 of the tongue)
2. Lateral wall: palatine tonsil, tonsillar fossa, fauces, and glossotonsillar groove
3. Posterior wall
4. Superior wall: inferior surface of soft palate and uvula

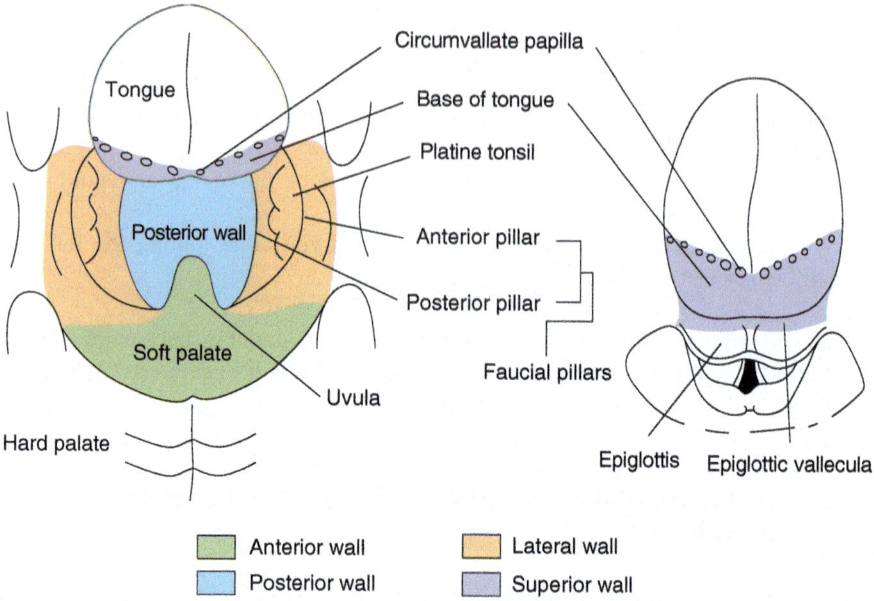

Fig. 3.6 Diagram of oropharyngeal subsites (revised UICC TNM classification)

Fig. 3.7 Diagram of hypopharynx as visualized from the oropharynx (revised UICC TNM classification)

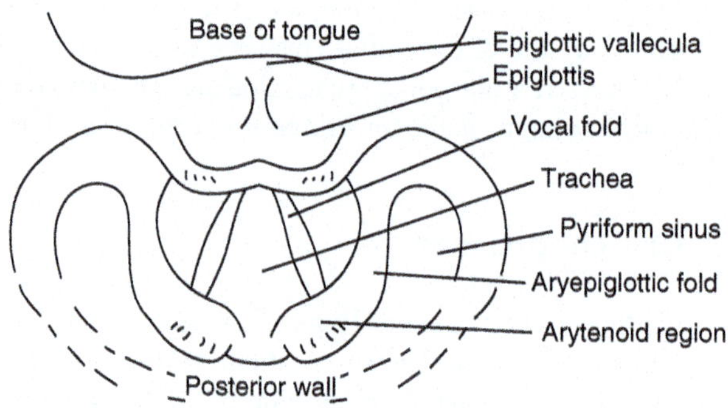

3.3.2 Hypopharynx

3.3.2.1 Subsites

The hypopharynx extends from the upper margin of the hyoid bone (or the base of the epiglottic valleculae) to the level of the lower margin of the cricoid cartilage and is divided into the following subsites (Figs. 3.7 and 3.8):

1. Pharyngoesophageal junction (postcricoid area (PC)): from the level of the arytenoid cartilage and interarytenoid region to the lower margin of the cricoid cartilage (forms the anterior wall of the hypopharynx)
2. Piriform sinus (PS): from the pharyngoepiglottic fold to the upper margin of the esophagus (lateral boundary is the thyroid cartilage, medial border the

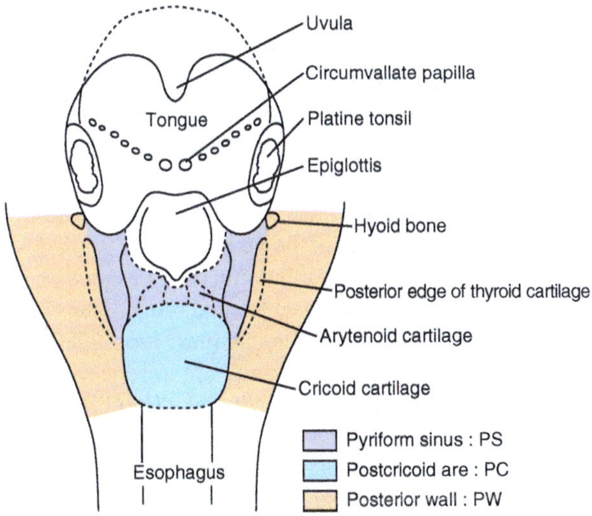

Fig. 3.8 Diagram of oropharynx and hypopharynx opened up left and right from the middle of the posterior wall

hypopharyngeal face of the aryepiglottic fold, and the arytenoid and cricoid cartilages)

3. Posterior pharyngeal wall (PW): from the level of the upper margin of the hyoid bone (base of the epiglottic valleculae) to the lower margin of the cricoid cartilage and from the apex of one PS to the apex of the other

3.3.2.2 Boundaries of Subsites

The boundaries of the subsites are defined as follows:

1. Boundary between PW and PC: lateral margin of the cricoid cartilage below the apex of the PS
2. Boundary between PW and PS: lateral margin of the thyroid cartilage
3. Boundary between PS and PC: lateral margin of the cricoid cartilage
4. Boundary between larynx and PS: ridge of the aryepiglottic fold (however, the arytenoid area, including the posterior aspect, is part of the larynx)

3.3.3 Difficulty Delineating the Pharyngeal Subsites

It is no easy matter for a gastrointestinal endoscopist to understand the anatomical positions of the subsites of the pharynx. This is because, unlike ENT surgeons, they only examine the mucosal surface and are unable to grasp the anatomical relationships between the cartilages and bones, used so often in defining the boundaries between subsites (particularly in the hypopharynx). The best course is to make contact with our ENT colleagues to assist us in improving our understanding.

3.4 Images of the Vasculature of the Esophageal Squamous Epithelium (1): IPCL Classification Using Magnifying Endoscopy

3.4.1 Magnifying Image of Normal Esophageal Mucosa

A schematic drawing of the superficial vascular network of the normal esophageal mucosa and submucosa is shown in Fig. 3.9 [1]. With a non-magnifying endoscope, as we draw close to the normal mucosa, we can discern the branching vascular network. Most of this network is located immediately above the muscularis mucosae.

The intraepithelial papillary capillary loops (IPCLs), rising perpendicularly from the branching vascular network, are rarely discernible during non-magnifying examinations. Using a scope such as the H 260Z, with magnification up to 70 times, we can discern the ICPLs in the normal mucosa as red dots. The recent advent of NBI has enabled us to distinguish ICPLs even more clearly as brownish dots. With M-NBI, the esophageal superficial vascular network appears green and the ICPLs as brownish looping lines.

Intraepithelial papillary capillary loops (IPCLs) can be seen within the epithelial papillae.

3.4.2 Use of the IPCL Pattern Classification in Evaluation of the Endoscopic Degree of Atypia

In regions with squamous epithelium, such as the pharynx and esophagus, with magnifying endoscopy, we can evaluate the endoscopic degree of atypia of a lesion through observation of changes in the IPCL pattern (Fig. 3.10 red box). IPCLs are blood vessels situated adjacent to the basal layers of the epithelium and are considered to exhibit characteristic changes that correlate with structural atypia of the parabasal and basal

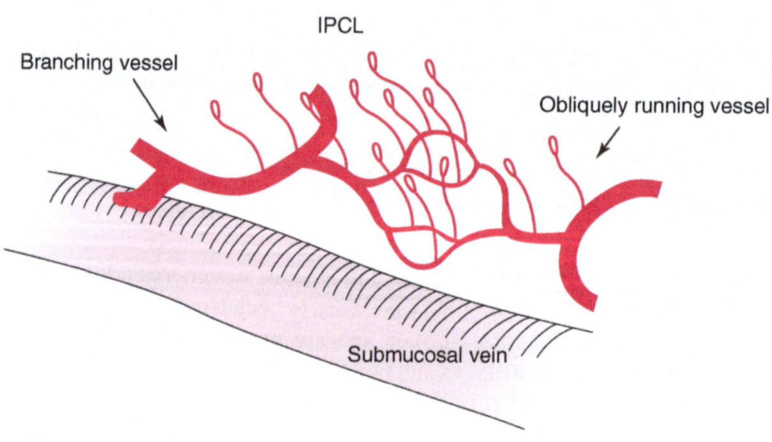

Fig. 3.9 Schematic drawing of the superficial vascular network of the normal esophageal mucosa

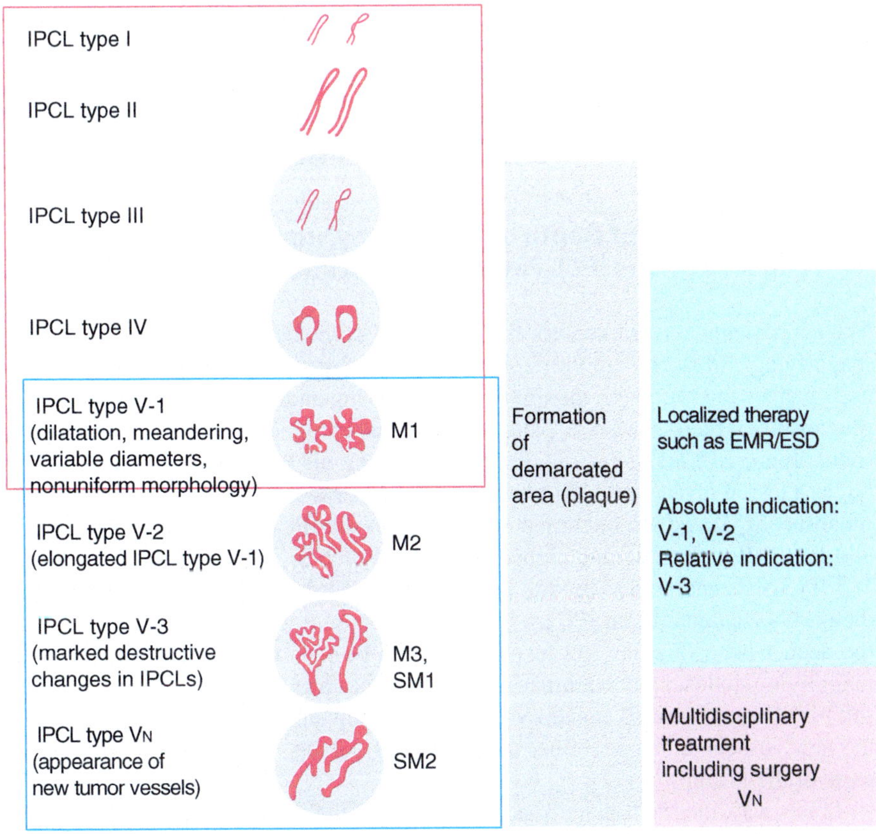

Fig. 3.10 IPCL pattern classification. The morphology of IPCLs located within epithelial papillae reflects changes in the epithelial papillary structure. IPCL pattern types I to V 1 are characteristic of flat lesions (*red box*), whereas IPCL pattern types V-1 to V_N reflect the depth of invasion by a superficial cancer (*blue box*) (Modified from Inoue et al. [4])

layers. We accordingly anticipate the IPCL pattern classification will be useful in the evaluation of the endoscopic degree of atypia of squamous epithelium.

Within the areas of intraepithelial cancers that do not stain with iodine, four elements of IPCL changes are often seen: (1) dilatation, (2) meandering, (3) variable diameters, and (4) nonuniform morphology [2]. These IPCL changes correlate with the degree of atypia of the lesion. In evaluating of the endoscopic degree of atypia, we first delineate the lesion as an area not staining with iodine, or a brownish area using NBI, and then perform a qualitative analysis using the IPCL pattern. The classification extends from type I (normal mucosa) to type V (intraepithelial cancer). Types II and III often correspond to inflammatory or reactive changes, type III to inflammatory changes or low-grade intraepithelial neoplasia (LGIN), types IV and V to high-grade intraepithelial neoplasia (HGIN), and type V-1 to M1 cancer. We can infer that morphological changes in IPCLs reflect the histological degree of structural atypia.

In this way, we can evaluate the endoscopic degree of atypia to a certain extent using the IPCL pattern classification. Importantly, we can be confident that watchful expectation is indicated for type III lesions, whereas treatment such as endoscopic mucosal resection (EMR) or endoscopic submucosal dissection (ESD) is indicated for IPCL type IV or V lesions.

3.4.3 Evaluation of Depth of Invasion by Superficial Cancers Based on the IPCL Pattern Classification

The main diagnostic markers for the evaluation of the depth of invasion using non-magnifying endoscopy are the degree of concavity or protuberance, color changes, and changes in shape with insufflation. Magnifying endoscopy provides additional diagnostic markers, the IPCL pattern and the appearance of tumor vessels [3]. M1 (epithelium, EP) lesions show changes including all four characteristic features, but as a lesion invades to M2 (lamina propria mucosae, LPM) and M3 (muscularis mucosae, MM), we see increased destruction of the IPCLs seen in the M1 lesions, and the IPCLs also become elongated in the direction of the deeper layers. Type V-3 IPCLs (irregular vessels) run horizontally, completely different to the perpendicularly oriented normal IPCLs. This is a common finding in M3 cancers (and in the deeper parts of some M2 lesions) and can be seen near the surface layers on magnifying endoscopic examination. On the other hand, type V_N (new tumor vessels) is characteristic of cancers invading the deep submucosal (SM) layers, with the new vessels larger in caliber than type V-3 vessels, and located in the deeper parts of the lesion.

In this way, the IPCL pattern indirectly reflects the changes in the epithelial papillary structure and is useful in qualitative histological evaluation and evaluation of the depth of invasion of superficial cancers.

3.5 Images of the Vasculature of the Esophageal Squamous Epithelium (2): Microvascular Classification of Superficial Esophageal Lesions Using Magnifying Endoscopy

The advent of magnifying endoscopy has enabled endoscopic histopathological imaging, differentiation between benign and malignant superficial esophageal lesions, and accurate evaluation of the depth of invasion of superficial esophageal cancers. Combination with NBI or flexible spectral imaging color enhancement (FICE) increases the diagnostic accuracy, as well as increasing the reliability of diagnoses of EP and LPM cancers. This makes it possible to proceed to the next treatment step without the need for biopsies. I will now explain the microvascular classification of superficial esophageal lesions using magnifying endoscopy.

3.5.1 Microvascular Pattern Classification of Superficial Esophageal Lesions Visualized Using Magnifying Endoscopy

Magnified examination of the normal esophageal mucosa reveals intraepithelial papillary capillaries branching from the subepithelial vascular network. The intraepithelial papillary capillaries are capillaries located within the subepithelial papillae, with a vessel diameter of 10–15 μm. The spaces between papillae are approximately 100 μm.

The microvascular pattern (MVP) classification (updated version) as visualized using magnifying endoscopy is shown in Fig. 3.11. Microvascular patterns are broadly divided into four types, each closely reflecting a histopathological type. With type 3 and type 4 vascular pattern as diagnostic markers for cancer, the accuracy for distinguishing between benign and malignant lesions is 95 %. The corresponding endoscopic findings are shown in 3.11.

3.5.2 Characteristics of Each Type

3.5.2.1 Type 1

Narrow straight intrapapillary vessels, similar to the normal mucosa, can be seen, so this is histologically esophageal epithelium with no atypia in almost its entirety.

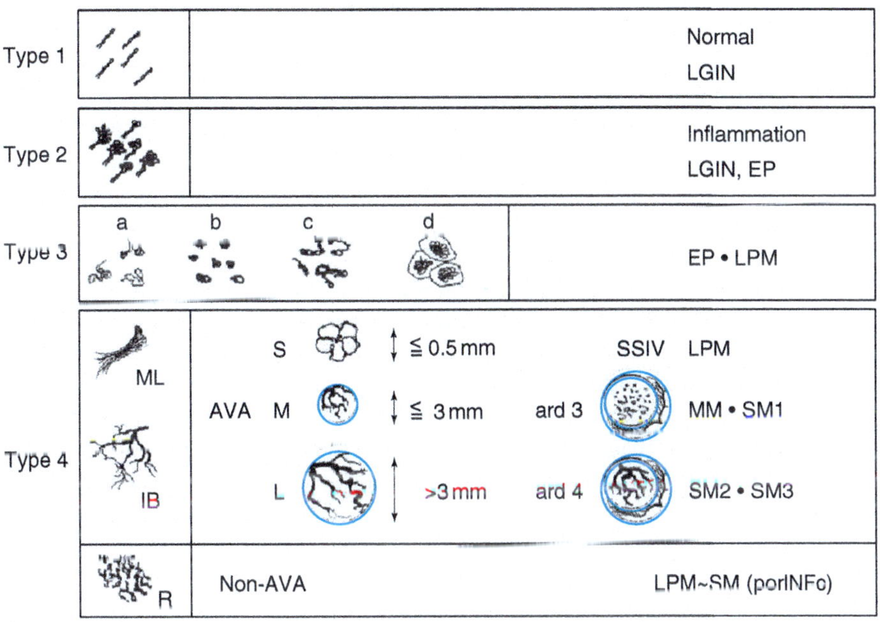

Fig. 3.11 Schematic diagram of a microvascular pattern classification of superficial esophageal lesions visualized using magnifying endoscopy (Arima classification). *LGIN* low-grade intraepithelial neoplasia, *HGIN* high-grade intraepithelial neoplasia, *ML* multilayered, *IB* irregularly branching, *R* reticular, *AVA* avascular area (Arima et al. [7], revised in part)

However, there is a small likelihood that it may include an area of low-grade intraepithelial neoplasia (LGIN).

3.5.2.2 Type 2

Despite findings of elongated vessels, dilated vessels, branching or spiral-shaped swellings, and increased vascular density, the vascular structure is preserved with a relatively regular arrangement. Although this vascular pattern is typical of inflammatory changes without atypia, type 2 also includes small numbers of lesions difficult to distinguish from LGIN or EP cancers. Areas repeatedly subjected to chronic inflammation can be difficult to distinguish from cancers.

3.5.2.3 Type 3

This vascular pattern is characteristic for EP and LPM cancers, with destruction of the intrapapillary vascular structure and irregularly arranged vessels with nonuniform diameters. It is further divided into the following four subtypes: 3a: vessels resembling broken threads; 3b: vessels resembling crushed red spots; 3c: 3b vessels that are elongated or anastomosing with each other; 3d: salmon roe appearance, with aggregations of fine spiral vessels within the papillary prominences.

3.5.2.4 Type 4

The basic morphologies of vessels appearing in areas of LPM to SM invasion are multilayered (MV, Fig. 3.12a), irregularly branching (IB, Fig. 3.12b), and reticular (R, Fig. 3.12c).

The invasive part of the cancer appears as an avascular area (AVA), an area lacking in hypertrophic vessels, surrounded by stretched type 4 vessels. The size of the AVA correlates closely with the depth of tumor invasion, so even in LPM cancers type 4 vessels can be seen surrounding a 200–300 μm decolored AVA. Based on the size of the AVA, this type is divided into three subtypes: 4S, <0.5 mm (Fig. 3.12d); 4M, <3 mm (Fig. 3.12e); and 4L, ≥3 mm. 4S lesions correspond to LPM cancer, 4M to MM or SM1 cancers, and 4L to SM2 and SM3 cancers.

Saucer-shaped lesions with raised edges form a surrounding area with stretched irregular vessels (SSIVs). The depth of invasion can be evaluated using the vessels enclosed by the SSIV; if they are type 3, it is type 4 around type 3 (ard 3), and if they are type 4, it is type 4 around type 4 (ard 4, Fig. 3.12f).

On the other hand, non-AVA type 4R lesions that do not form an AVA are often poorly differentiated cancers that do not form a distinct tumor mass, lesions that exhibit infiltrative growth pattern c (INFc), or cancers of a specific histological type with fine honeycomb pattern of invasion. They tend to have a gently sloping thickened surface or an SMT-like morphology but sometimes appear as part of a IIc surface.

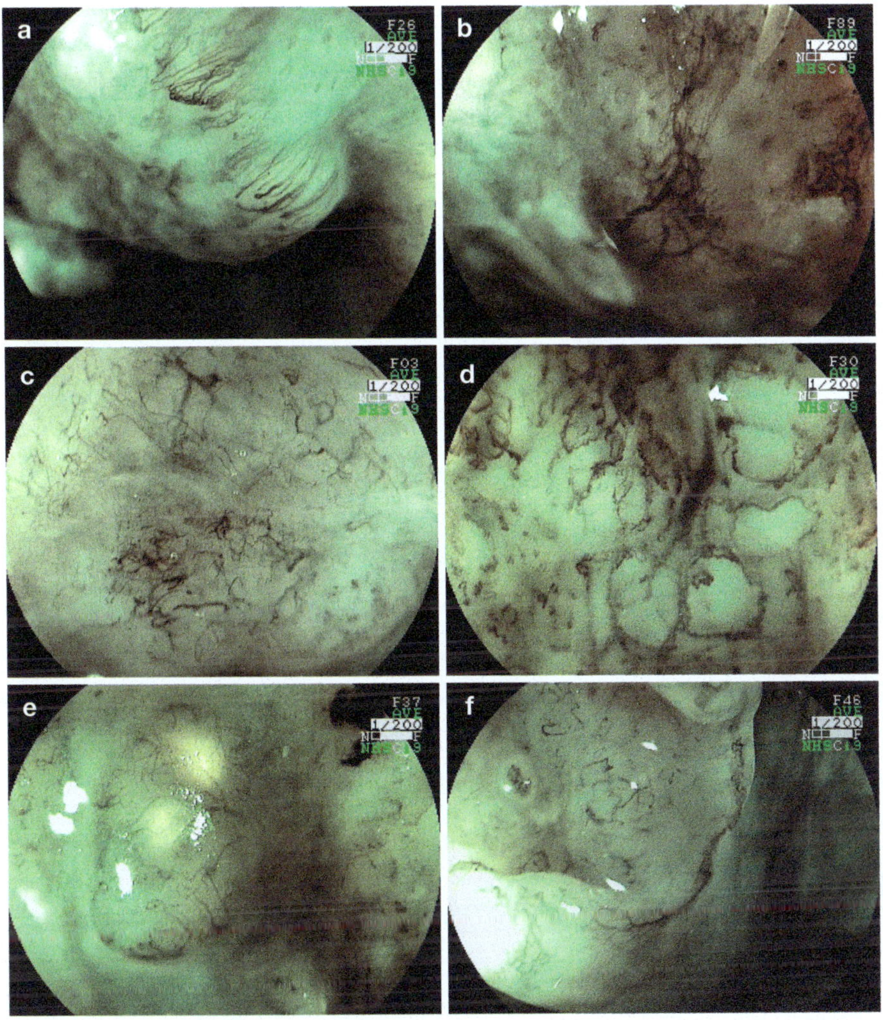

Fig. 3.12 Magnifying endoscopy with FICE images. (**a**) Multilayered vessels (MV), (**b**) irregularly branching vessels, (**c**) reticular vessels (R), (**d**) 4S, (**e**) 4M, (**f**) ard 4

References

1. Japan Society for Head and Neck Cancer (eds). General Rules for Clinical Studies on Head and Neck Cancer (4th edition), Kanehara Shuppan, 2005.
2. Inoue H, et al: Dig Endosc 8: 134–138, 1996
3. Inoue H, et al: Dig Endosc 9: 16–18, 1997
4. Inoue H, et al: Stomach and Intestine 41:19–205, 2006
5. Arima H, et al: Gastroenterol Endosc 39:1557–1565, 1997
6. Arima M, et al: Esophagus 4: 191–197, 2005
7. Arima M, et al: Stomach and Intestine 44: 1675–1687, 2009

4 Atlas of Normal Appearance: Normal Squamous Epithelium

Manabu Muto

The mucosal surface of the pharynx and esophagus comprises stratified squamous epithelium, and NBI examination is extremely useful in this region.

M. Muto
Department of Therapeutic Oncology,
Kyoto University Graduate School of Medicine,
54 Kawahara-cho, Syogoin, Sakyo-ku, Kyoto 606-8507, Japan
e-mail: mmuto@kuhp.kyoto-u.ac.jp

M. Muto et al. (eds.), *Atlas of Endoscopy with Narrow Band Imaging*,
DOI 10.1007/978-4-431-54243-8_4

4.1 Explanation

The squamous epithelial surface of the pharynx and esophagus is visualized using WLI as a smooth light pinkish surface, and blood vessels appear red (Fig. 4.1a, c). With NBI, the mucosa itself is seen as greenish white, with blood vessels in the more superficial layers appearing rather brownish and vessels in deeper layers rather greenish (Fig. 4.1b, d). The smooth surface can sometimes appear quite glossy. Blood vessels in the subepithelial layers branch like the veins in a leaf, whereas microvessels that cannot be discerned with WLI can be visualized using NBI. Furthermore, M-NBI examination reveals intraepithelial papillary capillary loops (IPCLs) more clearly than with M-WLI (Fig. 4.1c, d).

4.2 Characteristics Under NBI Examination

Optical principles dictate that the light intensity of NBI is less than that of WLI, so the images obtained with the former tend to appear darker than with the latter. However, for SCCs of the pharynx and esophagus, the detection power and diagnostic power are considerably superior for NBI than WLI.

NBI uses an optical filter matched to the absorptive properties of hemoglobin, so tumors rich with vascular proliferation are readily seen as brownish areas. Lesions lacking vascular proliferation or lesions with a strong tendency to keratinization are difficult to recognize. The same applies to WLI examinations; so for these lesions, previously developed WLI diagnostic systems are extremely important.

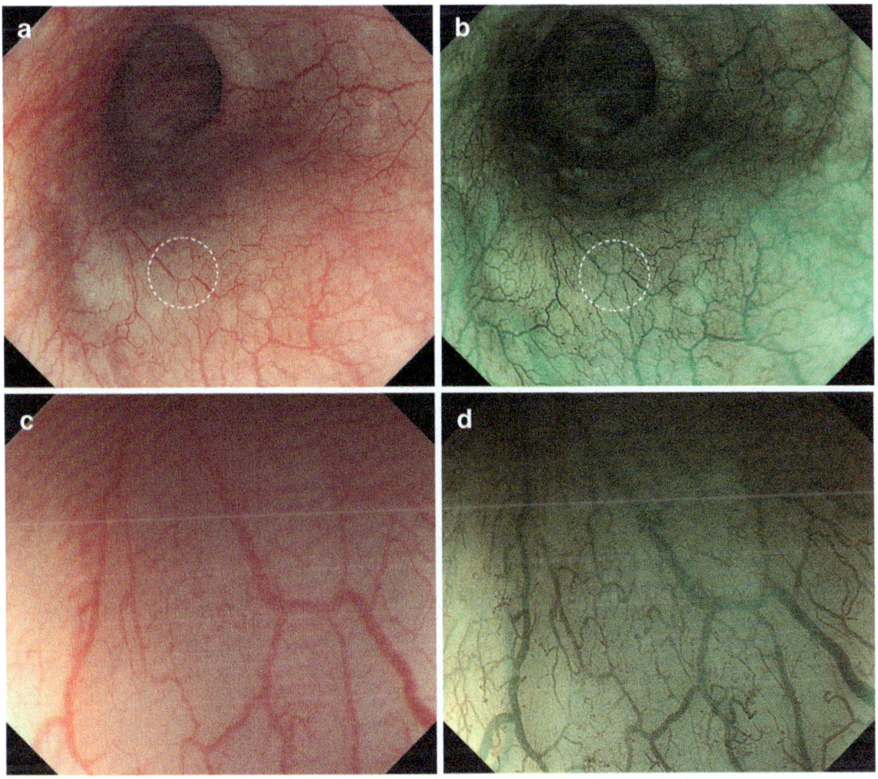

Fig. 4.1 WLI and NBI images of vascular network of esophagus, (**a**) nonmagnifying WLI, (**b**) magnifying NBI image, (**c**) magnifying WLI, (**d**) magnifying NBI

References

1. Muto M, et al: J Clin Oncol 28:1566–1572, 2010
2. Muto M, et al: Cancer 101:1375–1381, 2004
3. Muto M, et al: Clin Gastroenterol Hepatol 3: S16–20, 2005
4. Inoue H, et al: Dig Endosc 9:16–18, 1997
5. Kumagai Y, et al: Endoscopy 34:369–375, 2002
6. Muto M, et al: J Gastroenterol Hepatol 24:1333–1346, 2009

Atlas of Nonneoplastic Lesions

5

Yasumasa Ezoe, Manabu Muto, Kenichi Goda, Masahiro Ikegami, and Hisao Tajiri

Y. Ezoe (✉)
Department of Multidisciplinary Cancer Treatment, Kyoto University Graduate School of Medicine, 54 Kawahara-cho, Shogoin, Sakyo-ku, Kyoto 606-8507, Japan
e-mail: yasuzoe@kuhp.kyoto-u.ac.jp

M. Muto
Department of Therapeutic Oncology, Kyoto University Graduate School of Medicine, Kyoto, Japan

K. Goda
Department of Endoscopy, The Jikei University School of Medicine, Tokyo, Japan

M. Ikegami
Department of Pathology, The Jikei University School of Medicine, Tokyo, Japan

H. Tajiri
Department of Gastroenterology and Hepatology, The Jikei University School of Medicine, Tokyo, Japan

M. Muto et al. (eds.), *Atlas of Endoscopy with Narrow Band Imaging*,
DOI 10.1007/978-4-431-54243-8_5

5.1 Telangiectasia

Telangiectasias are dilated subepithelial blood vessels, endoscopically appearing as red dots or patches from a distance. They can occur in any part of the gastrointestinal tract. Almost all lesions in the oropharynx, hypopharynx, and esophagus are asymptomatic, whereas telangiectasias in the small and large intestines can hemorrhage repeatedly and are a cause of gastrointestinal bleeding.

Because telangiectasias are a morphological abnormality of blood vessels, they are now relatively easy to diagnose with increased endoscopic resolutions and the advent of M-NBI. Biopsy is generally contraindicated, as they are essentially vascular malformations.

5.1.1 Explanation

In this case, non-magnifying WLI examination reveals a 2 mm reddened patch on the posterior wall of the hypopharynx (Fig. 5.1a). Non-magnifying NBI examination shows this as a brownish area (Fig. 5.1b). With M-WLI, we see that this area is a collection of dilated microvessels (Fig. 5.1c). M-NBI shows this collection of dilated microvessels even more clearly, and we can confirm no variability in vessel diameter or direction (Fig. 5.1d). Based on these findings, we made the diagnosis of telangiectasia.

5.1.2 Characteristics Under NBI Examination

Because telangiectasias are abnormalities of blood vessels, from a distance using non-magnifying NBI, they may appear as brownish areas. However, there are epithelial morphological or color changes, as seen in neoplastic lesions.

M-NBI examination reveals that this lesion is a collection of dilated microvessels, with no epithelial changes in the background mucosa. We can also clearly see that the microvessels show no variation in caliber or irregularity of their paths.

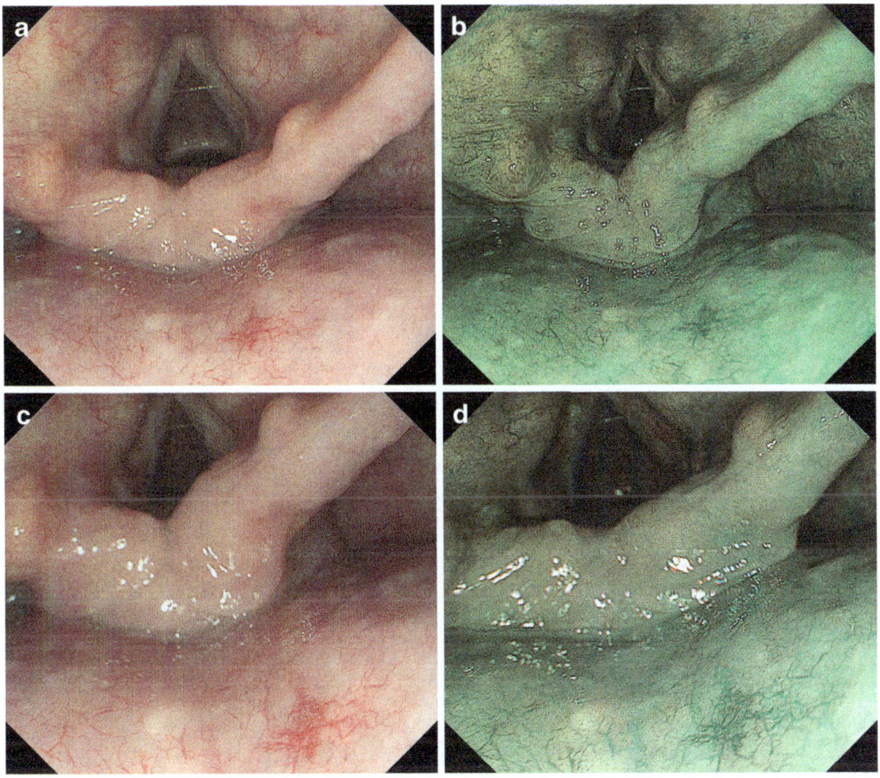

Fig. 5.1 Teleangiectasia of the posterior wall of hypopharynx, (**a**) nonmagnifying WLI, (**b**) magnifying NBI image, (**c**) magnifying WLI, (**d**) magnifying NBI

5.2 Melanosis

Melanosis refers to intraepithelial deposits of brown melanin pigment, visualized endoscopically as dark brownish lesions. It has been reported that when melanosis is detected in the pharyngeal or esophageal mucosa, it is highly likely that an SCC will also be present in the pharynx or esophagus, so melanosis should be considered a biomarker of malignancy [1].

5.2.1 Explanation

Melanosis is easily diagnosed using WLI, appearing as dark brownish lesions (Fig. 5.2a, b). On the other hand, caution is required during NBI examinations, as melanosis is visualized as brownish areas, similar to cancers. Magnified examination, whether WLI or NBI, reveals no proliferation of abnormal blood vessels, with intraepithelial deposition of brown pigment unrelated to any blood vessels (Fig. 5.2b–d). The diagnosis of melanosis is not difficult, but it is important to be prepared to switch over to WLI examination when necessary for simple confirmation.

In this case, biopsy confirmed the diagnosis of melanosis, with deposition of melanin pigment in the basal layers of the stratified squamous epithelium (Fig. 5.2e, f).

5.2.2 Characteristics Under NBI Examination

Caution is required because using NBI examination melanosis is visualized as brownish areas, similar to cancers.

When a brownish area is detected during an NBI examination, no IPCL changes will be seen within the lesion, as long as the melanosis is not associated with atypia or cancer. However, even at higher magnification, lesions will often appear blurred and difficult to focus.

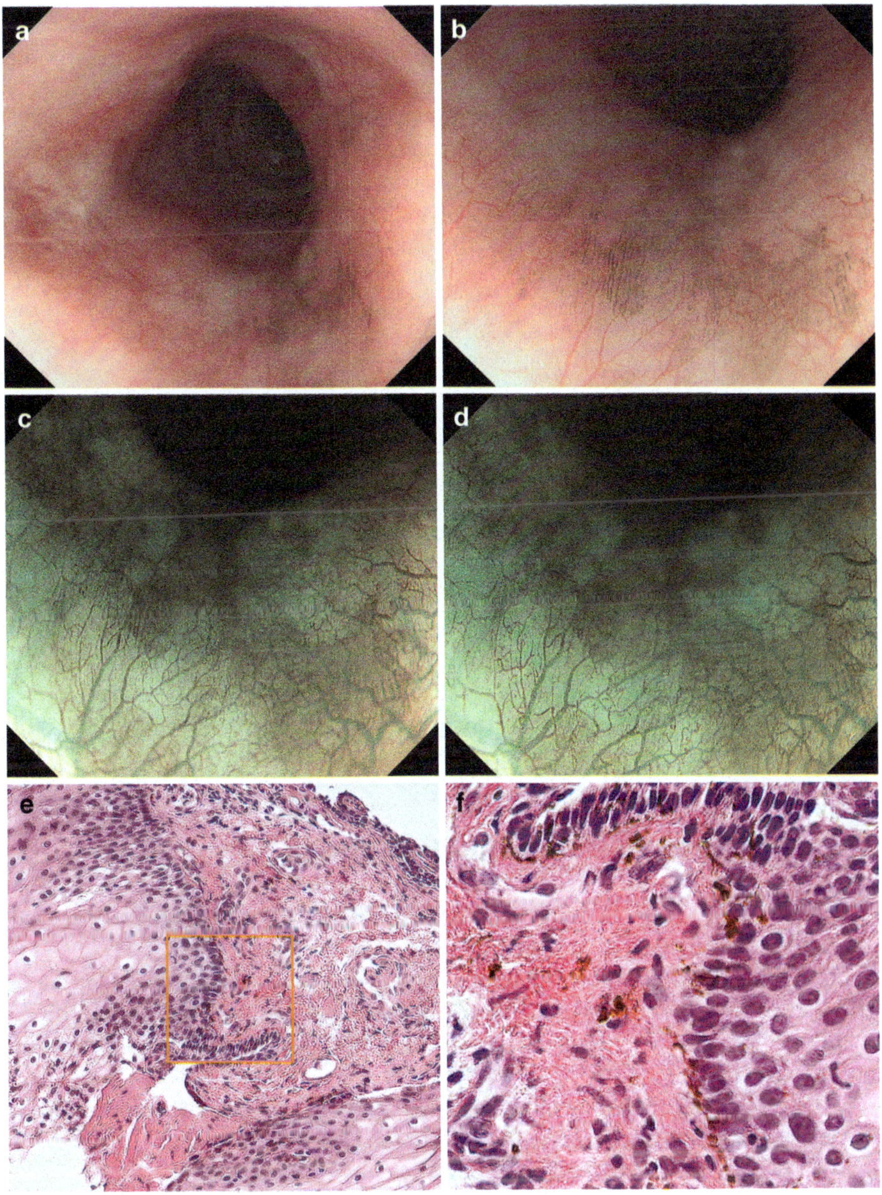

Fig. 5.2 Melanosis of the esophagus, (**a**, **b**) nonmagnifying WLI, (**c**, **d**) nonmagnifying NBI image, (**e**) HE image, (**f**) high-power view, melanin was deposited at baseline membrane

5.3 Inflammatory Changes

These lesions are experienced relatively frequently in the clinical practice. Although inflammatory changes may be seen in any part of the oropharynx or hypopharynx, they most often present as mild redness in the tonsillar region, with its abundant lymphoid follicles, as well as the epiglottis and the left and right piriform sinuses. Inflammatory changes are sometimes associated with erosions. The degree and extent of inflammation varies, so the endoscopic appearance is also highly variable.

5.3.1 Explanation

In this case, non-magnifying WLI examination of the left piriform sinus of the hypopharynx shows loss of visibility of the blood vessels, a small yellowish-white projection, and redness of the apex (Fig. 5.3a). Non-magnifying NBI examination reveals a brownish area with indistinct margins (Fig. 5.3b). M-WLI examination reveals a ground-glass surface appearance, with a scattering of very mildly dilated microvessels (Fig. 5.3c). M-NBI shows the ground-glass appearance of the mucosal surface more clearly, and we can clearly see that the blood vessels within the lesion are only mildly dilated, with no variability in vessel diameter or irregular proliferation and no proliferation of atypical vessels (Fig. 5.3d).

In this case, biopsy confirmed the diagnosis of inflammatory changes, with infiltration of inflammatory cells (Fig. 5.3e).

5.3.2 Characteristics Under NBI Examination

Areas of inflammatory change often appear reddened in color with WLI, so with NBI they are visualized as brownish areas, similar to cancers.

M-NBI examination shows more distinctly that the boundary between the lesion and the surrounding mucosa is unclear. Only mild changes are seen in the IPCLs within the lesion, often visualized as minor vascular changes giving a ground-glass appearance.

Pointers for differentiating inflammatory changes from neoplastic lesions are the unclear margins and the absence of proliferation of atypical vessels.

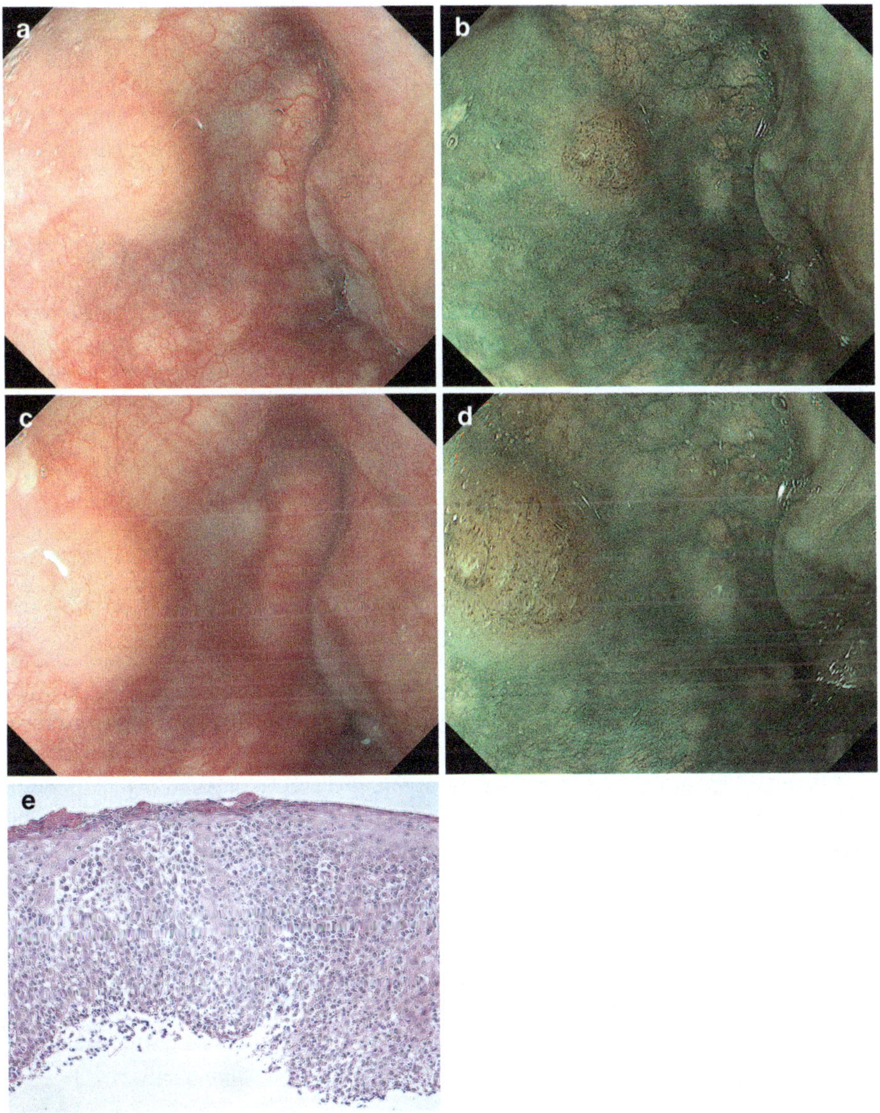

Fig. 5.3 Inflammatory change of left piriform sinus, (**a**) nonmagnifying WLI, (**b**) nonmagnifying NBI, (**c**) close view of WLI, (**d**) close view if NBI, (**e**) HE image

5.4 Squamous Papilloma

Squamous papillomas are lesions with proliferation of squamous epithelium with a papillary structure and are considered reactive rather than neoplastic in nature. They are classified into the following three subtypes based on the histological findings [2]:

1. Exophytic type: stratified squamous epithelium lines the branching surface of the lamina propria.
2. Endophytic type: branching stratified squamous epithelium lines the inverted globular surface of the lamina propria.
3. Spiked type: spikes of narrow-based lamina propria protrude into the epithelial layer.

Endoscopically, the appearances of the different subtypes are described as (1) a sea anemone, (2) a pine cone, and (3) verrucoid or a low flat protuberance.

5.4.1 Explanation

Under non-magnifying WLI examination, most squamous papillomas are visualized as white lesions, either a protuberance resembling a sea anemone (Fig. 5.4a) or a pine cone (Fig. 5.4b). These characteristic appearances make a relatively easy diagnosis.

Magnified examination reveals narrow atypical vessels elongated in the direction of the lesion surface (Fig. 5.4c, d). Characteristic of these elongated vessels is that they are not "tightly coiled like corkscrews" as seen in cancers but rather "smoothly elongated, with little twisting." No variability in diameter is seen. Both the surface structure and the microvascular pattern are better visualized using M-NBI than M-WLI.

In both these lesions, biopsy confirmed the diagnosis of papillomatous proliferation of stratified squamous epithelium (Fig. 5.4e, f).

When a lesion does not show the typical endoscopic appearance of a squamous papilloma, biopsy may be necessary to distinguish it from a neoplastic lesion.

5.4.2 Characteristics Under NBI Examination

Squamous papillomas are usually visualized as a protuberance resembling either a sea anemone or pine cone.

Smoothly elongated atypical blood vessels, with no variability in diameter or irregularity, are seen within the papillary structure.

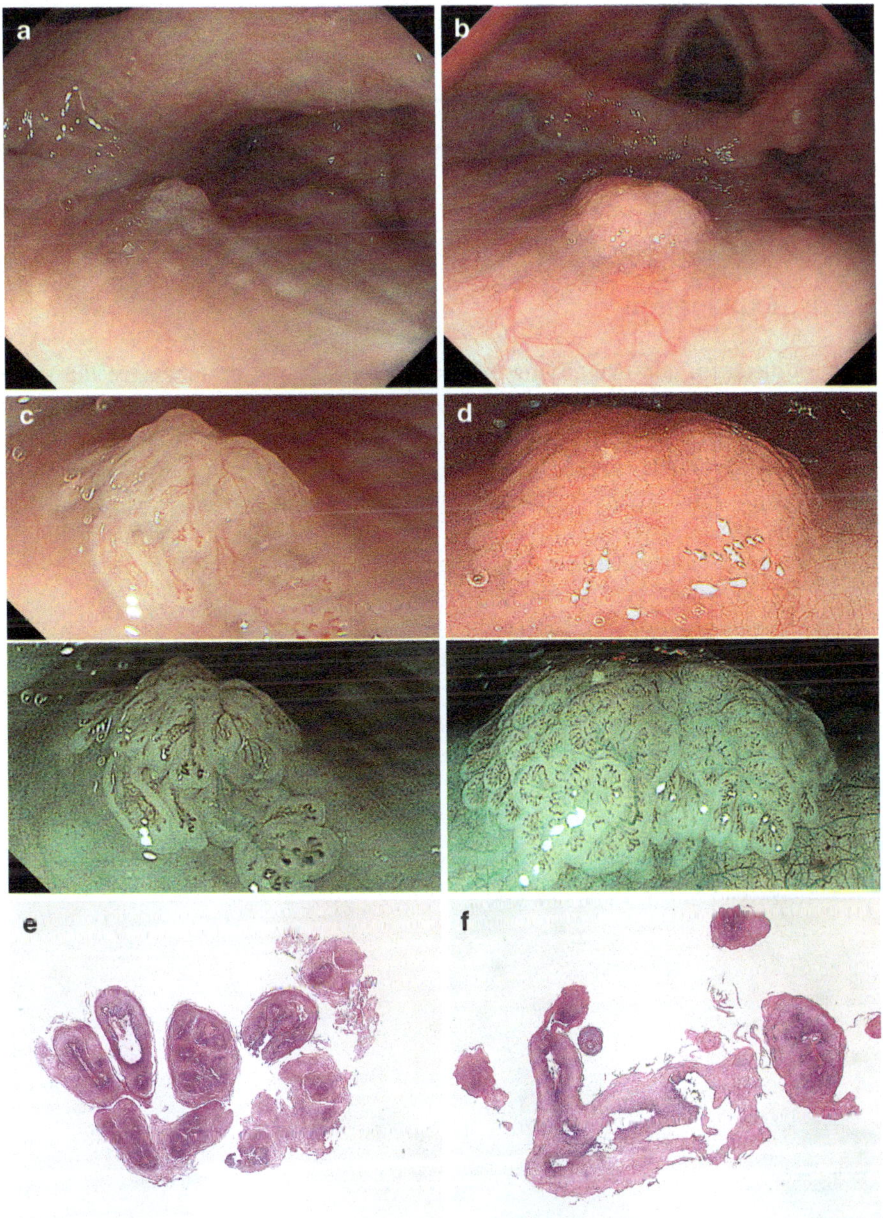

Fig. 5.4 Papilloma, (**a**, **c**, **e**) exophytic type, (**b**, **d**, **f**) endophytic typea, (**a**, **b**) nonmagnifying WLI, (**c**, **d**) close view of WLI and NBI, (**e**, **f**) HE image

5.5 Flat Squamous Papilloma

Squamous papillomas are classified into (1) a sea anemone, (2) a pine cone, and (3) verrucoid, or a low flat protuberance, with most either type (1) or (2). However, since endoscopic examination of the pharynx has become possible, verrucoid squamous papillomas presenting as a low flat protuberance are also frequently encountered.

5.5.1 Explanation

From a distance, non-magnifying WLI reveals a low flat protuberance the same color as the surrounding mucosa (Fig. 5.5a). With non-magnifying NBI from a distance, we are still only able to identify a low flat protuberance, with no difference in color to its surrounds (Fig. 5.5b). Magnified examination reveals proliferation of vessels with mild atypia within the substance of the papillary protuberance (Fig. 5.5c, d).

In this case, biopsy confirmed the diagnosis of squamous papilloma.

5.5.2 Characteristics Under NBI Examination

Common to all subtypes of squamous papilloma, within the mucosa showing a papillary structure run blood vessels with a low degree of atypia.

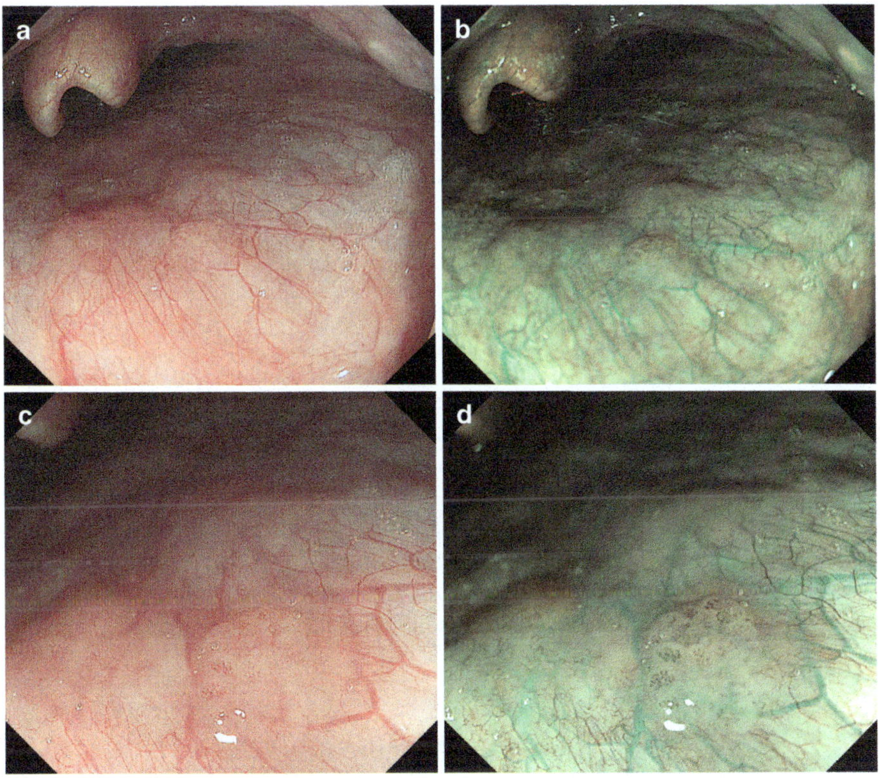

Fig. 5.5 Flat type papilloma, (**a**) nonmagnifying WLI, (**b**) nonmagnifying NBI, (**c**) close view of WLI, (**d**) close view of NBI

5.6 Post-radiotherapy Changes

Radiotherapy may be indicated for organ preservation in cancers of the pharynx, larynx, or esophagus, even in the operable stages. Cures can be achieved in cases of pharyngeal and esophageal cancer through radiotherapy in combination with anticancer chemotherapy. Laryngeal cancers tend to become symptomatic at an early stage, so radiotherapy is often indicated for organ preservation (preservation of function of speech).

5.6.1 Explanation

Figures 5.1, 5.2, 5.3, 5.4, 5.5, and 5.6 are photographs of the oropharynx of a case of laryngeal cancer in which complete response to radiotherapy was achieved. Non-magnifying WLI examination reveals blood vessels of varying diameters and irregular paths (Fig. 5.6a). Non-magnifying NBI examination shows these blood vessels with variable diameters and directionality even more distinctly (Fig. 5.6b). Magnified examination reveals vessels with nonuniform diameters spreading out in a winding irregular manner (Fig. 5.6c, d). In particular, vessels running horizontally are characterized by "curliness," and in certain places, dilatation of vessels is seen (Fig. 5.6c, d).

5.6.2 Characteristics Under NBI Examination

Post-radiotherapy changes are characterized by "curly" vessels with different diameters running horizontally and irregularly. Localized irregular dilatation can also be seen, producing an easily recognized "sludge worm" (*Tubifex tubifex*) morphology.

Even following radiotherapy, if a metachronous lesion occurs, it will be visualized as a brownish area, so the differential diagnosis between neoplastic and non-neoplastic lesions is relatively easy to make.

5.6.3 For Reference: Mucosa That Has Not Been Irradiated

In normal pharyngeal mucosa that has not undergone irradiation, we can see blood vessels that taper neatly like the veins of a leaf, and we can see they are not "curly" (Fig. 5.6e, f).

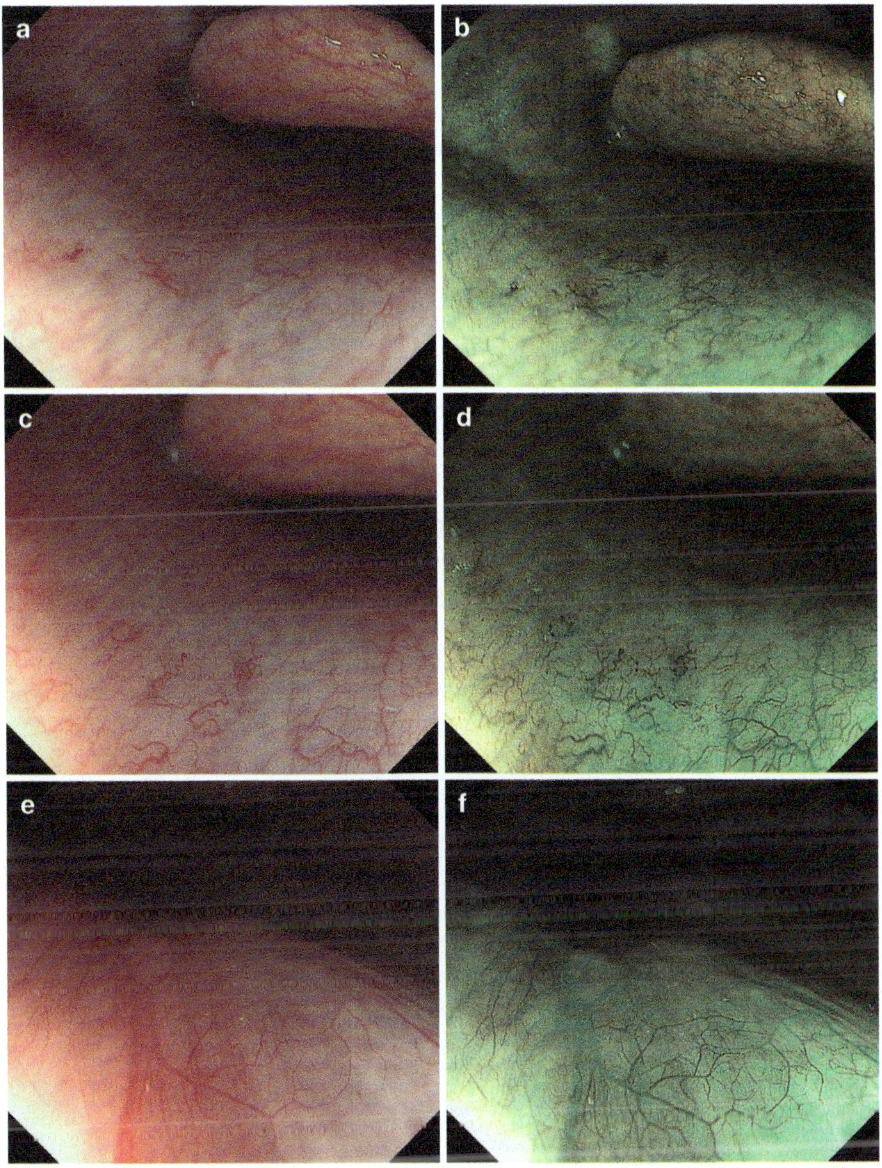

Fig. 5.6 Post radiotherapy changes, (**a**) nonmagnifying WLI, (**b**) nonmagnifying NBI, (**c**) close view of WLI, (**d**) close view of NBI, (**e**) WLI image of non-irradiated pharyngeal mucosa, (**f**) NBI image of non-irradiated pharyngeal mucosa

5.7 Post-ESD Scar

Endoscopic submucosal dissection (ESD) has also become widely used as an endoscopic treatment for early esophageal cancers [3]. As NBI becomes more widely used, we can anticipate that more early cancers and superficial cancers of the esophagus will be detected and expect that ESD will be indicated in more cases.

5.7.1 Explanation

Non-magnifying WLI reveals "puckering" associated with the (Fig. 5.7a). Similarly, non-magnifying NBI examination shows scar-associated "puckering" (Fig. 5.7b). Magnified examination clearly shows blood vessels gather within the scar toward its center (Fig. 5.7c, d).

5.7.2 Characteristics Under NBI Examination

Similar to inflammatory changes, nonneoplastic regenerative changes are associated with a degree of regularity to the vessel paths, along with a uniform directionality, in particular a tendency to travel in a horizontal direction.

On the other hand, neoplastic lesions will show a derangement of polarity, with irregular vessels running perpendicular to the mucosal surface (see Chap. 6).

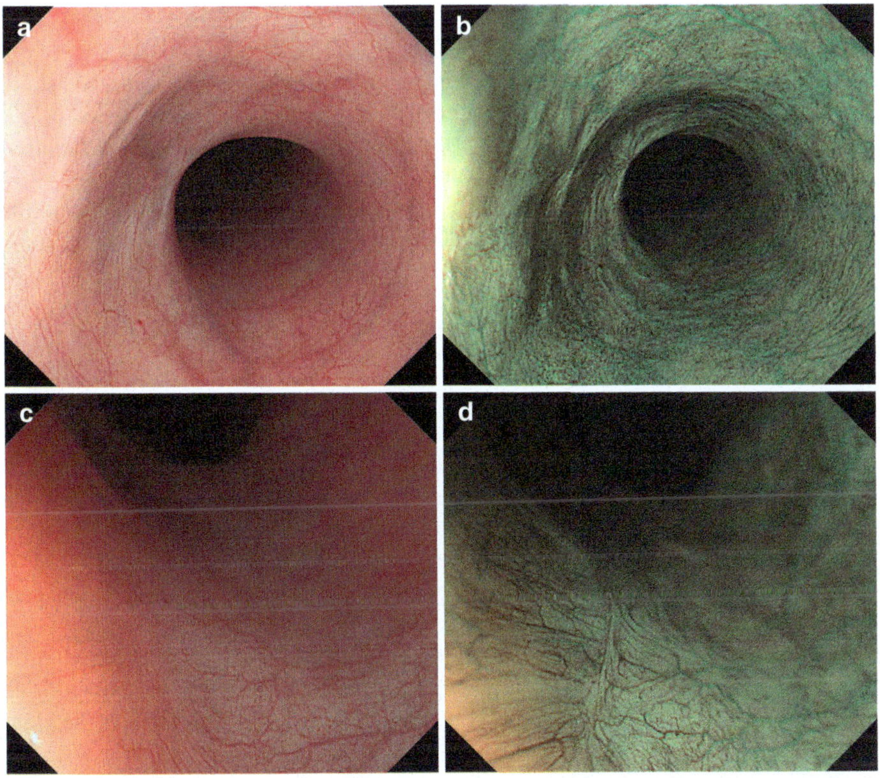

Fig. 5.7 Post ESD scar of the esphagus, (**a**) nonmagnifying WLI, (**b**) nonmagnifying NBI, (**c**) magnifying WLI, (**d**) magnifying NBI

5.8 Ectopic Gastric Mucosa

Ectopic gastric mucosa is an area of columnar epithelium often seen near the esophageal introitus, thought to be a mucosal remnant from the embryonic period [4, 5]. Ectopic gastric mucosa is detected in 10–14 % of patients undergoing WLI examinations. Endoscopically, lesions often present as oval patches, but they range in size from very small to circumferential. There may also be a single lesion or multiple lesions. Histologically, they resemble fundic glandular epithelium, although some resemble pyloric glands.

5.8.1 Explanation

When examining the cervical and upper esophagus, from the esophageal introitus to around 20 cm from the incisors, a clearer field of vision is obtained as the endoscope is withdrawn. Accordingly, patient discomfort is also minimized by examining the proximal part of the esophagus during scope withdrawal rather than insertion. If this area is to be examined during the first part of the examination, the scope should be first inserted as far as 20 cm from the incisors, and then examine the esophageal mucosa as the scope is withdrawn.

Non-magnifying WLI examination reveals discrete oval-shaped reddened areas (Fig. 5.8a), whereas non-magnifying NBI examinations show these lesions to be brownish areas with distinct margins (Fig. 5.8b). M-NBI (Fig. 5.8c) shows the glandular epithelial structure more clearly than M-NBI (Fig. 5.8d).

In this case, biopsy confirmed the diagnosis of ectopic gastric mucosa (Fig. 5.8f). Ectopic gastric mucosa is unstained by iodine staining (Fig. 5.8e), necessitating differentiation from cancer, although the diagnosis is easily made using M-NBI.

5.8.2 Characteristics Under NBI Examination

When a brownish area with distinct margins is detected in the cervical esophagus using non-magnifying NBI, we should immediately change over to M-NBI to confirm whether a glandular epithelial structure is present.

If a glandular epithelial structure is seen, the diagnosis of ectopic gastric mucosa can be made without the need for biopsy. On the other hand, if a glandular epithelial pattern cannot be seen, but proliferation of atypical vessels is seen within the brownish area, cancer should be suspected and biopsy performed.

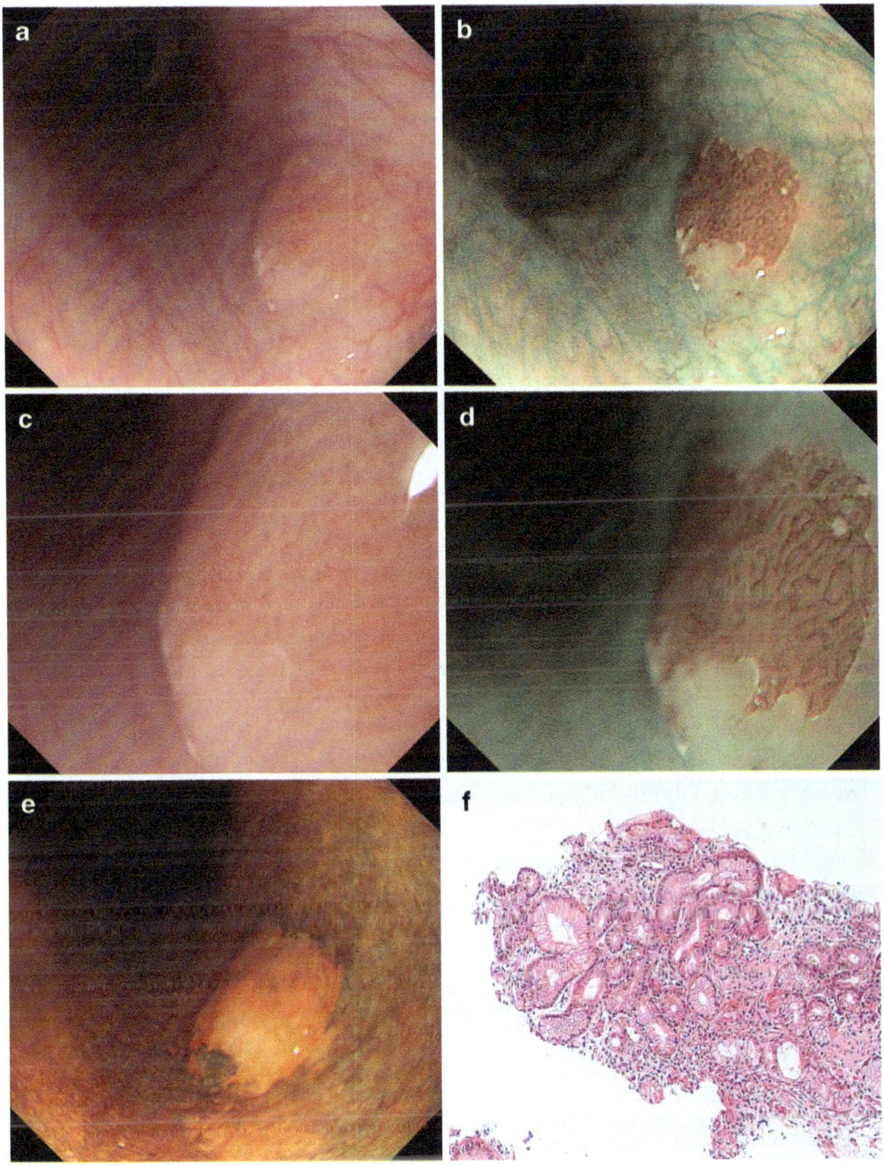

Fig. 5.8 Ectopic gastric mucos, (**a**) nonmagnifying WLI, (**b**) nonmagnifying NBI, (**c**) magnifying WLI, (**d**) magnifying NBI, (**e**) lugol staining, (**f**) HE image

5.9 Reflux Esophagitis

Gastroesophageal reflux disease (GERD) is defined as a condition that develops when the reflux of the gastric contents into the esophagus causes symptoms such as heartburn and complications including damage to the esophageal mucosa [6]. Although formerly considered relatively uncommon in Japan, recently the number of patients with GERD has increased, associated with an increasingly Westernized diet, aging of the population, and reduced *Helicobacter pylori* infection rates [7].

The manifestations of GERD are broadly classified into the esophageal and extraesophageal syndromes. The esophageal syndrome includes reflux esophagitis (RE), with endoscopic findings of mucosal damage (mucosal breaks, reddened areas with distinct margins, erosions, ulceration). A widely used endoscopic classification of RE is the Los Angeles (LA) classification [8], although the modified LA classification proposed by Hoshihara et al. [9] is the standard in Japan.

5.9.1 Explanation

We can see two long narrow reddened depressed areas (mucosal breaks), approximately 10 mm in length, between 12 and 2 o'clock at the gastroesophageal junction. The surrounding mucosa has a turbid white, mildly thickened appearance, with fewer visible vessels (Fig. 5.9a). This is consistent with RE of LA classification grade B.

Non-magnifying NBI examination delineates the reddened depressed areas as dark brown areas with distinct margins (Fig. 5.9b). Low-magnification NBI examination reveals linear microvessels in areas adjacent to the depressions, with densely packed, slightly dilated microvessels within the depressed areas, in places resembling a string of beads (Fig. 5.9c). Raising the magnification even further, the dilated microvessels within the depressed areas are relatively uniform in morphology, and the punctate and linear vessels in the surrounding mucosa do not show any definite atypia (Fig. 5.9d). Iodine does not stain, or only lightly stains, the reddened depressed areas, and the surrounding mucosa shows a fuzzy staining pattern [10], the typical chromoendoscopic findings for RE (Fig. 5.9e).

In this case, biopsy revealed intraepithelial and subepithelial inflammatory cell infiltration, the findings of papillomatous proliferation of RE (Fig. 5.9f).

5.9.2 Characteristics Under NBI Examination

Under NBI examination, the areas of mucosal damage appeared dark brown, with linear microvessels arranged in palisades seen in the surrounding cloudy white, mildly thickened mucosa.

Under strong magnification, we can see proliferation of dilated microvessels within the areas of damaged mucosa and their marginal areas, although their morphology is relatively uniform, with a regular arrangement.

Almost all cases of RE can be diagnosed on regular light (ALI) examination alone. However, although they are uncommon, some cases of superficial cancer are difficult to distinguish from RE. When such lesions are encountered, the diagnosis can be made easier by iodine staining, NBI examination, or following changes over time with administration of a proton pump inhibitor (PPI).

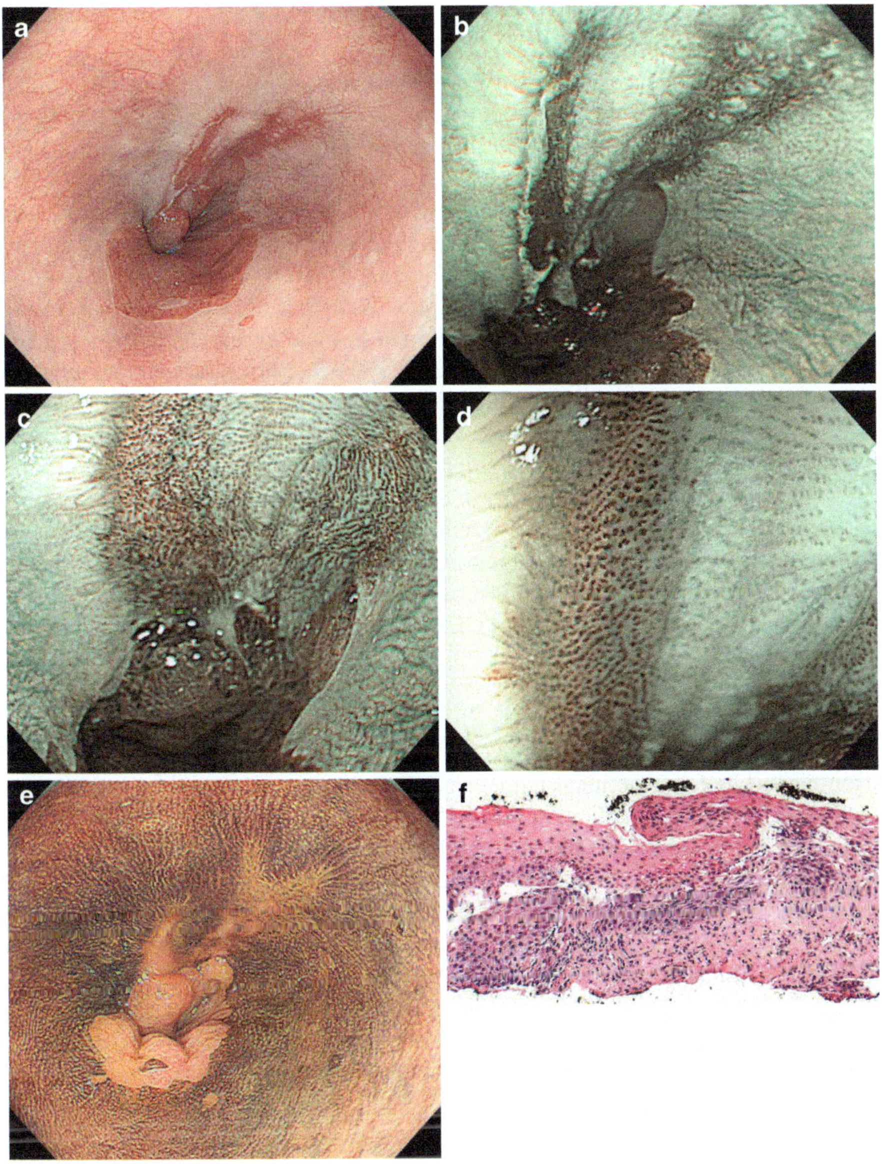

Fig. 5.9 Reflux esophagitis, (**a**) nonmagnifying WLI, (**b**) nonmagnifying NBI, (**c**) close view of NBI, (**d**) magnifying NBI, (**e**) lugol staining, (**f**) HE image

5.10 Nonerosive Reflux Disease (NERD)

The condition that develops when the reflux of the gastric contents into the esophagus causes symptoms such as heartburn and complications including damage to the esophageal mucosa is known as gastroesophageal reflux disease (GERD) and is broadly classified into the esophageal and extraesophageal syndromes [6]. When the esophageal syndrome is associated with no endoscopic findings of mucosal damage (mucosal breaks, reddened areas with distinct margins, erosions, ulceration), the diagnosis is nonerosive reflux disease (NERD).

Causative factors for NERD are complex, including not only reflux of gastric acid, but also esophageal contractile abnormalities and hypersensitivity. Although the majority of Japanese patients with GERD with heartburn symptoms are reported to have NERD [11], there are no endoscopic findings corresponding to NERD in the Los Angeles (LA) classification [8], which rates the degree of mucosal damage. NERD may correspond to grade M color changes (minimal change: whitish turbidity with reduced visibility of vessels) in the modified LA classification proposed by Hoshihara et al. [9]. Sharma et al. examined the lower esophagus near the gastroesophageal junction using M-NBI, reporting significantly increased numbers, tortuosity, and dilatation of intraepithelical papillary capillary loops (IPCLs) in patients with NERD than in controls without GERD [12].

5.10.1 Explanation

Non-magnifying conventional light (WLI) examination reveals white turbid areas with indistinct margins radiating in the 1, 5, 7, and 11 o'clock directions. This corresponds not to mucosal damage but to grade M changes (Fig. 5.10a). Non-magnifying NBI examination shows the white turbid areas more clearly (Fig. 5.10b). Low-magnification NBI examination reveals a marked increase in the number of IPCLs (Fig. 5.10c). Raising the magnification even further, we can see dilatation (Fig. 5.10d) and tortuosity (Fig. 5.10e) of the IPCLs.

In this case, biopsy revealed infiltration of inflammatory cells, with aggregation of lymphocytes and small numbers of neutrophils (Fig. 5.10f lower left) and IPCL hyperplasia (Fig. 5.10f arrows) and dilatation (Fig. 5.10g arrows). These findings correspond to esophagitis.

5.10.2 Characteristics Under NBI Examination

As seen in this case, grade M changes are easily diagnosed using NBI, even with non-magnifying examination.

In cases with suspected NERD, the lower esophagus near the gastroesophageal junction should be examined using M-NBI to identify morphological changes in the IPCLs.

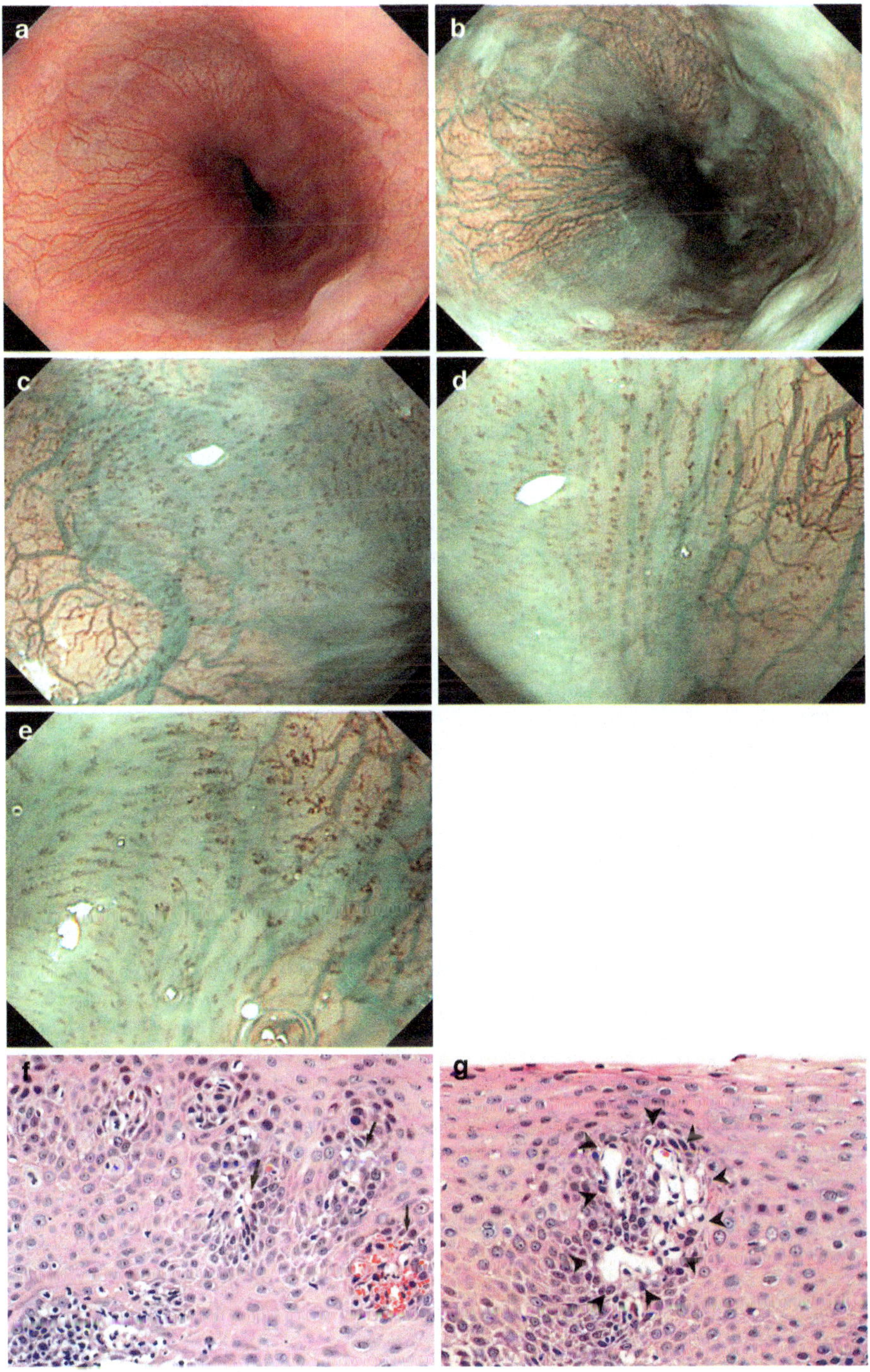

Fig. 5.10 Nonerosive Reflux Disease (NERD) (**a**) nonmagnifying WLI, (**b**) nonmagnifying NBI, (**c**–**e**) magnifying NBI, (**e**, **f**) HE image

5.11 Barrett's Epithelium

In Japan, Barrett's epithelium is defined as columnar epithelium continuous with the stomach extending into the esophagus, irrespective of whether intestinal metaplasia is present [13]. In Western countries, the term Barrett's is used only in cases with intestinal metaplasia.

Identification of the gastroesophageal junction is extremely important in the endoscopic diagnosis of Barrett's epithelium. In Japan, the lower margin of the lower esophageal palisade vessels (LEPVs) is emphasized in determining the site of the gastroesophageal junction, whereas in Western countries the oral termination of the vertical gastric rugae is considered more important [14].

In Japan, when Barrett's epithelium is circumferential and 3 cm or greater in length, it is called long-segment Barrett's esophagus (LSBE), and if less than 3 cm, short-segment Barrett's esophagus (SSBE) [13]. Pathognomic findings of Barrett's epithelium include: (1) esophageal glands beneath the columnar epithelium, (2) islands of squamous epithelium within the columnar epithelium, and (3) duplication of the muscularis mucosae [13]. Only (2) can be discerned endoscopically, and particular attention should be given to this finding when diagnosing SSBE.

Although areas of intestinal metaplasia within Barrett's epithelium are considered to be the carcinogenic foci, the two cannot be differentiated during conventional light (WLI) examinations. In recent years, however, studies have been conducted to clarify the characteristic appearance of intestinal metaplasia using magnifying endoscopy, with favorable results reported [15–17].

5.11.1 Explanation

In the region of the gastroesophageal junction, we can see Barrett's epithelium with a petallike appearance and confirm the lower margin of the LEPVs (dotted line) and the oral termination of the gastric rugae (arrows) (Fig. 5.11a). With NBI (non-magnifying) examination, we can identify the LEPVs, although they are darker and slightly less easily discernible than with conventional light (WLI) (Fig. 5.11b).

Figure 5.3 shows the WLI, and Fig. 5.4 the NBI images at medium magnification. The squamocolumnar junction (SCJ) is more clearly delineated using NBI than with WLI (Fig. 5.11c, d arrowheads). Small islands of squamous epithelium within the columnar epithelium, difficult to discern using WLI, are easily detected using NBI (Fig. 5.11d arrows). The mucosal microsurface pattern is also more clearly delineated with NBI than with WLI.

NBI examination with strong magnification further improves the visibility of mucosal microsurface pattern (villous structure) and microvessels (dark brown curves within the villous structure) (Fig. 5.11e, f).

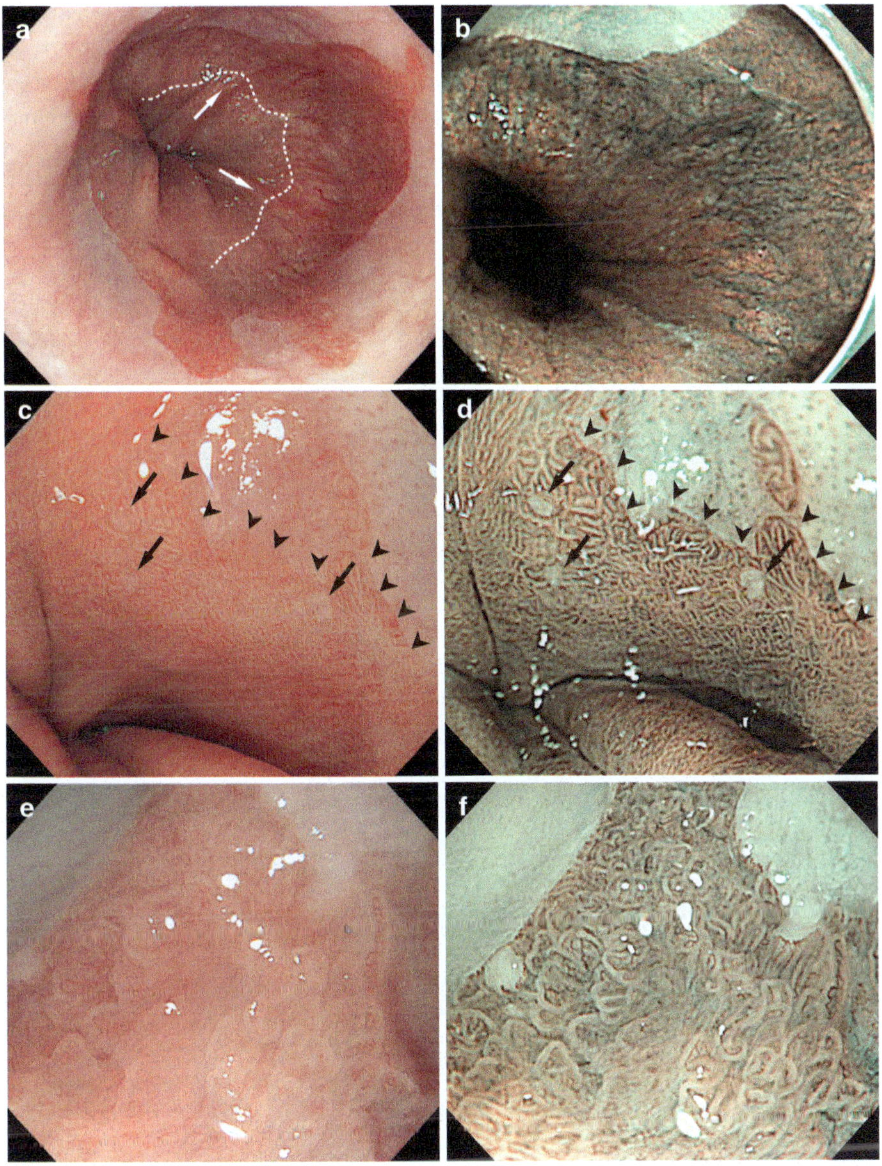

Fig. 5.11 Barrett's esophagus, (**a**) nonmagnifying WLI, (**b**) nonmagnifying NBI, (**c**) magnifying WLI, (**d**, **f**) magnifying NBI

5.11.2 Characteristics Under NBI Examination

Although not particularly useful in identifying the lower edge of the LEPVs or the oral margin of the gastric folds, NBI improves the visibility of the SCJ and small islands of squamous epithelium.

NBI is most useful in combination with magnified endoscopy, where without the need for staining, it can delineate both the mucosal microsurface pattern and the microvascular architecture.

References

1. Yokoyama A, et al: Cancer Sci 40:676–684, 2006
2. Odze R, et al: Am J Surg Pathol 17: 803–812, 1993
3. Fujishiro M, et al: Clin Gastroenterol Hepatol 4:688–694, 2006
4. Borhan-Manesh F, et al: Gut 32:968–972, 1991
5. Kumatani Y, et al: Prog Dig Endosc 66: 19–21, 2005
6. Vakil N, et al: Am J Gastroenterol 101:1900–1920, 2006
7. Ohara H et al: J Gastroenterol 102: 1010–1024, 2005
8. Armstrong D, et al: Gastroenterology 111: 85–92, 1996
9. Hoshihara Y: Clinical Gastroenterology 11: 1563–1568, 1996
10. Makuuchi H: Gastroenterology 11: 589–595, 1989
11. Furukawa N, et al: J Gastroenterol 4: 441–444, 1999
12. Sharma P, et al: Gastroenterology 133: 454–464, 2007
13. Japan Esophageal Society (eds). Japanese Classification of Esophageal Cancer (Revised 10th edition), Kanehara Shuppan, pp 40–42, 2008.
14. Lambert R, et al: Endoscopy 37: 879–920, 2005
15. Endo T, et al: Gastrointest Endosc 55: 641–647, 2002
16. Toyoda H, et al: Gastrointest Endosc 59: 15–21, 2004
17. Goda K, et al: Gstrointest Endosc 65: 36–46, 2007

Atlas of Neoplastic Lesions

6

Manabu Muto, Haruhiro Inoue, Shuko Morita, Kuniko Monma, Tomonori Yano, Chikatoshi Katada, Kenichi Goda, Hisao Tajiri, and Junko Fujiwara

M. Muto (✉)
Department of Therapeutic Oncology, Kyoto University Graduate School of Medicine, 54 Kawahara-cho, Syogoin, Sakyo-ku, Kyoto 606-8507, Japan
e-mail: mmuto@kuhp.kyoto-u.ac.jp

H. Inoue
Digestive Disease Center, Showa University Koto Toyosu Hospital, Tokyo, Japan

S. Morita
Department of Gastrointestinal Medicine, Kobe City Medical Center General Hospital, Kobe, Japan
e-mail: mmuto@kuhp.kyoto u.ac.jp

K. Monma • J. Fujiwara
Department of Endoscopy, Tokyo Metropolitan Komagome Hospital, Tokyo, Japan

T. Yano
Division of Digestive Endoscopy and Gastrointestinal Oncology, National Cancer Center Hospital East, Kashiwa, Japan

C. Katada
Department of Gastroenterology, Kitasato University School of Medicine, Sagamihara, Japan

K. Goda
Department of Endoscopy, The Jikei University School of Medicine, Tokyo, Japan

H. Tajiri
Department of Gastroenterology and Hepatology, The Jikei University School of Medicine, Tokyo, Japan

M. Muto et al. (eds.), *Atlas of Endoscopy with Narrow Band Imaging*,
DOI 10.1007/978-4-431-54243-8_6

6.1 Multiple Lugol-Voiding Lesions

Lugol-voiding lesions are the lesion not staining with iodine when sprayed with iodine solution. Lesions that do not stain with iodine include areas of inflammation, atypical epithelium, intraepithelial cancers, and invasive cancers, whereas squamous cell carcinoma is extremely likely with a positive pink color sign, a pink color change following iodine staining. Multiple Lugol-voiding lesions are seen in individuals with ALDH2 deficiency who habitually consume alcohol, and they are at an increased risk of multiple cancers of the esophagus and laryngopharyngeal region.

6.1.1 Explanation

There are often no particular abnormalities seen with non-magnifying WLI examination (Fig. 6.1a). When there are strong inflammatory changes, these may present as a pattern of thickened mucosa with marked whitish coloration, or mucosal areas with no visible vasculature. There are similarly often no particular abnormalities seen with non-magnifying NBI examination (Fig. 6.1b). Areas containing atypical epithelium may appear as brownish areas with indistinct, difficult to identify margins. It is often the case that spraying of iodine stain reveals for the first time multiple non-iodine staining lesions of varying sizes (Fig. 6.1c).

6.1.2 Characteristics Under NBI Examination

Some might tend to think that NBI is not suited to the detection of multiple Lugol-voiding lesions; however, it can also be said that with NBI we can detect lesions with high-grade intraepithelial neoplasia (HGIN) or higher, for which treatment is indicated, but not detect inflammatory changes or low-grade intraepithelial neoplasia (LGIN) or greater, for which treatment is not indicated (Fig. 6.1d–f).

Brownish areas with distinct margins detected using NBI (Fig. 6.1e) are clearly delineated as Lugol-voiding lesions following iodine staining (Fig. 6.1f). This is clinically highly significant because we may be uncertain which of many non-iodine staining lesions should be biopsied, but with NBI we can more accurately identify which should be biopsied.

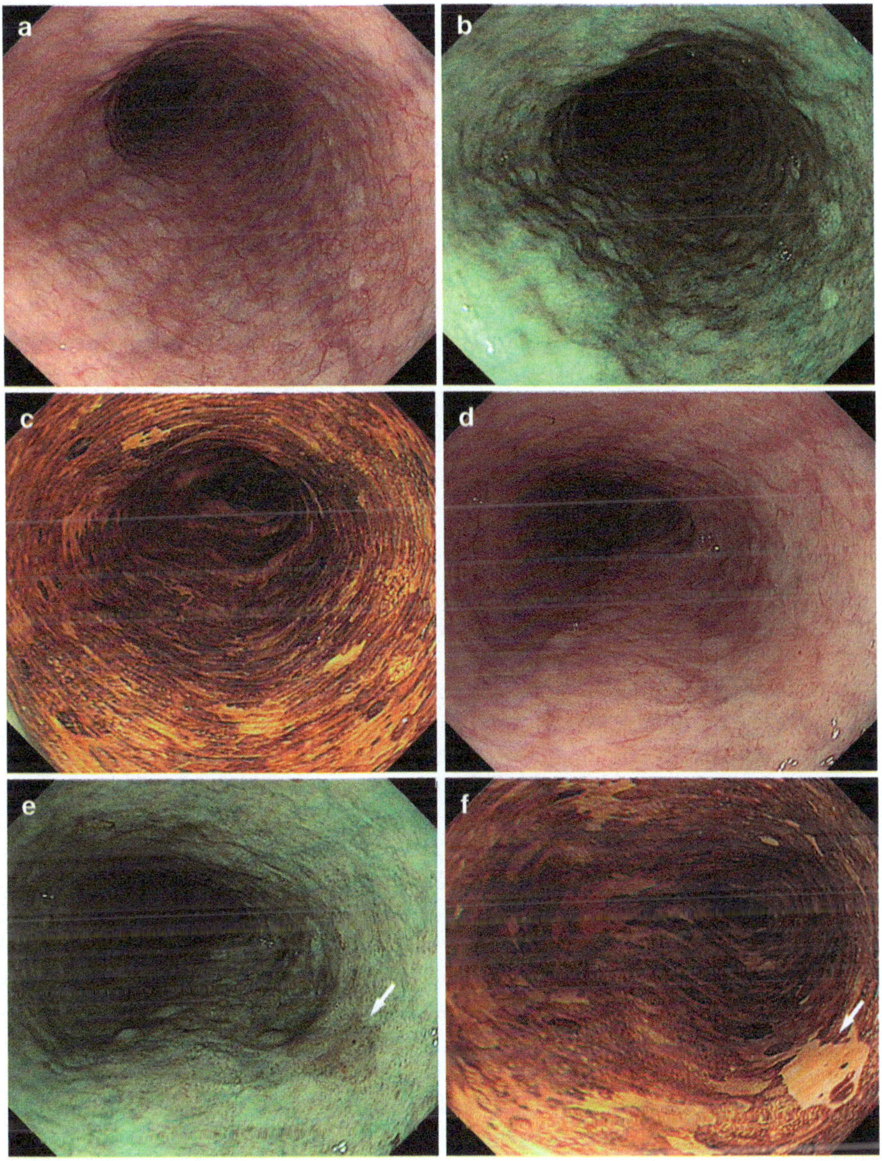

Fig. 6.1

6.2 Small Intraepithelial Neoplasia (Pharynx)

Small brownish areas are often seen in the pharynx during screening endoscopies. Small flattish lesions are also often seen on the posterior wall of the oropharynx that M-NBI shows to be IPCL type IV or V lesions, with vascular proliferation within the lesion.

These lesions are often intraepithelial tumors, but consideration should also be given to the possibility of low-grade intraepithelial neoplasia (LGIN). In particular, the presence of background coloration (BC) increases the likelihood of malignancy. A BC (+) IPCL type IV lesion has a 69 % probability of being high-grade intraepithelial neoplasia (HGIN) or higher. On the other hand, a BC (−) lesion has a 77 % probability of being low-grade intraepithelial neoplasia (LGIN) or lower. These lesions do not necessarily increase rapidly in size, and an overall approach to management should be taken with consideration of the patient's general condition.

6.2.1 Explanation

Non-magnifying WLI examination reveals a gently sloping reddened protuberance on the posterior wall of the oropharynx (Fig. 6.2a). Non-magnifying NBI examination of the same site shows a brownish area (Fig. 6.2b). Magnified examination shows an area of proliferation of abnormal vessels (Fig. 6.2c, d).

Histological examination of the endoscopic mucosal resection (EMR) specimen demonstrated HGIN or intraepithelial carcinoma with moderate to severe atypia, associated with the subepithelial aggregation of lymphoid follicles (Fig. 6.2e, f).

6.2.2 Characteristics Under NBI Examination

M-NBI demonstrated marked proliferation of IPCLs within the lesion in comparison with the background mucosa (IPCL type V-1). Examination of the individual vessels within the lesion reveals dilatation, tortuosity, variable diameters, and non-uniform morphologies on the basis of which we strongly suspect HGIN or intraepithelial carcinoma.

In general, color changes within a lesion increase the likelihood of malignancy, but even in BC (−) lesions such as this, marked vascular abnormalities also increase the likelihood of malignancy. BC can be considered a supplementary parameter to be evaluated along with vascular changes.

The gently sloping reddened protuberance seen in this case was considered to be the result of subepithelial aggregation of lymphoid follicles.

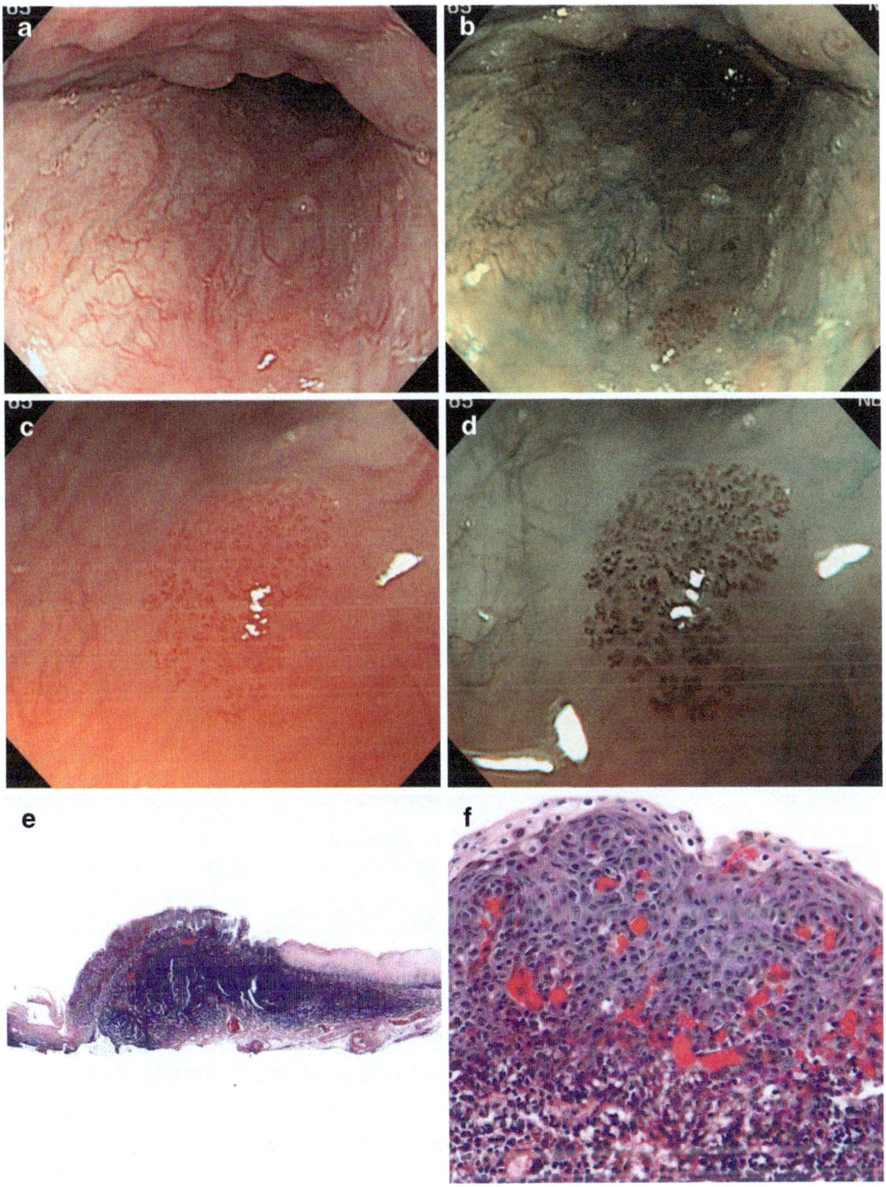

Fig. 6.2

6.3 Small Intraepithelial Neoplasia (Esophagus)

The advent of high-resolution endoscopes and NBI has made it relatively easy to detect small flat intraepithelial tumors. IPCL type IV lesions are roughly 50 % in each low-grade intraepithelial neoplasia (LGIN) and high-grade intraepithelial neoplasia (HGIN). Clinically, treatment (endoscopic mucosal resection (EMR) or endoscopic submucosal dissection (ESD)) is indicated for lesions of IPCL type IV or higher. Small lesions less than 5 mm in diameter can be surgically resected using cap-assisted EMR.

Because small flat IPCL type IV intraepithelial tumors do not usually grow rapidly, there are no problems with watchful waiting. Endoscopic complete resection biopsy is required in IPCL type V lesions, or lesions with an uneven surface.

6.3.1 Explanation

This lesion is a small flat esophageal intraepithelial tumor. Careful observation using non-magnifying WLI shows a lesion with light coloration impairing visualization of the dendritic vascular network (normal vascular network) (Fig. 6.3a). With non-magnifying NBI examination, the lesion is easily identified as a brownish area (brown spot) (Fig. 6.3b). With M-NBI we can further see that this is an IPCL type IV lesion (Fig. 6.3c). Endoscopic measurement indicates a diameter of approximately 1 mm.

Pathohistological examination of the endoscopic mucosal resection (EMR) specimen (Fig. 6.3d) yielded the diagnosis of HGIN with tumor tissue occupying the full thickness of the epithelium (Fig. 6.3e).

6.3.2 Characteristics Under NBI Examination

In this small but well-demarcated lesion, we can see proliferation of IPCLs within the lesion in comparison with the background mucosa (IPCL type IV). Abnormalities of the individual vessels within the lesion are not as severe as those typically seen in an intraepithelial carcinoma (dilatation, tortuosity, variable diameters, and nonuniform morphologies), but the lesion margin is clearly delineated in white.

6.3.3 For Reference: Endocytoscopy Findings

Figure 6.3f shows the ultramagnified endoscopic findings (endocytoscopic images). The lesion has clearly defined margins. The endocytoscope shows an increased cellular density on the lesion surface but no increase in nuclear size in comparison with the background mucosa (ECA-3). It is accordingly possible to determine endoscopically that this is a neoplastic lesion with a low degree of atypia, at least on the surface.

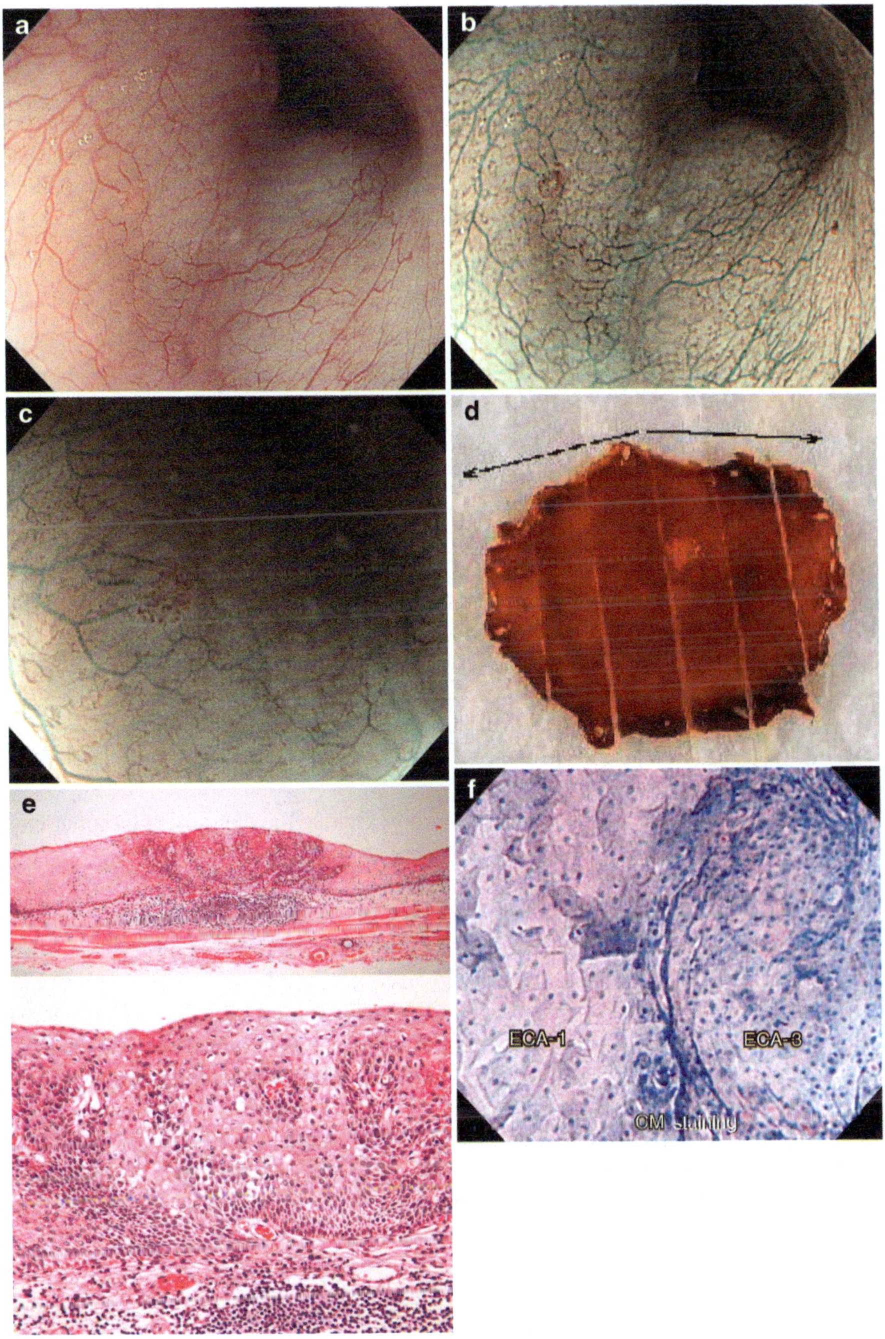

Fig. 6.3

6.4 Reddened Type IIa Lesion (Pharynx)

Type IIa lesions are reported to comprise 46.6 % of superficial elevated lesions [5]. A height of approximately 1 mm is considered a yardstick for esophageal cancers, but no such yardstick exists for the pharynx. The depth of invasion is no deeper than the subepithelial for low protuberances with almost no unevenness. Higher lesions with marked unevenness may have invaded deeper layers [6].

6.4.1 Explanation

Non-magnifying WLI reveals a slightly protruding reddened lesion in the shows a lesion in the laryngeal side of the right piriform sinus in the hypopharynx, although the extent of the lesion is unclear (Fig. 6.4a). With non-magnifying NBI examination, the lesion is identified as a brownish area with distinct margins. In contrast to the surrounding mucosa, the lesion shows an overall dark brownish coloration (Fig. 6.4b).

With M-WLI we can identify a slightly protruding lesion but cannot delineate the margins, and we cannot definitely see any proliferation of atypical vessels within the lesion (Fig. 6.4c). On the other hand, with M-NBI we can discern a brownish area with a definite color difference to the surrounding mucosa, and we can clearly see proliferation of atypical vessels (Fig. 6.4d). The mucosa visualized between the individual atypical vessels is also brown in color, so in addition to the vascular atypia, the color change of the mucosa itself is an important finding indicative of malignancy.

Pathohistological examination (HE staining) yielded the diagnosis of a squamous cell carcinoma confined to the epithelium (Fig. 6.4e).

6.4.2 Characteristics Under NBI Examination

The term "brownish area" refers to a lesion showing color changes in the mucosa seen between atypical vessels, but careful examination is required because the margin with the nontumorous mucosa may be clearly delineable in its entire circumference or it may only be distinct in part.

The lesion margins may be distinctly visible at a distance with non-magnifying NBI, or they may be discernible for the first time with M-NBI. When a brownish area is detected, if magnified examination reveals dilated atypical vessels in addition to a distinct lesion margin, cancer should be strongly suspected.

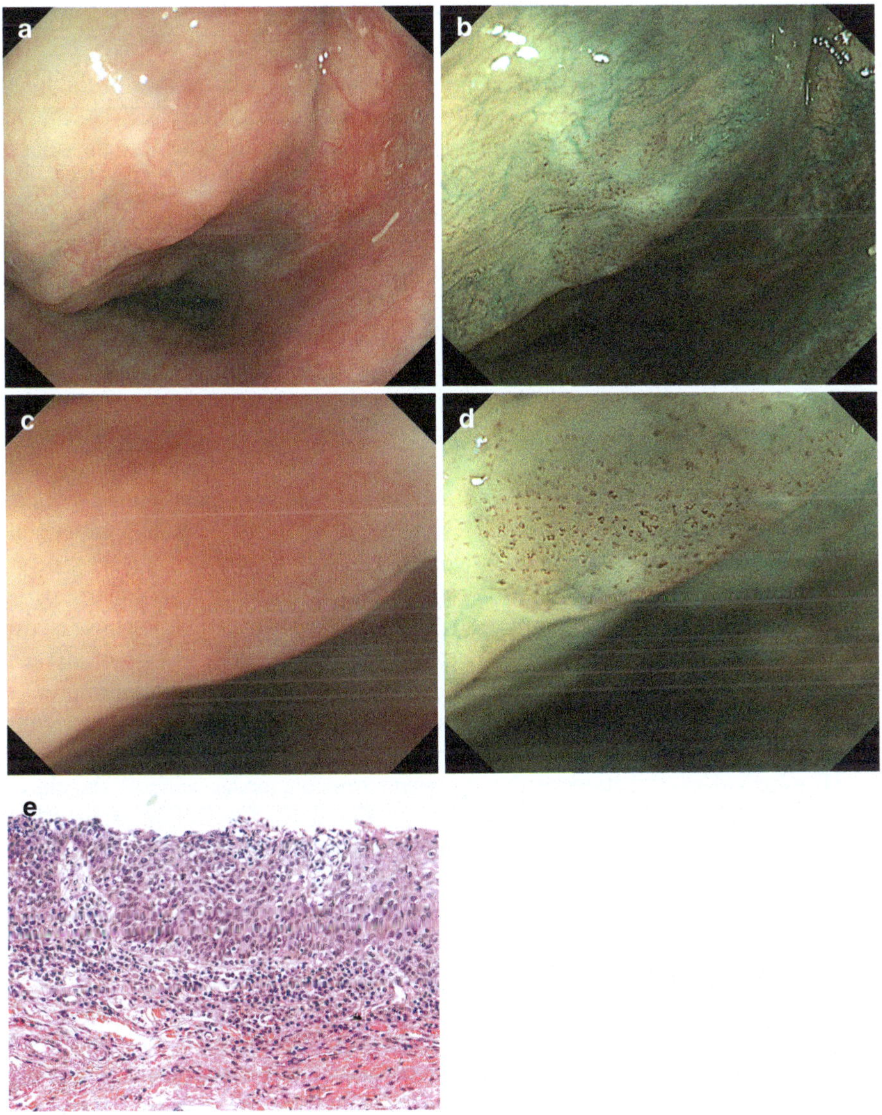

Fig. 6.4

6.5 Whitish Type IIa Lesion (Pharynx)

Whitish lesions are relatively rare among superficial elevated lesions of the pharynx. Histologically, lesions with a strong tendency to keratinize are seen as whitish. Low prominences with almost no surface unevenness tend to grow into the lumen, with the depth of invasion often confined to the subepithelial layer. Histologically, these lesions do often show downward growth, but there is no consensus as to whether this should be termed invasive or noninvasive. At present it is recommended that the thickness as measured from the surface of the lesion should be recorded.

6.5.1 Explanation

With non-magnifying WLI examination, we can just discern a slightly protruding whitish lesion in the right piriform sinus in the hypopharynx, although the extent of the lesion is unclear (Fig. 6.5a). With non-magnifying NBI examination, we can identify a whitish superficial elevated lesion (Fig. 6.5b). Iodine staining under general anesthesia reveals this lesion to be a distinct non-iodine staining area (Fig. 6.5c).

With M-NBI we can see that proliferation of atypical vessels is very sparse in the oral part of the lesion, and the difference in color to the surrounding mucosa is also slight (Fig. 6.5d). However, in the anal part of the lesion, proliferation of atypical vessels is rather marked, although they only show slight dilatation. Furthermore, the anal part of the lesion is seen as a distinct brownish area due to the difference in color to the surrounding mucosa (Fig. 6.5e).

Histological examination of the specimen resected under general anesthesia yielded the diagnosis of intraepithelial cancer (Fig. 6.5f). The lack of proliferation of atypical vessels within the lesion was thought to be the reason why it was difficult to detect atypical vessels within the lesion endoscopically.

6.5.2 Characteristics Under NBI Examination

The differential diagnosis for whitish elevated lesions of the pharynx is between a papilloma and hyperplastic changes. The surface of papillomas usually shows a papillary structure, making differentiation relatively easy.

Some cancers also show a papillary surface structure, but this can often be distinguished by its so-called "frog's eggs" appearance.

It can sometimes be difficult to differentiate between hyperplastic changes and cancer, but it can be identified as the latter if a brownish area with a distinct margin, and proliferation of atypical vessels, can be seen somewhere within the lesion. Vessel dilatation is often the only vascular abnormality to be seen.

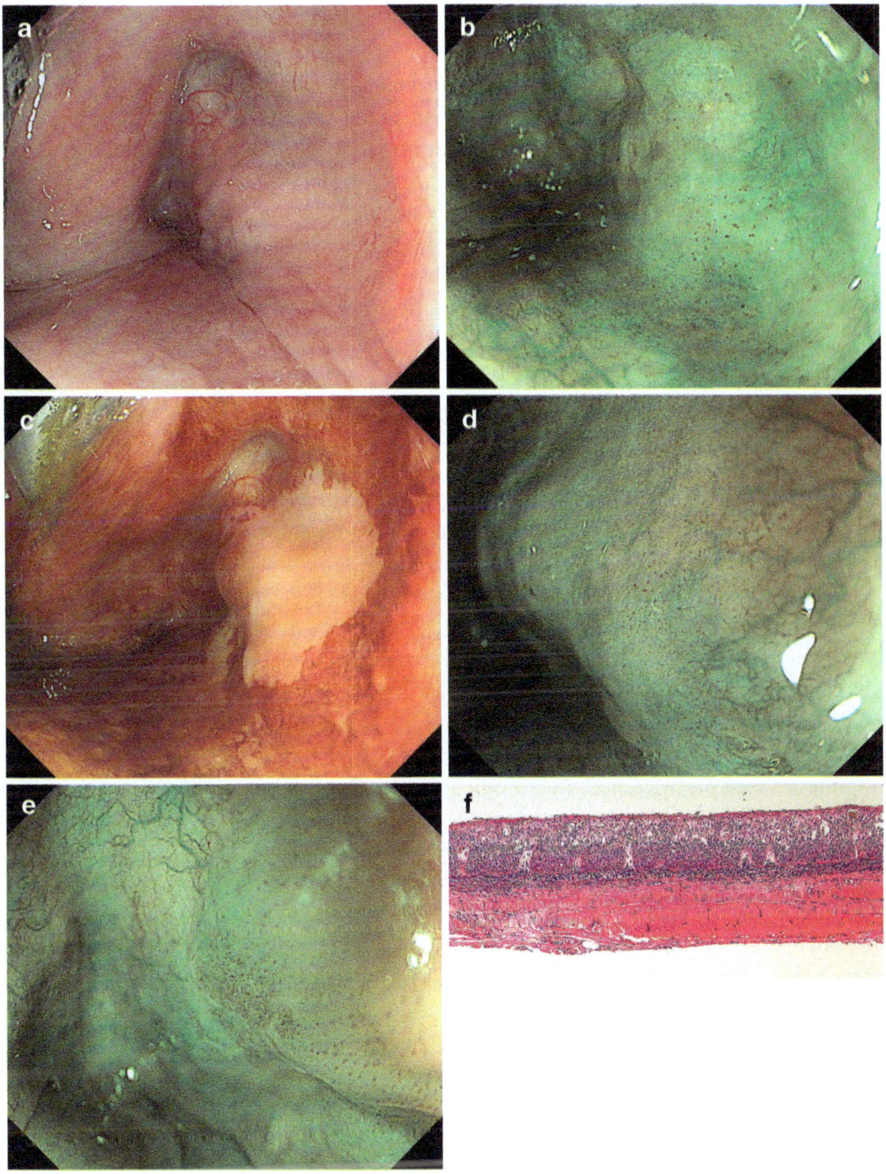

Fig. 6.5

6.6 Intraepithelial Neoplasia (Esophagus): Type 0-IIa

The "Japanese Classification of Esophageal Cancer" classifies surface type superficial cancers protruding slightly to less than 1 mm as type 0-IIa lesions. Type 0-IIa lesions are reportedly the next most common after 0-IIc and 0-IIb, accounting for approximately 15 % of superficial esophageal cancers [7]. Type IIa lesions that appear whitish on WLI examination often show upward growth into the esophageal lumen. Histologically, they show a strong tendency toward differentiation, and the depth of invasion is often no greater than T1a-EP or LPM. In contrast, reddened lesions tend to invade the deeper layers of the esophageal wall, with a depth of invasion often greater than T1a-MM [8].

6.6.1 Explanation

Non-magnifying WLI examination reveals a whitish flat-topped elevated lesion which has lost the normal vascular pattern. Some unevenness is evident in the center of the lesion, but it is small in magnitude (Fig. 6.6a). Non-magnifying NBI examination shows a brownish area with distinct margins (Fig. 6.6b). With M-NBI we can see dark brownish coloration within the lesion, with a dense proliferation of dilated atypical vessels (Fig. 6.6c). These atypical vessels correspond to IPCLs, characteristic vessels for neoplasia as described by Arima, Inoue, etc., and in conjunction with their non-staining with iodine, we can diagnose this lesion as a carcinoma (Fig. 6.6d).

Figure 6.6e shows a pathohistological image from the resected specimen.

6.6.2 Characteristics Under NBI Examination

Reddened lesions are visualized as brownish areas using NBI. Whitish lesions may be seen as either whitish or brownish areas using NBI.

If M-NBI shows a distinct area as well as atypical vessels as described by Arima, Inoue, etc., then the diagnosis of SCC can be made easily and with a high sensitivity [9].

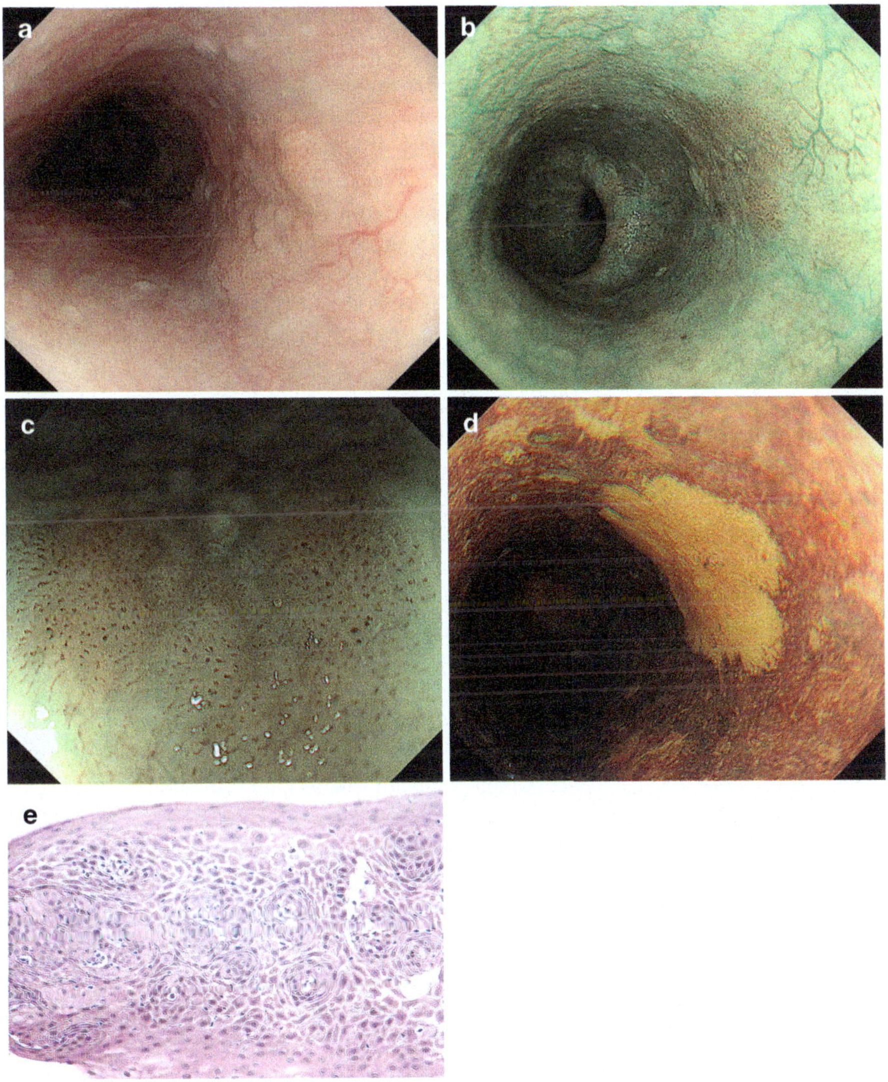

Fig. 6.6

6.7 Intraepithelial Neoplasia (Pharynx): Type 0-IIb

Although the mucosa of the oropharynx and hypopharynx is squamous epithelium as in the esophagus, the lack of muscularis mucosae means that at the time of their detection, lesions are often progressive cancers, making detection at the earliest possible stage desirable in this region. Now that superficial cancers of the oropharynx and hypopharynx can be detected endoscopically, follow-up examinations of patients after endoscopic resection of early esophageal cancers have changed: now the examination commences at the moment the endoscope enters the oral cavity. NBI is useful in this area, where iodine staining is difficult, in detecting lesions that might otherwise be missed.

The risk of developing SCCs is particularly high in people deficient in enzymes that metabolize acetaldehyde, whose faces go red when they drink alcohol, and a thorough examination commencing in the oral cavity is important in this group. A careful examination of the esophagus is required in these high-risk groups, as they also have an increased risk of esophageal cancer, and synchronous pharyngeal and esophageal cancers are common. The ratio of cancers of the oropharynx and hypopharynx to esophageal cancer is of the order of 10:1, so many more esophageal cancers will be detected at endoscopy.

The classification of superficial esophageal cancers in the "Japanese Classification of Esophageal Cancer" is followed in typing superficial cancers [10].

6.7.1 Explanation

WLI examination reveals a pale reddened area of mucosa, through which vessels cannot be visualized, in the posterior wall of the oropharynx/hypopharynx (Fig. 6.7a, c). From the absence of unevenness within the lesion, and no difference in height to the surrounding mucosa, this was classified as a 0-IIb lesion. NBI examination shows the lesion as a brownish area, with proliferation of intraepithelial papillary vessels, visualized as a pattern of dots (Fig. 6.7b, d). Iodine staining of the same region delineates the lesion as an irregularly shaped non-staining area (Fig. 6.7e).

Based on the endoscopic diagnosis of a 0-IIb intraepithelial cancer, the lesion was resected in one piece using the EMR method. The histological findings were as follows: lesion size 6×5 mm and depth of invasion Tis, ly0, v0 (Fig. 6.7f).

6.7.2 Characteristics Under NBI Examination

Non-magnifying NBI examination shows a brownish area, with proliferation of intraepithelial papillary vessels, enabling a qualitative diagnosis and delineation of the lesion margins.

The M-NBI findings show dilated tortuous intraepithelial papillary vessels.

No agreement has been reached in how to evaluate the microvasculature using magnified endoscopy in the oropharynx and hypopharynx, where under the epithelium lies the subepithelial layer, unlike the structure of the esophageal wall. To what extent the microvascular pattern reflects the depth of invasion is also a subject for future studies.

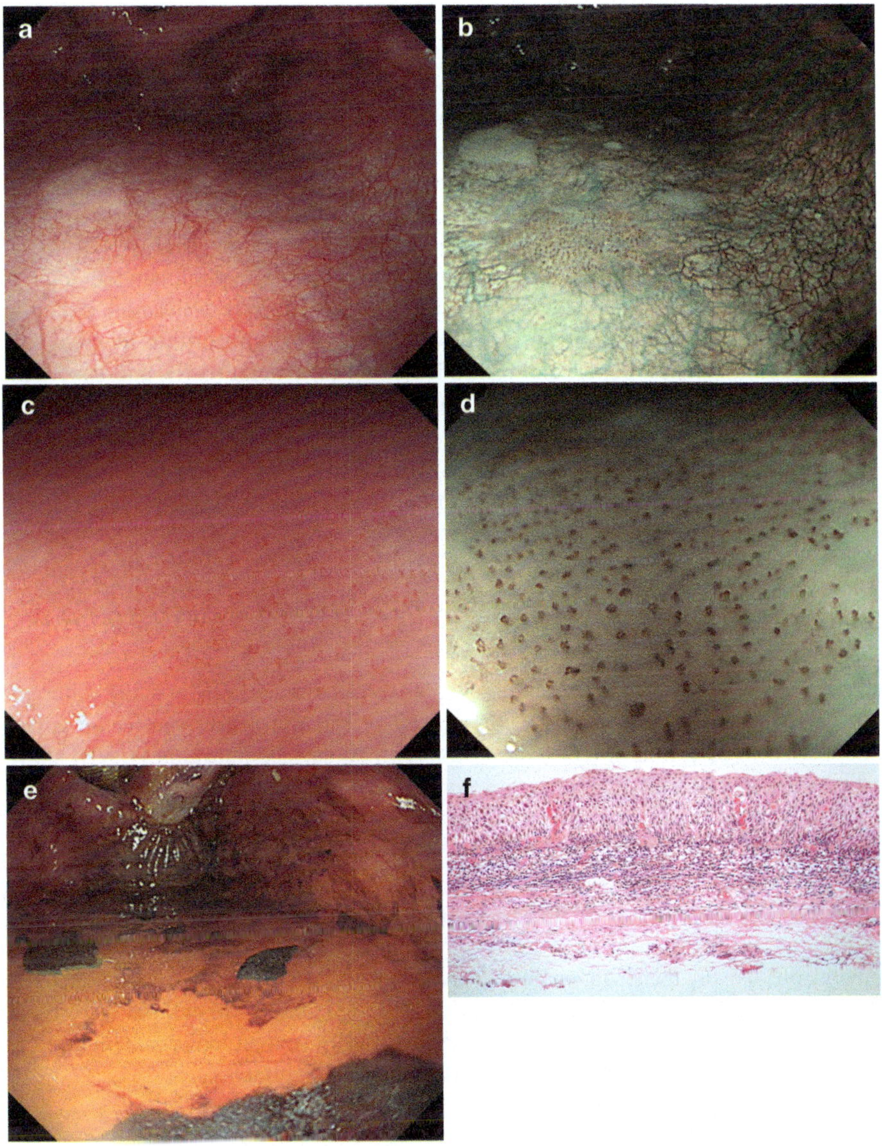

Fig. 6.7

6.8 Intraepithelial Neoplasia (Esophagus): Type 0-IIb

Iodine staining was previously thought indispensible in the detection of early esophageal cancers, particularly lacking in symptoms even among superficial esophageal cancers. However, the advent of NBI has changed the screening method for esophageal cancer. During introduction we examine the esophageal mucosa using WLI, looking for changes in color, unevenness of the surface, and changes in the vascular network. If an abnormality is detected, we immediately change over to NBI to confirm the presence and extent of any lesions. Even if no abnormalities are detected during insertion of the scope, during withdrawal we use NBI to examine the entire esophagus. Superficial esophageal cancers are classified according to their morphology into 3 types: superficial protruded (0-I), superficial (0-II), and superficial excavated (0-III) [11]. Type 0-II is further subdivided into superficial elevated (0-IIa), superficial flat type (IIb), and superficial shallow depressed type (0-IIc). The majority of type 0-I and 0-II lesions are submucosal cancers. Most mucosal cancers are type 0-II, but 0-IIc lesions range from EP to SM3, necessitating accurate assessment of the depth of invasion [12].

6.8.1 Explanation

WLI examination reveals a pale reddened area of the mucosa (Fig. 6.8a). Although increased glycogen acanthosis in the adjoining mucosa makes the lesion appear depressed in part, it is in fact a flat lesion with no surface unevenness. NBI shows the lesion as a brownish area, with no proliferation of intraepithelial papillary vessels visualized on non-magnifying examination (Fig. 6.8b). Iodine staining of the same region delineates the lesion as an irregularly shaped non-staining area, containing a small strongly staining area (Fig. 6.8c). This 5 mm non-iodine staining area is a flat lesion, with no unevenness, yielding an endoscopic diagnosis of type 0-IIb cancer, depth of invasion EP. The histological findings of the lesion, resected in one piece using the EMR method, were as follows: lesion size 5×3 mm and depth of invasion EP, ly0, v0 (Fig. 6.8d–f). Although the tendency to cellular differentiation toward the epithelial surface is preserved to some extent, enlargement and loss of polarity of the nuclei are seen, as well as increased cellularity.

6.8.2 Characteristics Under NBI Examination

During NBI examination, we examine changes in two factors, dark brown color changes in the background and changes in the vascular network. We can assess the degree of atypia using the combination of these two characteristics. In this case, no changes in the ICPLs within the brownish area were evident using non-magnifying NBI.

Histological examination of the resected specimen confirmed an intraepithelial carcinoma, with preservation of the tendency to cellular differentiation toward the epithelial surface, but minimal proliferation of ICPLs.

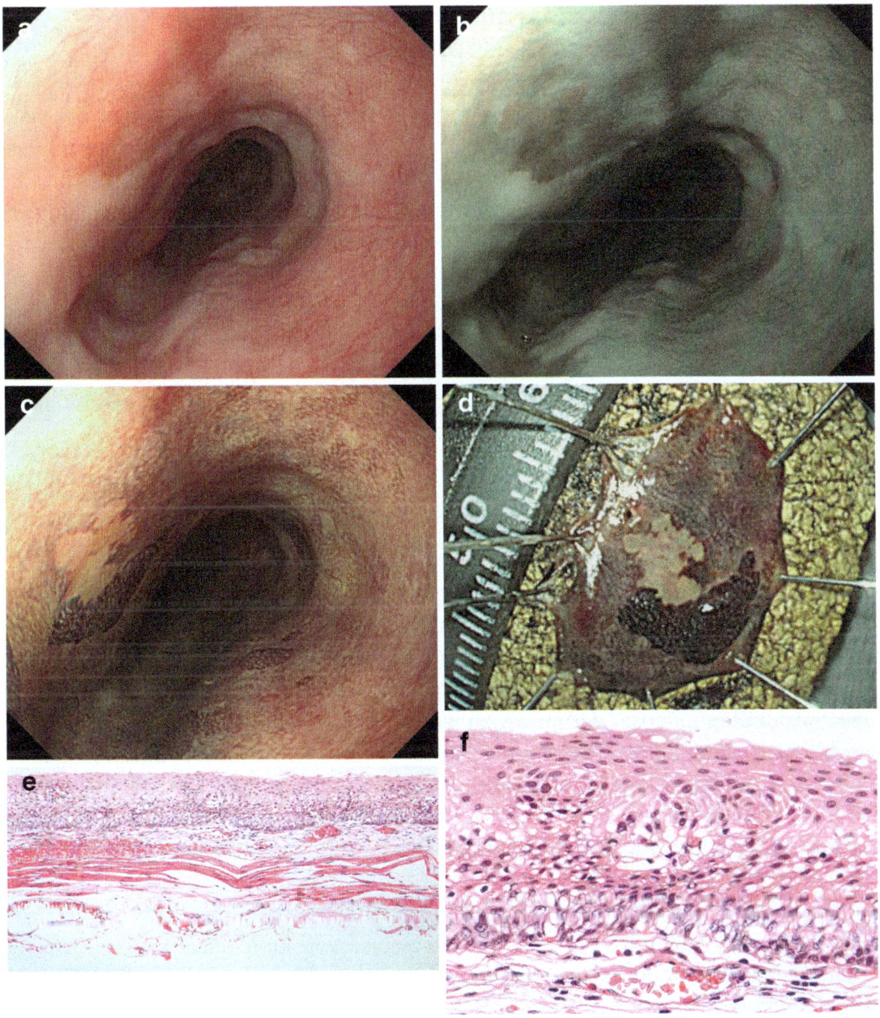

Fig. 6.8

6.9 Findings of the Margins of Superficial Cancers of the Pharynx and Esophagus

Most superficial squamous cell carcinomas of the pharynx and esophagus are visualized as a brownish area with distinct margins, with proliferation of atypical vessels within the lesion. The margins of the brownish area can sometimes be delineated over their entire circumference, but they may only be identifiable in part, making the diagnosis difficult. Furthermore, in some cases a brownish area is visualized but light in color, making us unsure whether we should suspect cancer or not.

In these cases, we should concentrate on the contrast between the smooth greenish white surface of the surrounding nonneoplastic mucosa and the rather dark brownish coloration and roughened mucosal surface within the lesion and the presence of a fine fuzzy white adherent furry substance. Squamous cell carcinoma is likely if these findings are present.

6.9.1 Explanation

From a distance, non-magnifying WLI examination reveals a light red-colored flat lesion with loss of visibility of the vasculature (Fig. 6.9a). On the periphery of the reddened area, we can see some adherent white substance. From a distance, non-magnifying NBI examination shows a brownish area with a distinct boundary with the surrounding mucosa, within which we can see a pattern of dots (Fig. 6.9b).

M-WLI examination reveals, in contrast to the smooth surfaced nonneoplastic mucosa, a reddened lesion with proliferation of atypical microvessels (Fig. 6.9c). With M-NBI we can see the boundary between tumor and nontumor even more clearly and confirm the fine fuzzy white furry substance adherent to the marginal area (Fig. 6.9d).

Raising the magnification even further, NBI shows the fine fuzzy white furry substance and the proliferating atypical vessels even more clearly (Fig. 6.9e, f). Within the lesion, submucosal translucency is reduced, as is visibility of the branching vascular network.

6.9.2 Characteristics Under NBI Examination

When a brownish area is identified in the esophagus or pharynx, we should be cognizant that in the case of a neoplastic lesion, there may be a fine fuzzy white furry substance adherent to the marginal area between the tumor and nontumor.

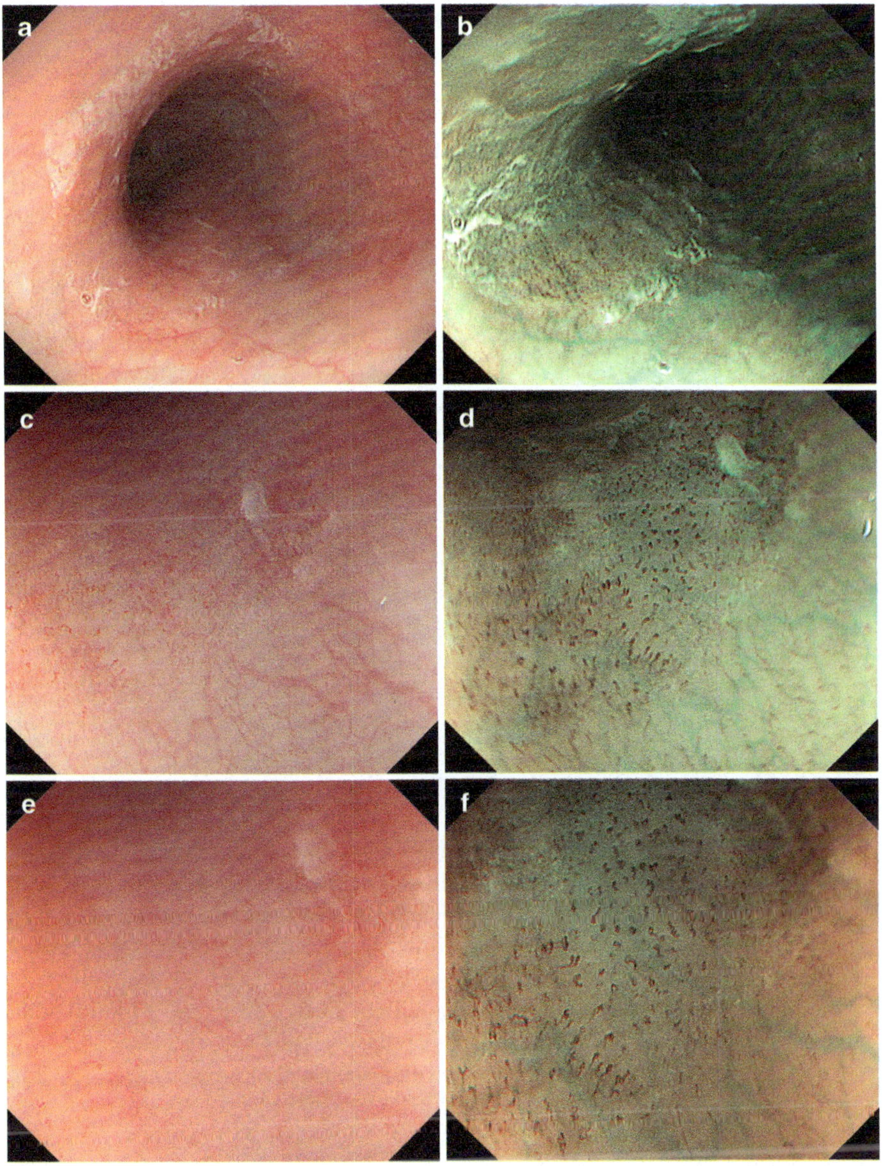

Fig. 6.9

6.10 Superficial Pharyngeal Cancer with Prominent Protrusion: Type 0-I

Type I lesions are relatively uncommon in the pharynx, accounting for 5.7 % of all cancers in one study. Invasive lesions, reaching the subepithelial layer, are common [1]. Although prominent protrusions make this type of lesion easy to detect, careful inspection of the surrounding area is required, because near the base there may exist an associated superficial lesion with little or no unevenness.

6.10.1 Explanation

Although type I lesions are easily detected using WLI due to their prominent protrusions, they are often associated with a flat lesion in the vicinity of their base, necessitating careful examination of the surrounds for accurate margin delineation. The surface has a wrinkled appearance like a mulberry, sometimes requiring differentiation from a papilloma (Fig. 6.10a, b).

Although it is difficult to discern any blood vessels in this protruding lesion using M-NBI (Fig. 6.10c), the flat lesion spreading out from its base is visualized as a brownish area with distinct margins and proliferation of dilated atypical vessels, typical of a squamous cell carcinoma (Fig. 6.10d).

Figure 6.10e shows a pathohistological image.

6.10.2 Characteristics Under NBI Examination

Whether using NBI or not, when we detect a protruding lesion with an irregular surface, we should suspect malignancy. In some cases proliferation of vessels cannot be visualized using M-NBI, but the diagnosis is easy if proliferation of atypical vessels or a brownish area can be identified in the area of superficial extension spreading out from the base of the protrusion.

Papillomas have a relatively uniform papillary surface structure, with little dilatation or atypia seen in the extended intrapapillary vessels.

On the other hand, dilated vessels are often seen within type I cancers, making differentiation possible.

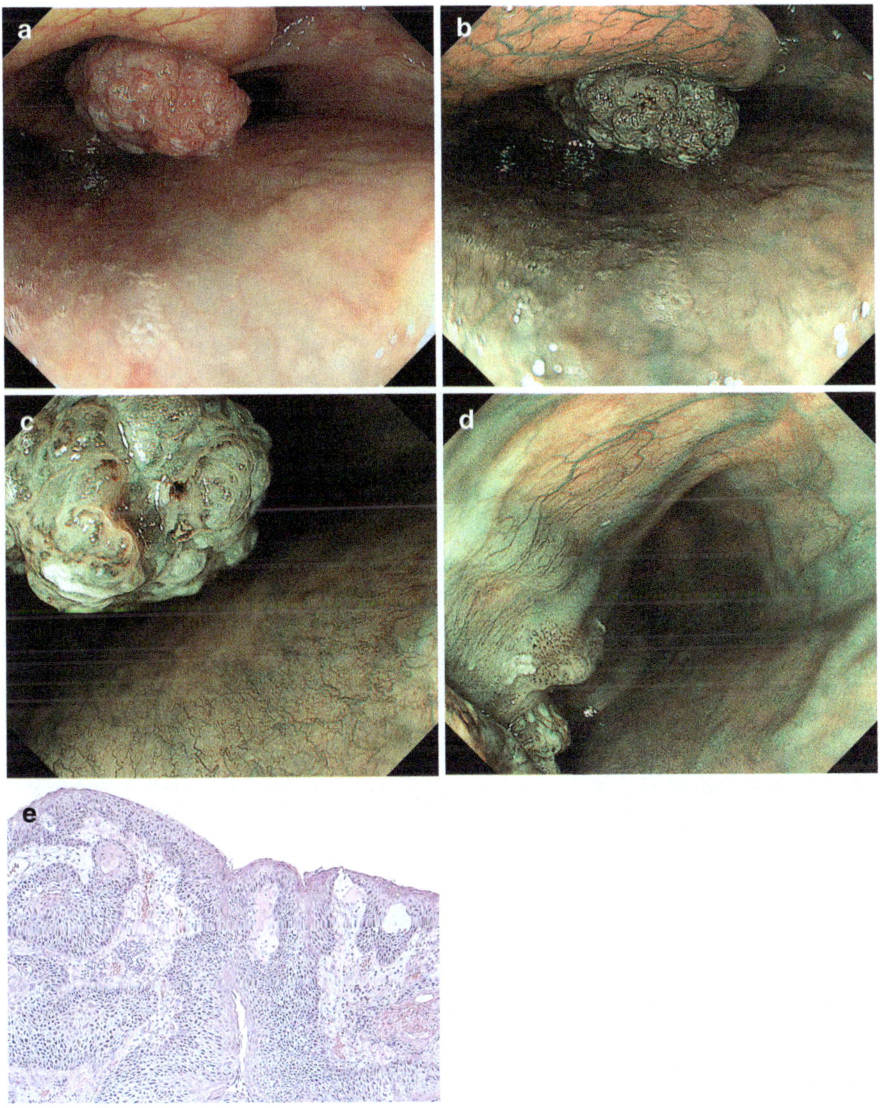

Fig. 6.10

6.11 Superficial Esophageal Cancer with Prominent Protrusion: Type 0-I

The macroscopic type and depth of invasion correlate closely for superficial esophageal cancers, so determination of the macroscopic type enables prediction of the depth of invasion to a degree. Prominently protruding lesions with a height ≥2 mm are classified as superficial protruded (type 0-I), further subdivided into type 0-Ip, with a narrow base (pedunculated polyps), and type 0-Is, with a broad base (sessile polyps).

In general, the depth of invasion of type 0-I lesions is considered deeper than the mid-layers of the submucosa (SM), with type 0-Ip including carcinosarcomas and pseudosarcomas. Of the type 0-I lesions, caution is required concerning the depth of invasion in type 0-Ip lesions, as some lesions with a narrow base reach only a shallow depth. When a type 0-Ip lesion is detected, while examining its morphology, attention should also be paid to the hardness of the protrusion.

6.11.1 Explanation

When we detect a protruding lesion in the esophagus, we should examine the protrusion to determine its height, size, morphology, hardness, and mobility. The height of this lesion sticking out into the esophageal lumen is at least 2 mm, with a narrow base, and as a lesion progresses its morphology changes, so we can classify this as a type 0-Ip lesion. The lesion surface shows a granular unevenness, but it is soft without any tension and mobile, indicating that the depth of invasion of this tumor is no greater than MM (Fig. 6.11a). A lower protruding lesion extends from the anal end of this lesion, yielding the diagnosis of a type 0-I+IIa lesion. NBI examination reveals proliferation of IPCLs within the brownish area, with the majority of vessels within the protruding lesion of type 3 using the Arima classification [13] (Fig. 6.11b, d). Iodine staining reveals a non-staining area as seen in Fig. 6.11c.

Based on the endoscopic diagnosis of a 0-I+IIa lesion with depth of invasion MM, this lesion was resected using the ESD method. The histological findings were as follows: lesion size 20×16 mm and depth of invasion MM, ly0, v0 (Fig. 6.11e, f). The 0-I portion was 11×10 mm in size and located on the anal side of the protruding part of the lesion, an MM cancer invading the muscularis mucosae.

6.11.2 Characteristics Under NBI Examination

Although NBI examination is useful in detecting lesions and determining their horizontal extent, WLI is more than adequate to detect type 0-I lesions with prominent protrusions.

Although M-NBI examination is useful for determining the depth of invasion, for 0-Ip protruding lesions, the hardness and mobility of the protrusion are the most useful predictive factors for the depth of invasion. When the invading part of the lesion is very narrow in horizontal extent, inability to visualize any vascular abnormalities can make determination of the depth of invasion difficult.

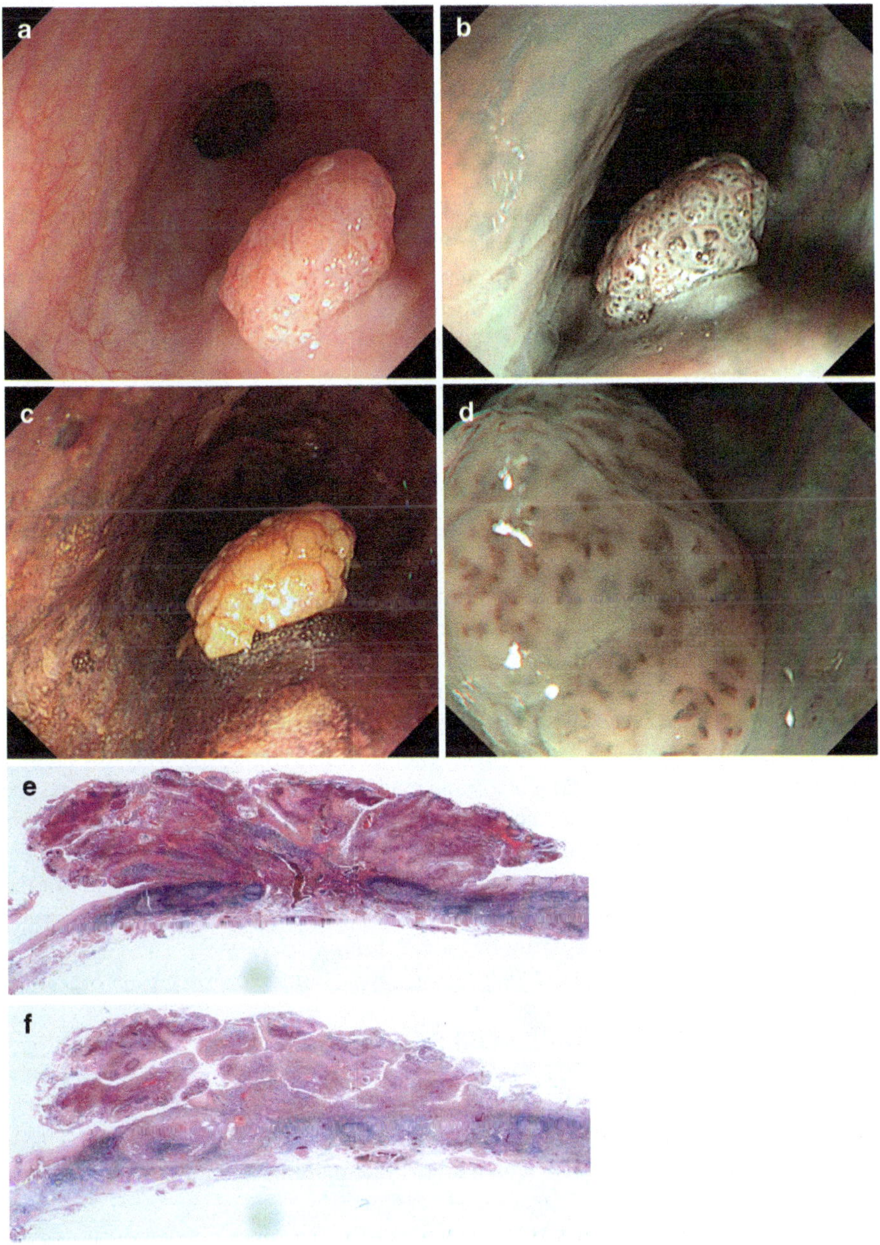

Fig. 6.11

6.12 Superficial Cancer of the Uvula

The development of NBI has made it possible to detect superficial cancers of the oropharynx and hypopharynx. Muto et al. conducted a multicentered comparative trial of NBI and WLI in patients with esophageal cancer, finding significant superiority for NBI over WLI in the detection of superficial cancers in the head and neck region. They found superficial cancers in the head and neck region in approximately 8 % of patients with esophageal cancer [9].

In the series of 140 superficial cancers of the oropharynx and hypopharynx detected in 98 patients using NBI between April 2002 and April 2008 at the National Cancer Center Hospital East, only 2 lesions (1.4 %) were superficial cancer of the uvula.

6.12.1 Explanation

As proximity of the tongue makes it difficult to examine the uvula, we ask the patient to say "Ah" to make it easier to see. Although there is considerable individual variation in uvular size, a large uvula may indicate involvement of the entire uvula in a disease process, so the surface should be examined carefully and thoroughly.

In this case, non-magnifying WLI examination revealed a light reddened area on the right side of the uvula (Fig. 6.12a), seen as a brownish area with distinct margins on non-magnifying NBI examination (Fig. 6.12b). In comparison with low magnification WLI (Fig. 6.12c), NBI at the same magnification (Fig. 6.12d) delineates the margins more clearly, and we can also see proliferation of dilated atypical vessels within the lesion. Higher-magnification M-NBI shows a dense network of atypical vessels with an irregular arrangement (Fig. 6.12e). Histological examination of the resected lesion showed a squamous cell carcinoma with intraepithelial invasion associated with epithelial hypertrophy (Fig. 6.12f).

6.12.2 Characteristics Under NBI Examination

NBI examination should be performed whenever a pale reddened area is detected using WLI. Superficial cancer should be suspected, and biopsies taken, if NBI examination reveals a brownish area with distinct margins and magnified examination shows densely proliferating atypical vessels.

Even for reddened areas on WLI examination, if NBI does not demonstrate proliferation of atypical vessels, inflammatory changes are likely.

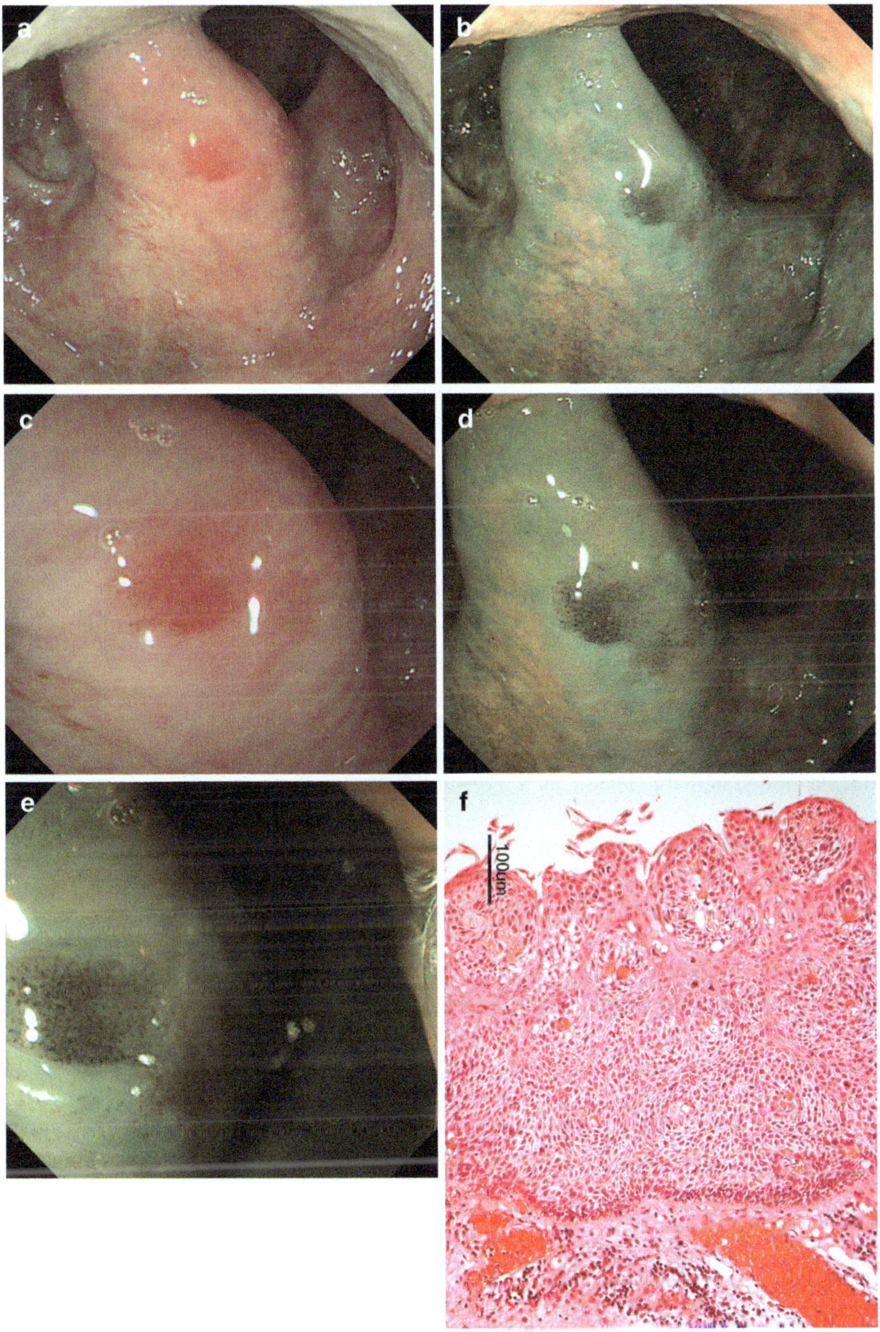

Fig. 6.12

6.13 Superficial Cancer of the Soft Palate

The oropharynx is anatomically divided into the anterior wall (base of the tongue), lateral walls (palatine tonsillar areas), superior wall (soft palate), and posterior wall (pharyngeal mucosa). Squamous cell carcinomas account for 90 % of oropharyngeal malignancies, with the lateral walls being the most common site, followed by the anterior wall, then the superior wall, and the posterior wall as the least common site [14]. Reported incidences of oral erythroplakia, or irreversible red patches on the oral mucosa, are of the order of 0.02–0.83 %, with alcohol and smoking identified as risk factors [15].

6.13.1 Explanation

From a distance, non-magnifying WLI examination of the superior wall of the oropharynx reveals a reddened patch around 1 cm in size, with poor visibility of the vasculature on the right side of the soft palate (Fig. 6.13a). Some melanosis is present. Non-magnifying NBI examination shows the lesion as a brownish area with a distinct boundary (Fig. 6.13b, c). With M-NBI we can discern dilated atypical vessels with variable diameters (Fig. 6.13c, d). The boundary between nontumor and tumor is distinct, and proliferation of atypical vessels within the tumor allows us to diagnose it as oropharyngeal cancer. Although a superficial elevated element is seen on the right side of the lesion, the overall flatness of the lesion indicates that the depth of invasion is intraepithelial. Iodine staining endoscopy under general anesthesia delineated the lesion as a non-iodine staining area with distinct margins (Fig. 6.13e).

This lesion was resected under general anesthesia using a peroral approach [16]. It was 12 × 8 mm in size (Fig. 6.13f). The histological diagnosis was of a squamous cell carcinoma confined to the epithelial layer (Fig. 6.13g).

6.13.2 Characteristics Under NBI Examination

Cancer should be suspected, and biopsies taken, if NBI examination reveals a brownish area with distinct margins and magnified examination shows proliferating atypical vessels. If still uncertain whether to biopsy on the basis of the NBI findings, iodine staining using a cotton tip applicator may assist in the decision.

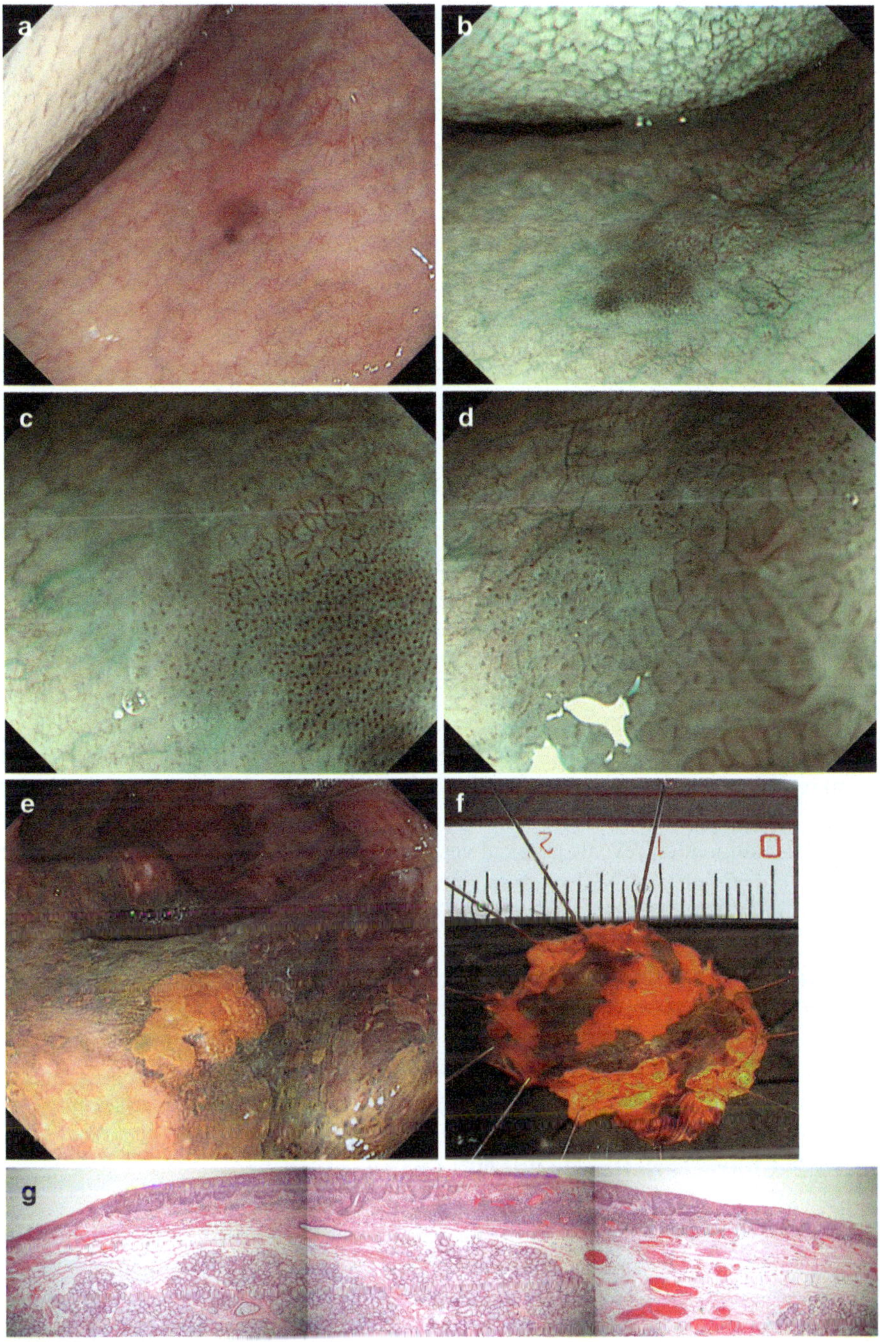

Fig. 6.13

6.14 Superficial Cancer of the Larynx

The age adjusted incidences of "oropharyngeal cancer," "laryngeal cancer," and "esophageal cancer" in Japan are in men 4.9, 3.3, and 9.5 per 100,000, respectively, and in women 1.7, 0.1, and 1.6 per 100,000 [17].

According to the National Register of Malignancies of the Head and Neck (initial diagnosis 1990–1999; 14,170 cases), published by the Japan Society for Head and Neck Cancer, the proportion of cancers according to subsite was 31.3 % for the supraglottis, 66.1 % for the glottis, and 2.6 % for the subglottis, with the glottis the most common. Of the 2,427 registered cases of glottal cancer, those diagnosed relatively early comprised 11 cases of intraepithelial cancer (Tis), 951 confined to one vocal cord (T1a), and 395 confined to both vocal cords (T1b) [10].

6.14.1 Explanation

Examinations of the larynx are routinely performed using a direct laryngoscope under general anesthesia. Endoscopic examination is often possible with the patient awake under laryngeal anesthesia, applied by spraying 4 % lignocaine solution (approximately 3 mL) using a spraying tube passed down the instrument channel. If a strong laryngeal reflex is seen despite application of an ample amount of laryngeal anesthetic, then observations and biopsies should be performed using a small-diameter endoscope.

In this case, from a distance, non-magnifying WLI examination of the left vocal cord reveals a protruding lesion slightly under 1 cm in size, whitish with a reddened tinge, toward the anterior commissure (Fig. 6.14a). Changing over to non-magnifying NBI examination reveals atypical vessels in the anterior commissure side of the lesion (Fig. 6.14b). M-NBI examination of this anterior commissure side of the lesion shows these atypical vessels to be irregularly tortuous (Fig. 6.14c). Near the center of the lesion, the epithelium has broken down, with disappearance of the atypical vessels (Fig. 6.14d). The posterior commissure side of the lesion is covered in a thick white adherent substance (Fig. 6.14e).

Pathohistological examination of the endoscopic biopsy specimen yielded the diagnosis of squamous cell carcinoma (Fig. 6.14f).

6.14.2 Characteristics Under NBI Examination

Identification of atypical vessels is difficult in areas with adherent white substance or keratinization. Laryngeal cancer can be diagnosed if irregular atypical vessels are identified within the lesion or at its margins.

Biopsies should always be taken for a tissue diagnosis due to the possibility that atypical vessels are obscured by adherent white substance or keratin plaques.

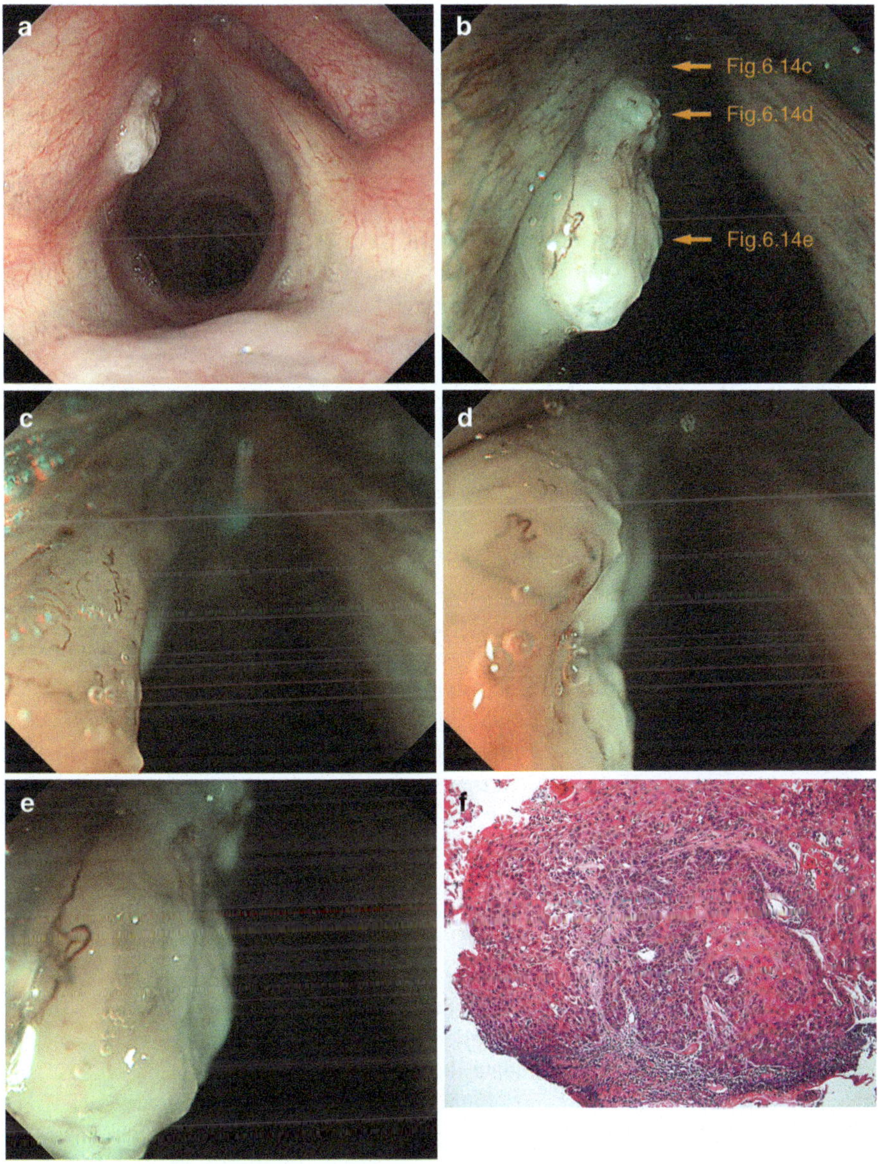

Fig. 6.14

6.15 Superficial Invasion in the Vicinity of a Polypoid Tumor (Pharynx)

Increased utilization of chromoendoscopy using iodine staining for the detection of esophageal cancer means that it is now well known that superficial invasion may be observed in the vicinity of polypoidal or ulcerated lesions. Furthermore, in the laryngeal area, the advent of NBI has allowed us to detect superficial invasion in the vicinity of polypoidal and ulcerated lesions. In recent times, determination of the extent of superficial invasion using NBI is considered necessary when deciding whether larynx-preserving partial resection is feasible.

6.15.1 Explanation

We carefully examine the vicinity of the main lesion. In this case, non-magnifying WLI examination revealed a lesion comprising protruding and ulcerated elements, with adherent white substance, extending from the right aryepiglottic fold to the piriform sinus (Fig. 6.15a). Non-magnifying NBI clearly shows a brownish area continuous with the left side of the main lesion (Fig. 6.15b). The brownish area crosses the midline, extending as far as the left aryepiglottic fold. Low-magnification WLI examination of the same region reveals proliferation of dilated atypical vessels (Fig. 6.15c). Low-magnification NBI delineates more clearly the distinctly dilated atypical vessels, as well as the border with the surrounding normal mucosa (Fig. 6.15d). With M-NBI, we can see the irregular arrangement of the elongated tortuous atypical vessels (Fig. 6.15e).

A biopsy specimen of this part of the lesion showed a squamous cell carcinoma with intraepithelial invasion (Fig. 6.15f).

6.15.2 Characteristics Under NBI Examination

Using NBI, we carefully examine the margins of the main lesion. When a brownish area is identified, we perform a magnified examination, confirming the presence of dilated atypical vessels. We delineate the border between the normal mucosa and the brownish area, identifying horizontal spread of the lesion. Without M-NBI, we cannot determine if superficial invasion by the lesion has extended as far as other subsites, across the midline, or as far as the esophageal introitus. These findings are extremely important in determining the extent of resection and the optimum therapeutic regimen.

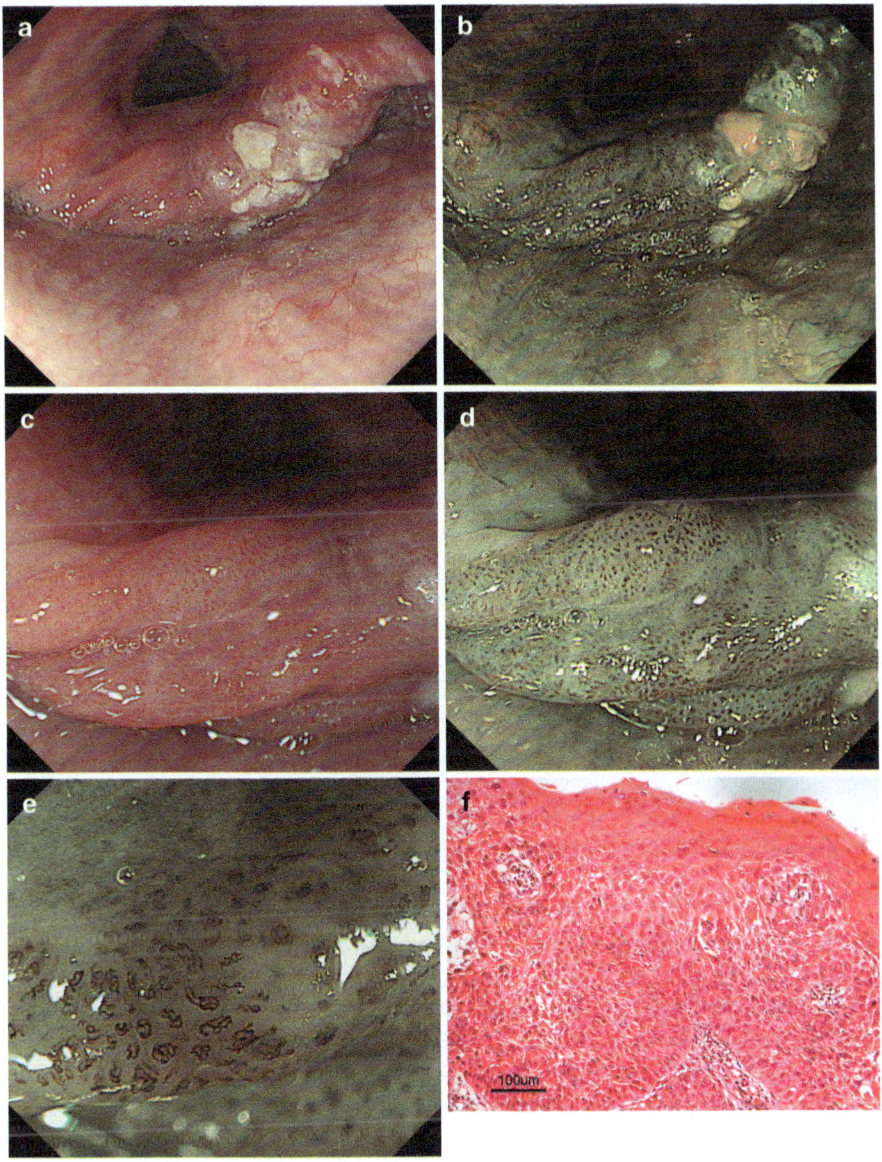

Fig. 6.15

6.16 Superficial Invasion in the Vicinity of a Polypoid Tumor (Esophagus)

Superficial invasion in the vicinity of esophageal cancers is often seen with both polypoid and ulcerated lesions. The true extent of this superficial invasion, as determined using chromoendoscopy with iodine staining, is an important finding when determining the target area for radiotherapy. It is becoming clear that NBI can also be used to determine the lateral extent of superficial invasion.

6.16.1 Explanation

Using non-magnifying WLI, we carefully examine, from the oral side, an area separate from the main lesion, using the visibility of the branching vascular network as a marker. In this case, a protruding lesion 1 cm in size can be seen on the left side of the middle thoracic (Mt) region of the esophagus. Around almost the complete circumference of this lesion can be seen area of light reddened mucosa with loss of visibility of the branching vessels (Fig. 6.16a). Non-magnifying NBI shows a brownish area corresponding to the area identified using WLI and delineates the boundary between the brownish area and the normal mucosa more clearly (Fig. 6.16b). M-NBI examination of the area of superficial invasion shows dilated, elongated, and tortuous atypical IPCLs, corresponding to type V-1 and V-2 vessels in the Inoue classification (Fig. 6.16c, d. Chromoendoscopy using iodine staining delineates the area of superficial invasion as a non-iodine staining area with distinct margins (Fig. 6.16e).

A biopsy specimen of this part of the lesion showed a squamous cell carcinoma with intraepithelial invasion (Fig. 6.16f).

6.16.2 Characteristics Under NBI Examination

Unlike with WLI, using NBI we can clearly discern the subepithelial branching vascular network in the normal mucosa. Carefully examining the vascular pattern in the normal mucosa on the oral side of the lesion, we take care not to miss the area where it becomes no longer visible. It is important to at the same time examine from the main lesion outwards, confirming the margin from both sides and thereby defining the extent of invasion. Classification of the vascular pattern using M-NBI is useful in determining the depth of invasion.

At present, however, chromoendoscopy using iodine is considered superior to NBI in detecting lesions and determining their horizontal extent, so where possible the two modalities should be used in combination.

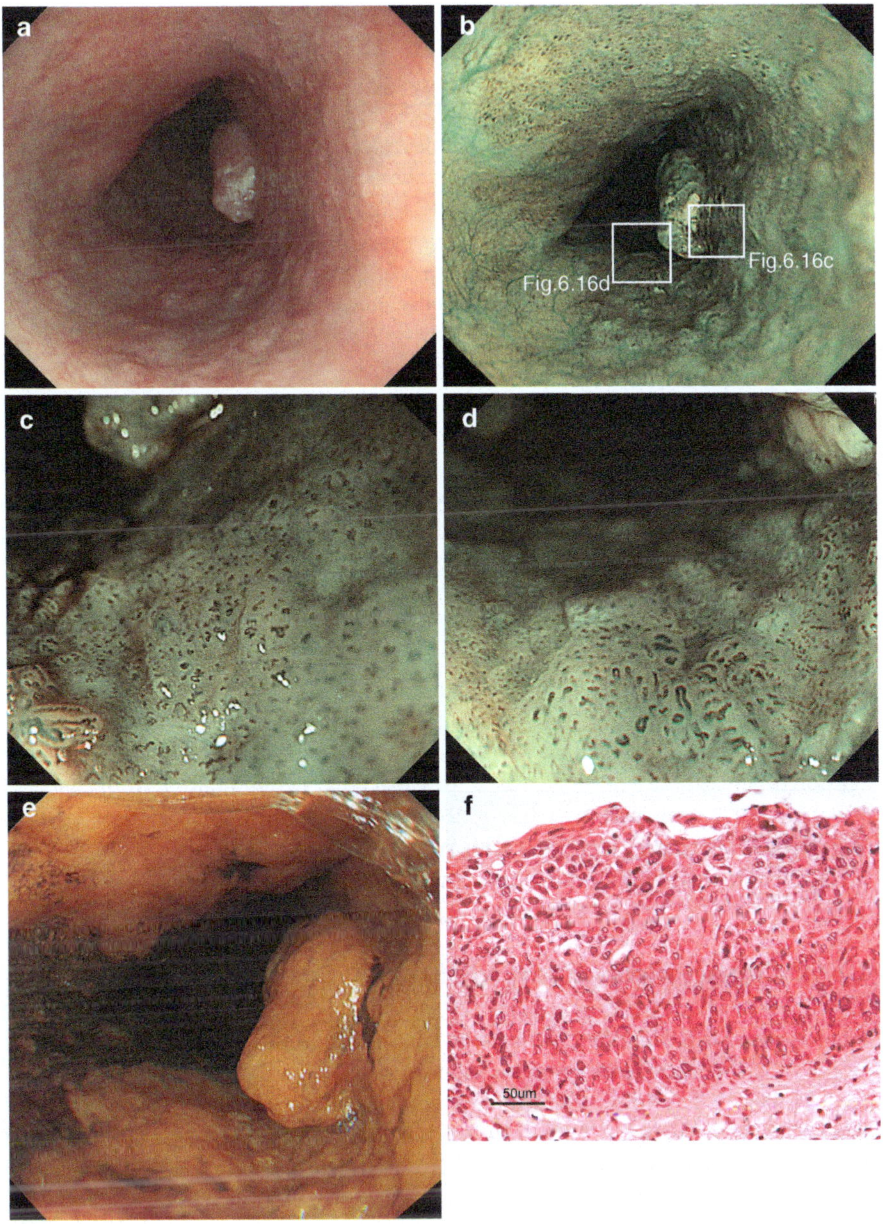

Fig. 6.16

6.17 Epithelial Tumor with Associated Melanosis (Pharynx)

Melanosis of the oral cavity, oropharynx, hypopharynx, and esophagus is commonly seen in alcohol-dependent individuals, in particular ALDH2 heterozygotes, and is thought to be related to acetaldehyde exposure. The presence of melanosis is known to correlate with an increased risk of esophageal dysplasia, esophageal cancer, and orolaryngopharyngeal cancer [18].

Pathologically, melanosis involves increased melanin granules, derived from melanocytes distributed within the mucosa, within the mucosal epithelial cells [19]. Melanosis is often observed in the vicinity of superficial pharyngeal cancers.

6.17.1 Explanation

Non-magnifying WLI reveals melanosis over a narrow extent on the right pillar of the fauces (Fig. 6.17a arrows), and on the left side of the melanosis, we can see an area in which the normal vascular pattern has become indistinct. Non-magnifying NBI shows the patch of melanosis as a brownish area with an indistinct border, to the left of which we can see an area of whitish and brownish mucosa, with dot-shaped vessels (Fig. 6.17b arrows). M-NBI examination reveals dense proliferation of threadlike dilated atypical vessels approaching the surface of the lesion (Fig. 6.17c). Iodine staining delineates a non-iodine staining area with distinct margins, indicative of squamous cell carcinoma (Fig. 6.17d).

Melanosis has a brownish appearance using NBI, and caution is required because a lesion of any extent will be seen as a brownish area. Differentiation from cancer is possible if the brownish area has indistinct margins, with no atypical vessels. Melanosis is also easily identified with WLI examination.

The histological findings are shown in Fig. 6.17e.

6.17.2 Characteristics Under NBI Examination

When melanosis is identified, a thorough examination should be performed looking for possible superficial cancers in the vicinity, or elsewhere in the pharynx or esophagus. Melanosis has the appearance of a light brownish area with indistinct margins using NBI, necessitating differentiation from cancer. Cancer can be easily excluded using M-NBI through the absence of atypical vessels. Changing over to WLI examination will also allow the easy identification of brown-colored melanosis.

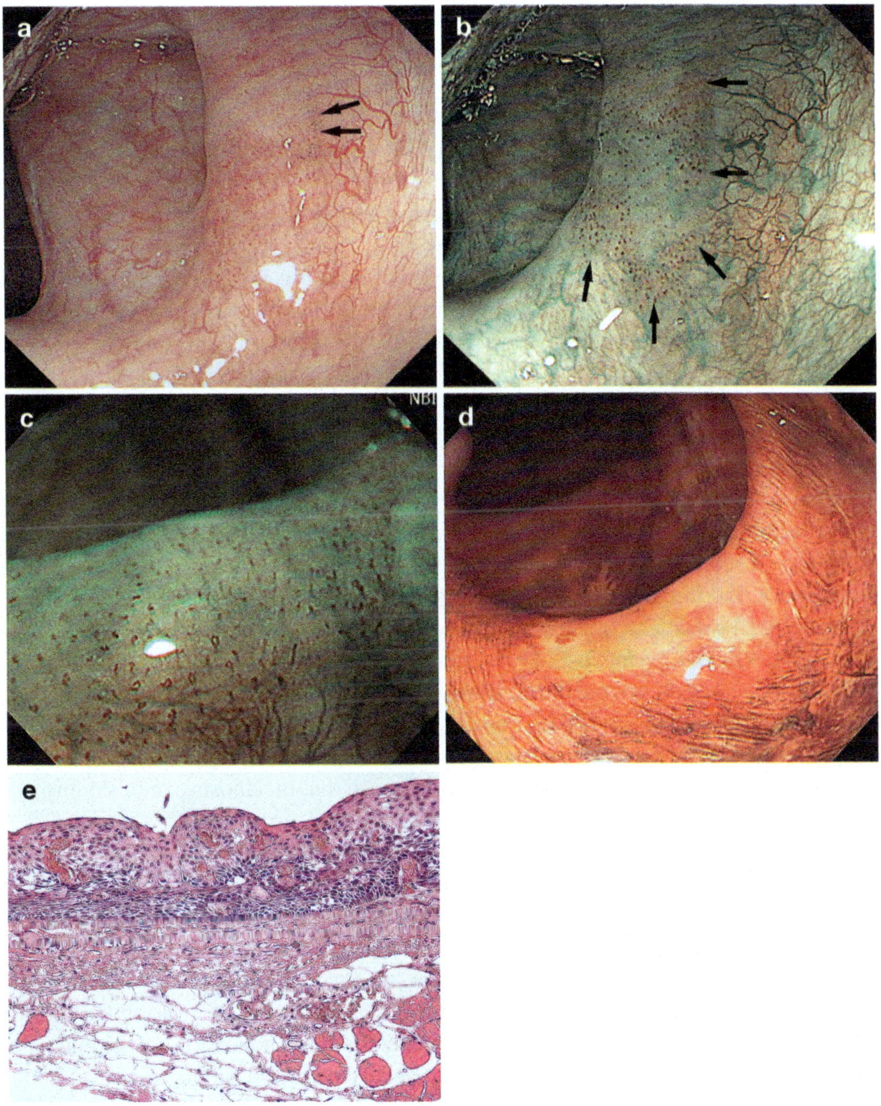

Fig. 6.17

6.18 Epithelial Tumor with Associated Melanosis (Esophagus)

A black patch on the esophageal mucosa, caused by a marked increase in melanin granules in the basal layer, is called melanosis. Apart from the esophagus, this also occurs on the soft palate and pharynx. The reported endoscopic prevalence was of the order of 0.1 % [20]; recent improvements in endoscopic equipment have made the detection of melanosis more common.

Melanosis may be seen as brown to light black using WLI when the quantity of melanin is not great or because of the epithelium lying superficial to the basal layer, with the whitish mucosa thinly covering the black surface.

6.18.1 Explanation

This mucosal lesion with a white substance adherent to its surface is visualized using non-magnifying WLI as white-clouded mucosa, through which the vascular pattern cannot be discerned (Fig. 6.18a, b). Although the lesion surface is slightly rough in appearance, the margins are indistinct with NBI alone. A patch of melanosis can be seen toward the anal end of the lesion, the oral part of which is near black, but the anal part is much lighter, somewhat like a sumi-e ink painting. NBI examination shows the lesion as a brownish area and delineates the margins more clearly than with WLI, although proliferation of IPCLs cannot be discerned using non-magnifying NBI (Fig. 6.18c). The presence of melanosis is difficult to detect using NBI alone, and it is only through comparison with the WLI appearance that melanosis can be confirmed; even then, the lightly colored anal part is difficult to discern.

Iodine staining shows an irregular non-iodine staining area corresponding to the part of the lesion discernible using NBI, although the lesion surface is lightly stained (Fig. 6.18d, e). This flat lesion with associated melanosis is therefore classified as type 0-IIb lesion, depth of invasion EP.

The histological findings of the specimen resected in one piece using the EMR method were of a type IIb lesion 15×11 mm in size and depth of invasion EP, ly0, v0 (Fig. 6.18f, g). In this intraepithelial cancer, cellular differentiation toward the epithelial surface is relatively well preserved, characterized by increased cellular density particularly in the basal half of the stratified squamous epithelium. Slightly enlarged melanocytes are seen within the lesion, associated with increased production of pigment.

6.18.2 Characteristics Under NBI Examination

NBI is not suited to the detection of melanosis. Comparison with the WLI findings enables confirmation that the more strongly pigmented areas are seen as a rather dark brown using NBI.

Detection of this intraepithelial cancer was difficult without NBI in this case. We were able to delineate the margins of this lesion using NBI, but there was no sign of proliferation of IPCLs within the lesion. Iodine staining showed a non-staining area, albeit with some light surface staining, indicating the lesion was mainly located in the basal layers.

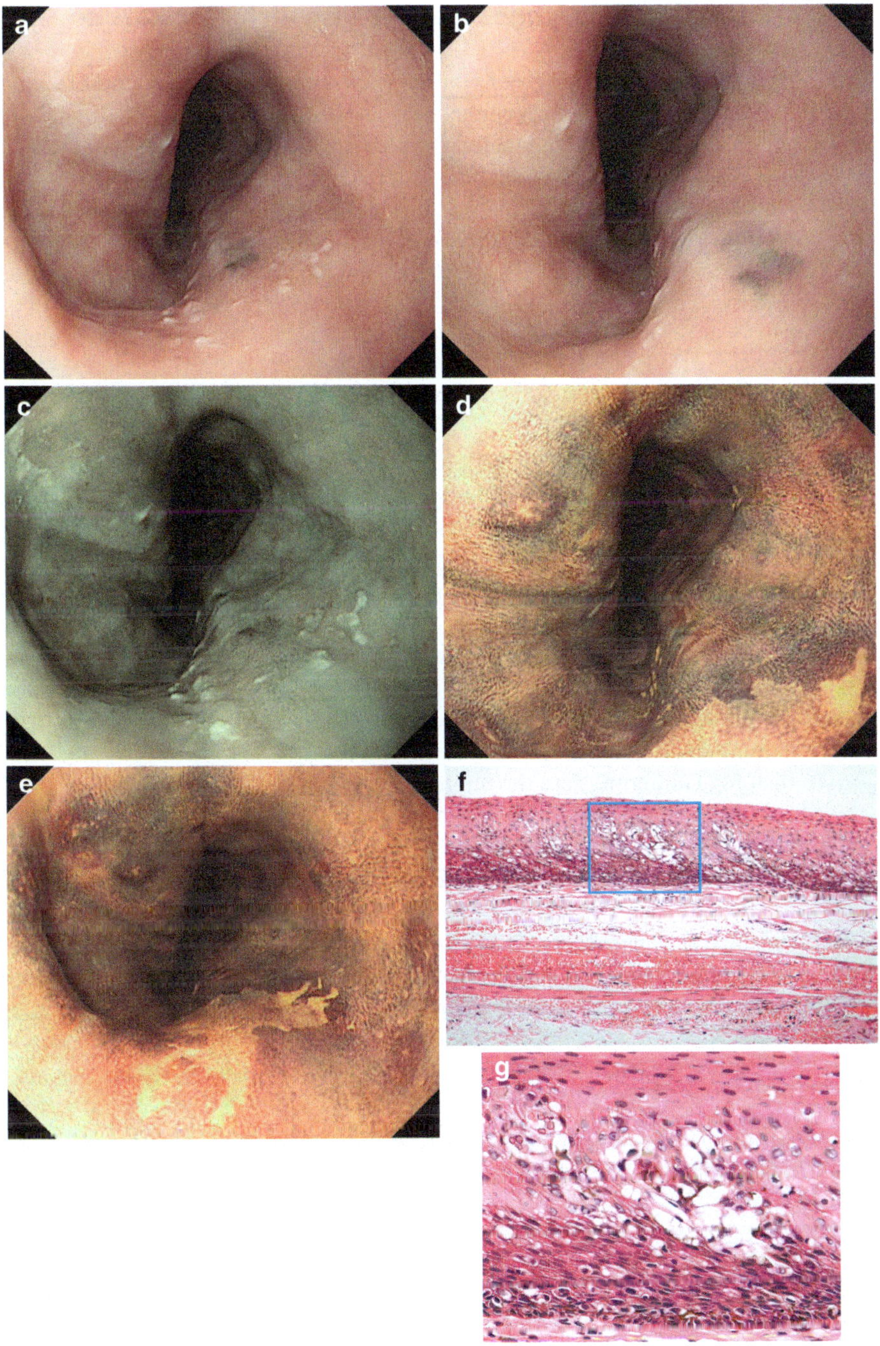

Fig. 6.18

6.19 Superficial Pharyngeal Cancer with Rich Vasculature

Proliferation of atypical vessels is found in association with most superficial cancers seen in sites with squamous epithelium. These atypical vessels are thought to arise in IPCLs located in the epithelial papillae and are visualized as vessels with irregular paths toward the luminal surface, unlike the branching vascular network running parallel to the mucosal surface in the nontumorous mucosa. Superficial cancers with a rich vasculature are easily discerned as reddened areas even with WLI due to their high red cell (hemoglobin) content. With NBI they are seen as brownish areas with distinct margins.

6.19.1 Explanation

From a distance, non-magnifying WLI reveals a reddened flat lesion with a protuberance in one part (Fig. 6.19a). At closer proximity, the reddened area has a rough surface and a distinct boundary with the surrounding area indicative of a neoplastic lesion (Fig. 6.19b). Close non-magnifying NBI examination shows the lesion as a brownish area with a distinct demarcation line with the surrounding mucosa (Fig. 6.19c). M-NBI reveals proliferation of irregularly dilated and elongated atypical vessels (Fig. 6.19d). The mucosa between the atypical vessels also has a different color to the surrounding mucosa and is visualized as a cloudy brownish area, in which the branching vascular network cannot be discerned (Fig. 6.19c, d). The iodine staining findings are as shown in Fig. 6.19e.

The histological findings are shown in Fig. 6.19f.

6.19.2 Characteristics Under NBI Examination

Superficial pharyngeal cancers with a rich vasculature are easily detected using WLI as vivid red-colored lesions. Visualized as brownish areas using NBI, they are easily recognized as typical superficial cancers due to the marked proliferation of atypical vessels.

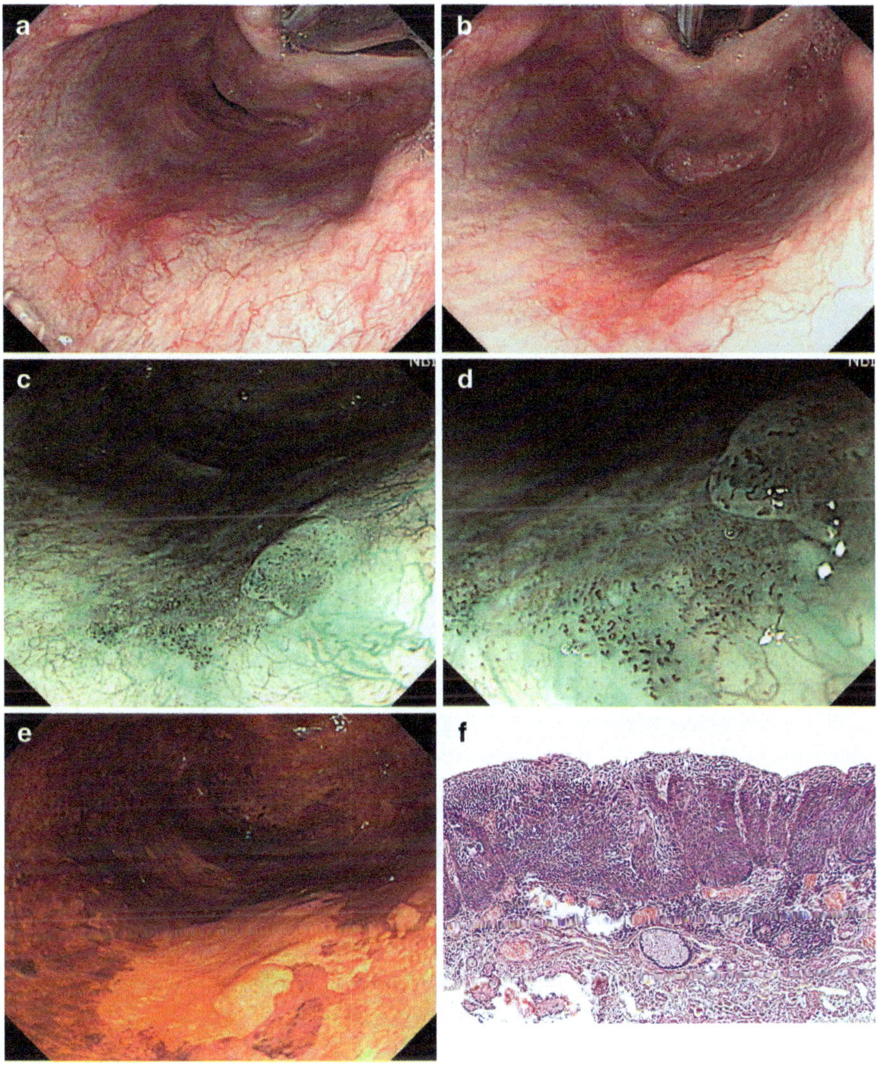

Fig. 6.19

6.20 Superficial Esophageal Cancer with Rich Vasculature

Proliferation of atypical vessels is found in association with most superficial cancers seen in sites with squamous epithelium. These atypical vessels are thought to arise in IPCLs located in the epithelial papillae and are visualized as vessels with irregular paths toward the luminal surface, unlike the branching vascular network running parallel to the mucosal surface in the nontumorous mucosa. Superficial cancers with a rich vasculature are easily discerned as reddened areas even with WLI due to their high red cell (hemoglobin) content. With NBI they are seen as brownish areas with distinct margins.

6.20.1 Explanation

From a distance, non-magnifying WLI reveals a reddened, low-protruding lesion (Fig. 6.20a). From a distance, non-magnifying NBI shows the lesion as a brownish area with a distinct boundary with the surrounding mucosa (Fig. 6.20b). M-NBI reveals proliferation of dilated atypical vessels within the granular protuberance (Fig. 6.20c). At the periphery of the lesion, dilated vessels can be seen within each granule, the so-called "frogs' eggs" appearance (Fig. 6.20c, vicinity of arrow). Iodine staining showed a non-staining area corresponding to the brownish area seen with NBI (Fig. 6.20d).

The histological findings were of aggregations of dilated vessels in the superficial layer of the lesion, in agreement with the endoscopic findings (Fig. 6.20e, f).

6.20.2 Characteristics Under NBI Examination

Superficial esophageal cancers with a rich vasculature are easily detected using WLI as vivid red-colored lesions. Visualized as brownish areas using NBI, they are easily recognized as typical superficial cancers due to the marked proliferation of atypical vessels.

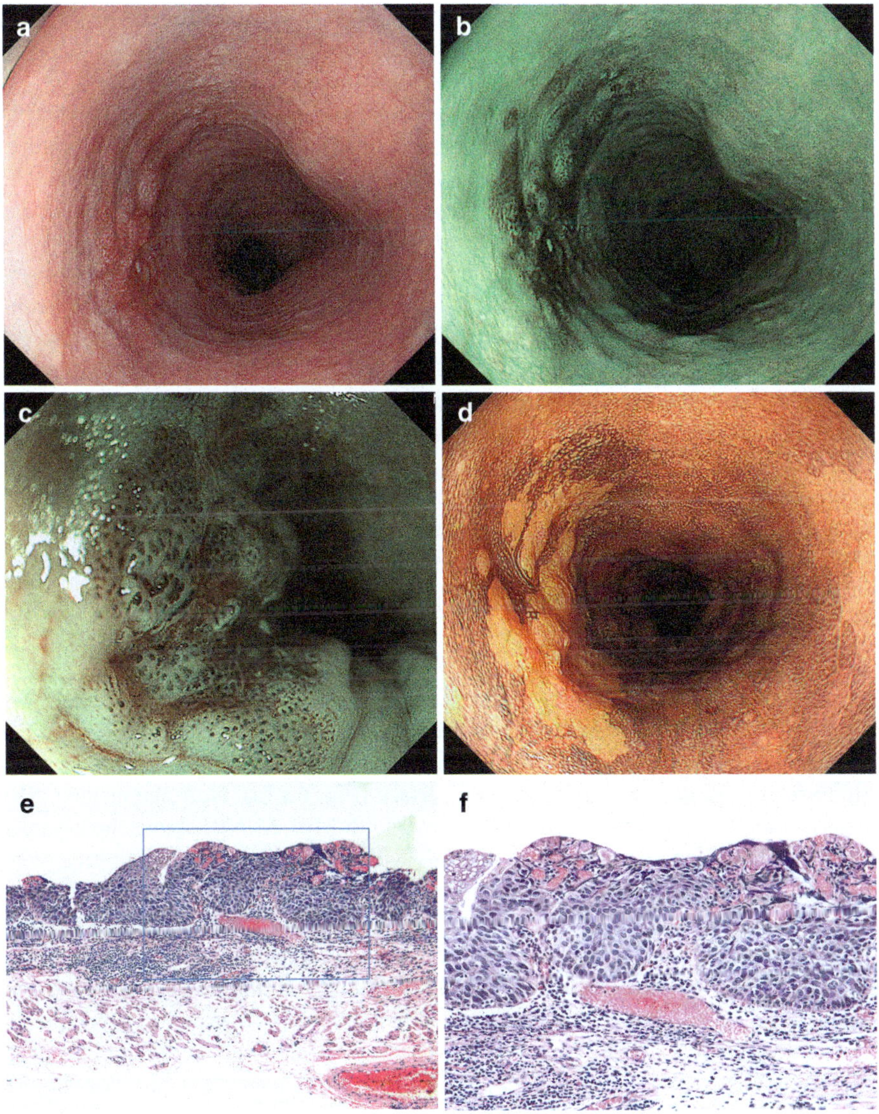

Fig. 6.20

6.21 Superficial Pharyngeal Cancer with Scant Vascular Proliferation

With increased use of chromoendoscopy has enabled the early detection of many esophageal squamous cell carcinomas (hereinafter esophageal cancers) and a marked improvement in outcomes. As a result, the incidence of cancers of the oropharynx and hypopharynx synchronous with esophageal cancers has increased, adversely affecting outcomes and quality of life in patients with esophageal cancer [22, 23].

Unlike the esophagus, iodine staining is unsuitable for screening in the pharyngeal region, making early cancer detection extremely difficult for many years. However, in recent years the advent of NBI has made early detection of oropharyngeal and hypopharyngeal intraepithelial cancers easy. Muto et al. reported that all intraepithelial cancers are delineated as brownish areas with distinct margins, accompanied by proliferation of dilated microvessels [24].

In the authors' study using M-NBI, only 1 out of 32 (3 %) superficial oropharyngeal and hypopharyngeal cancers was neither visualized as a brownish area nor showed proliferation of dilated microvessels [25]. When conducting NBI examinations, we should be aware that a small percentage of cancers will be difficult to detect, showing no vascular proliferation.

6.21.1 Explanation

Non-magnifying WLI examination reveals this protruding lesion, arising from the right epiglottic vallecula, to be the same color as the surrounding mucosa, with a shiny surface despite a slightly uneven surface (Fig. 6.21a). Non-magnifying NBI does not show the lesion as a brownish area (Fig. 6.21b). M-NBI shows the vascular network within the lesion to be continuous with that in the surrounding area, with no abnormal findings such as vascular proliferation, variable diameters, or nonuniform morphology (Fig. 6.21c). Vessels in the center of the lesion are similar to those at the periphery of the lesion and in the surrounding mucosa, with no signs of proliferation or other irregularities (Fig. 6.21d). Iodine staining showed a mixture of normal and light staining areas, with no distinct non-staining areas (Fig. 6.21e).

The histological findings were of nonneoplastic squamous epithelium covering the lesion (Fig. 6.21f). In the subepithelial layer we can see marked inflammatory cell infiltration (Fig. 6.21f) and findings of a squamous cell carcinoma proliferating in an alveolar fashion with keratinization (Fig. 6.21g).

6.21.2 Characteristics Under NBI Examination

The authors consider that brownish areas visualized using NBI are the result of three factors, color changes in the epithelium itself (between vessels) as well as microvessel dilatation and proliferation reported by Muto et al. [26]. This lesion did not appear as a brownish area, as it was lacking all three factors.

Lesions such as this one with predominantly subepithelial growth, covered by nonneoplastic epithelium, may be detectable only through distortion of the pharyngeal surface or anatomical differences between the left and right sides. Before NBI examinations, the authors examine the entire oropharynx and hypopharynx using WLI, looking for anatomical structural changes.

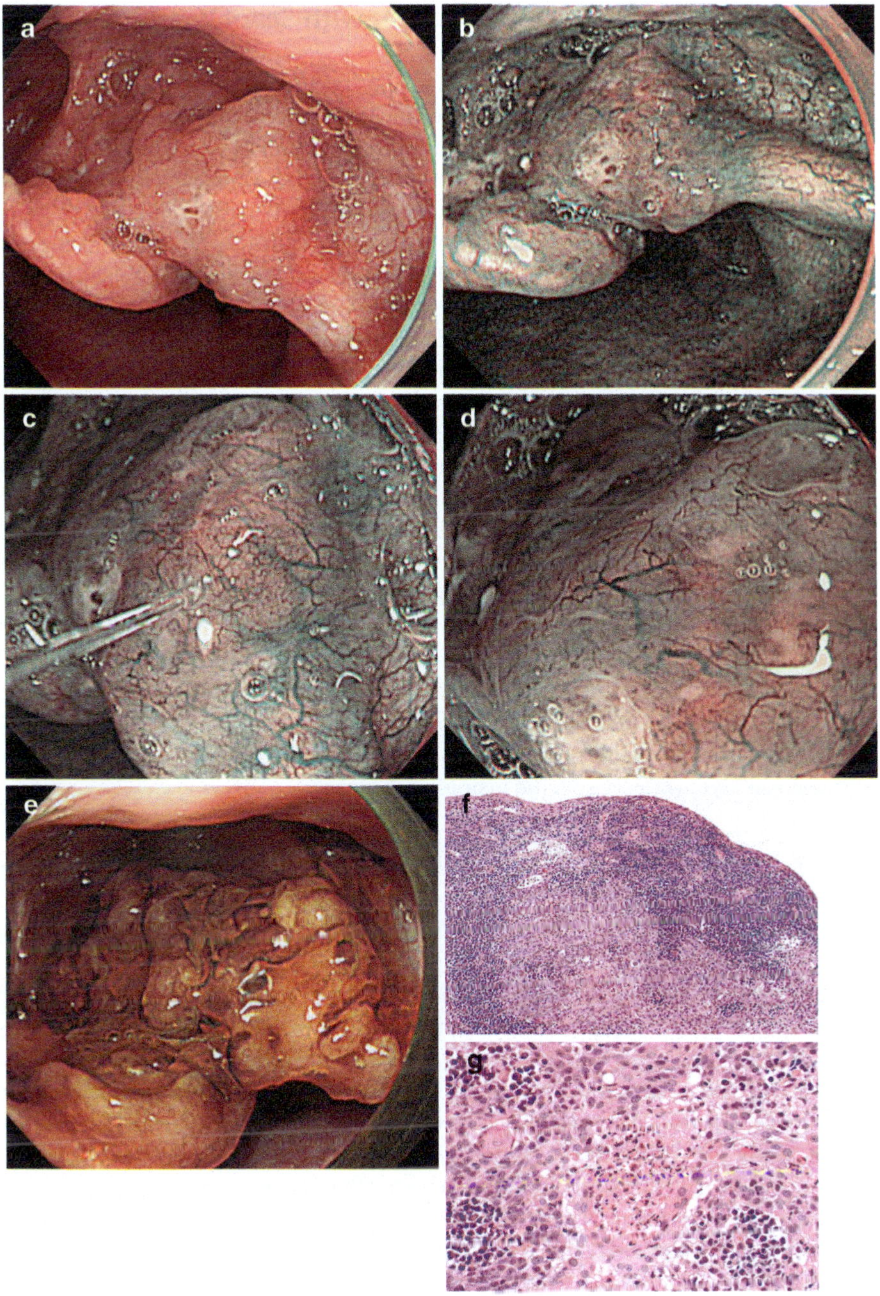

Fig. 6.21

6.22 Superficial Esophageal Cancer with Scant Vascular Proliferation

At our hospital, out of a series of 272 superficial esophageal cancers (squamous cell carcinomas), 239 (88 %), the great majority, were flat or excavated lesions. Most superficial esophageal cancers are flat or excavated and appear reddened when examined using conventional (WLI) endoscopy [27].

The latter half of the 1990s saw reports of the magnified endoscopic findings of microvessels in the esophageal mucosa and squamous cell carcinomas [28, 29], and the new century has seen great strides in diagnostic systems based on microvessel appearances, with the development of NBI and its clinical applications. Muto et al. have reported that many intraepithelial cancers of the oropharynx and hypopharynx, difficult to detect with WLI, are readily detected using NBI, and that all intraepithelial lesions present as a brownish area with distinct margins, associated with a proliferation of dilated microvessels [24]. These results have also been applied to the esophagus, where a multicentered prospective trial demonstrated detection rates and diagnostic accuracy for superficial esophageal cancers are both significantly better for NBI than for conventional (WLI) [9].

In this way, the reddened appearance exhibited by most superficial esophageal cancers is likely associated with proliferation of dilated microvessels. However, the authors have found that a low proportion of about 10 % of superficial esophageal cancers show scant vascular proliferation and are not visualized as a brownish area. Most of these lesions appear white or extremely lightly colored, with histological findings including cancers arising in the basal layers, cancers with surface parakeratosis or abnormal keratinization, and cancers growing and spreading mainly in the submucosal layer (mostly specific histological types).

6.22.1 Explanation

Non-magnifying WLI examination reveals an irregular white to translucent area with a rough surface in the lower esophagus (Fig. 6.22a arrowheads). Non-magnifying NBI delineates this lesion more clearly as a whitish slightly protruding lesion with a granular to platelike appearance (Fig. 6.22b arrowheads). Medium-magnification NBI shows dilated microvessels, resembling black sesame seeds, in one part of the rough whitish translucent lesion, but no vascular proliferation (Fig. 6.22c arrows). Microvessels cannot be clearly discerned in the thickened cloudy white part of the lesion (Fig. 6.22d). A distinct area of non-iodine staining corresponds to the whitish rough irregular area (Fig. 6.22e).

The histological findings were of a squamous cell carcinoma confined to the lamina propria (M2), the surface of which was covered in a thick layer of parakeratosis (Fig. 6.22f).

6.22.2 Characteristics Under NBI Examination

Esophageal cancers with associated parakeratosis will not be visualized as a brownish area using NBI, and delineation of the surface microvessels will often be difficult or impossible.

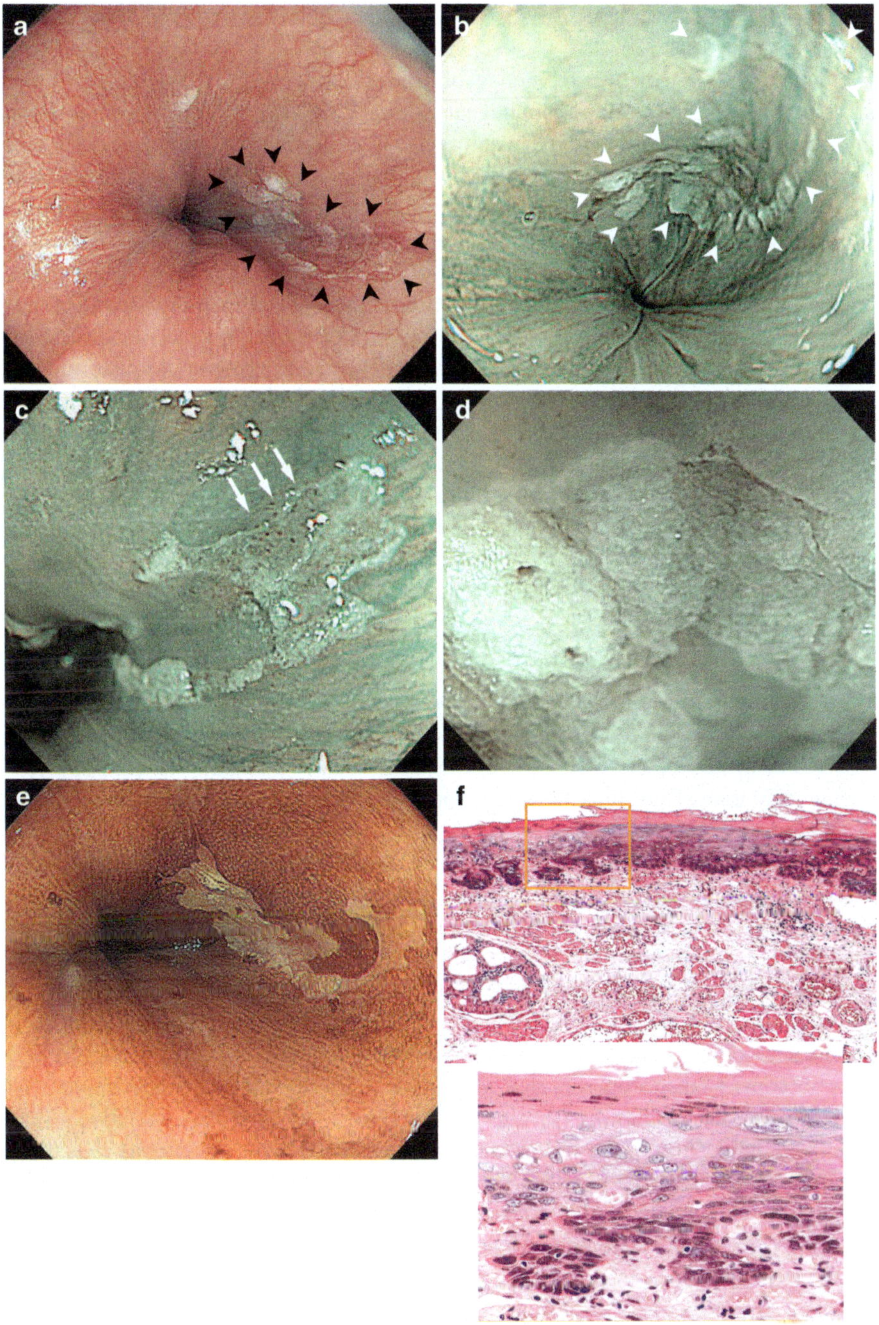

Fig. 6.22

6.23 Barrett's Adenocarcinoma (1)

A marked increase in the incidence of Barrett's adenocarcinoma means it now accounts for over half of all esophageal cancers [30]. On the other hand, in Japan more than 95 % of esophageal cancers are squamous cell carcinomas, and the incidence of Barrett's adenocarcinoma is low, albeit tending to increase in recent years [31]. In Western countries, the recommended method of surveillance for Barrett's adenocarcinoma (and dysplasia, the precursor lesion) has been to take multiple biopsies at intervals of 1–2 cm. In recent years, the usefulness of magnifying endoscopy in the early detection of Barrett's adenocarcinoma has been reported [3]. More recently, M-NBI has taken over the central role in Barrett's surveillance, clearly delineating the mucosal microsurface architecture and microvascular pattern, without the need for other modalities such as chromoendoscopy [32].

Japanese studies have found that most Barrett's adenocarcinomas are histologically well differentiated and usually appear as reddened areas or protrusions using conventional (WLI) endoscopy [33]. Accordingly, detection rates will improve with an initial thorough examination using WLI to identify areas requiring detailed examination using M-NBI.

6.23.1 Explanation

Non-magnifying conventional (WLI) endoscopy reveals a gently sloping protuberance associated with a light reddened area between 3 and 6 o'clock, as well as a light reddened area at 12 o'clock, within the Barrett's mucosa (Fig. 6.23a). We were unable to identify any areas of intestinal metaplasia following indigo carmine spraying (Fig. 6.23b).

NBI examination at low magnification showed a rough mucosal surface over a wide area distal to the border with the squamous epithelium, with loss of definition and miniaturization of the mucosal pattern (Fig. 6.23c). Further increasing the magnifying ratio, we can discern more clearly the loss of definition of the mucosal pattern and proliferation of irregular microvessels, allowing us to identify a neoplastic lesion and delineate its margins (Fig. 6.23d arrowhead). High-magnification NBI examination of the central part of the lesion reveals loss of the mucosal pattern and proliferation of tortuous abnormal vessels with variable diameters (Fig. 6.23e). The histological findings of biopsies taken from this area were of well-differentiated adenocarcinoma.

Following marking of the periphery of the lesion, based on the qualitative assessment and delineation of the lesion margins using M-NBI, the lesion was resected in one piece using the ESD method. The histological findings were of Barrett's adenocarcinoma with submucosal invasion, although the lateral and vertical margins were negative (Fig. 6.23f). The patient opted not to undergo adjuvant therapy despite a thorough explanation of the necessity was given. At the time of writing, the patient has survived free of recurrence for more than 3 years, with ongoing close follow-up.

6.23.2 Characteristics Under NBI Examination

When examined using M-NBI at low to medium magnification, Barrett's adenocarcinoma often shows irregularity or reduced visibility of the mucosal pattern. High magnification is likely to reveal abnormal vessels with irregular paths and variable diameters.

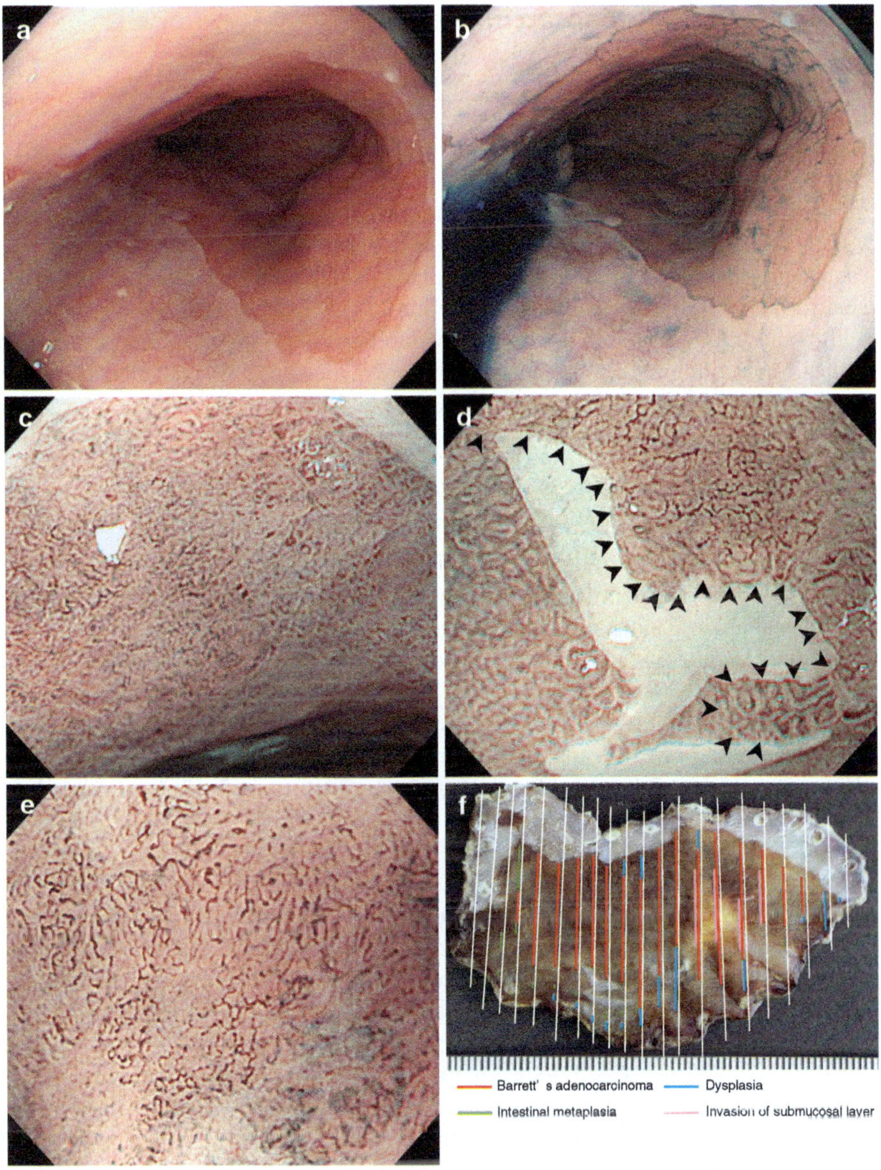
a
b
c
d
e
f
Barrett' s adenocarcinoma
Dysplasia
Intestinal metaplasia
Invasion of submucosal layer

Fig. 6.23

6.24 Barrett's Adenocarcinoma (2)

Columnar epithelium, extending from and continuous with the stomach, is known as Barrett's mucosa, and an area of esophagus with Barrett's mucosa is referred to as Barrett's esophagus. In comparison with Western countries, long-segment Barrett's esophagus (LSBE) ≥3 cm is much less common than short-segment Barrett's esophagus (SSBE) <3 cm or ultrashort-segment Barrett's esophagus (USBE).

The histological findings of Barrett's esophagus are one of the following: (1) esophageal gland ducts in the mucosa beneath the columnar epithelium, or esophageal glands beneath the columnar epithelium; (2) islands of squamous epithelium within the columnar epithelium; or (3) duplication of the muscularis mucosae beneath the columnar epithelium. The reported incidence of malignancy arising from Barrett's mucosa is approximately 0.5 % [34].

6.24.1 Explanation

In the background of Barrett's adenocarcinoma is the presence of GERD, and many patients also have an esophageal hiatal hernia. Reflux of gastric acid may give the esophageal mucosa in the vicinity of the lesion a white and cloudy appearance, with adherent mucous, so we rinse the mucosa well with a Gascon® solution containing Pronase® to remove any mucous before examinations. If the examination is performed with the patient awake, asking the patient to breathe deeply will open up the gastroesophageal junction and vicinity, making observation easier. In patients with an esophageal hiatal hernia, this maneuver is effective in facilitating retrograde examination of this region from the stomach.

Endoscopically, Barrett's mucosa refers to the area between the lower margin of the lower esophageal palisade vessels (LEPVs), or the oral termination of the gastric rugae, and the squamocolumnar junction (SCJ). A circumferential area of Barrett's mucosa ≥3 cm in length is termed long-segment Barrett's esophagus (LSBE) and if <3 cm short-segment Barrett's esophagus (SSBE). As cancers arising in Barrett's mucosa are adenocarcinomas, in principle their detection follows similar lines to those for gastric cancers, with careful examination of the mucosal surface for unevenness and color changes. Lesions with marked unevenness or strong red coloration will be easily detected during WLI examination, but flat lesions are difficult to detect even with spraying of dyes such as indigo carmine. In these cases, careful attention must be paid to the slightest redness or alteration in the shininess of the mucosal surface. M-NBI is useful in cases where a qualitative assessment is difficult using WLI alone.

This is a markedly protruding type 0-I lesion. The lesion narrows somewhat on its oral aspect, and the base is wider on the anal side of this well-differentiated adenocarcinoma invading to a depth of 700 μm into the sm layer (Fig. 6.24a–d). Examination of the protuberance under magnification reveals vessels with variable diameters and irregular paths (Fig. 6.24e).

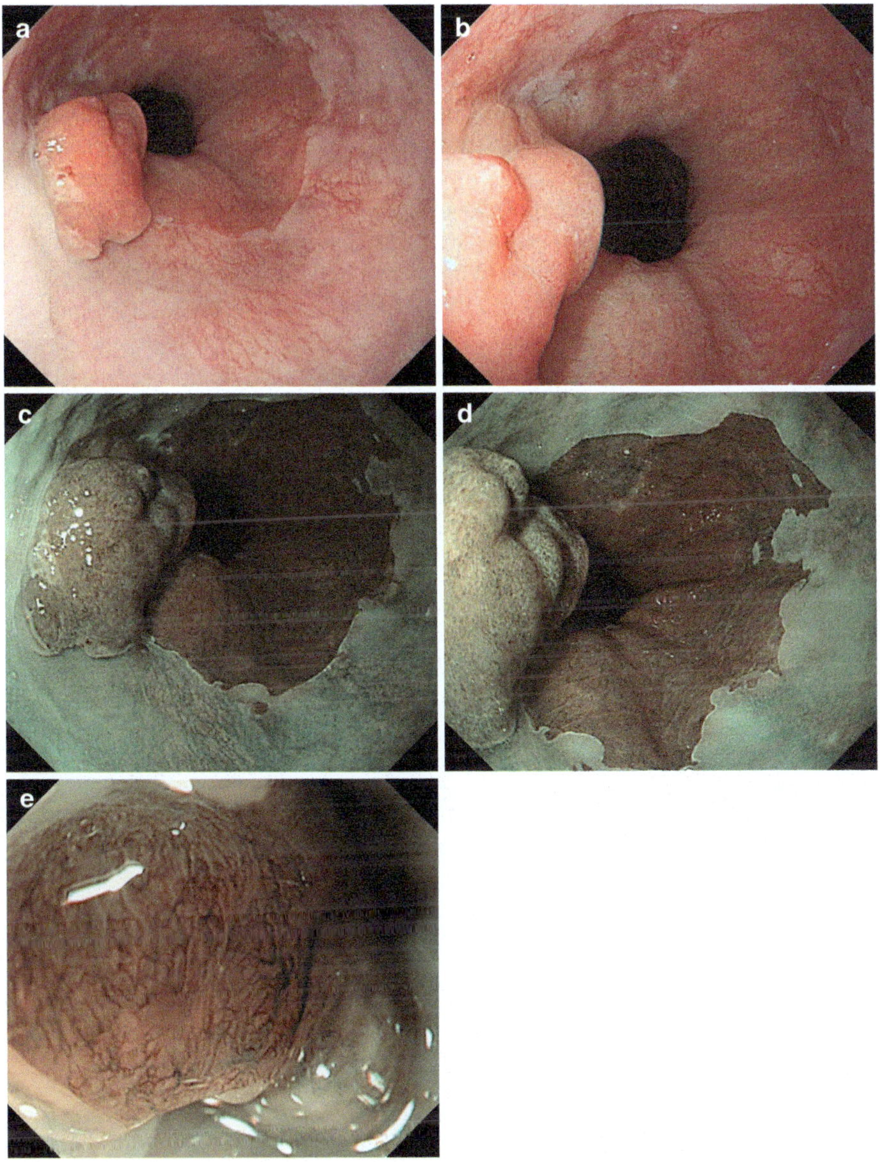

Fig. 6.24

6.24.2 Characteristics Under NBI Examination

M-NBI is useful for qualitative assessment and margin delineation.

Findings of the surface structure of the cancer include increased pit density and fused glands. In lesions forming high protrusions, adherence of necrotic substances is common, causing reduced visibility of the mucosal pattern. The surface pattern may be better visualized after spraying indigo carmine or acetic acid. The vascular pattern of this cancer shows vessels with variable diameters following irregular paths, showing the network pattern of a well-differentiated adenocarcinoma.

References

1. Shimizu Y, et al: Gastrointest Endosc 54: 190–194, 2001
2. Muto M, et al: Gastrointest Endos 56: 517–521, 2002
3. Muto M, et al: Carcinogenesis 26: 1008–1012, 2005
4. Shimizu Y, et al: J Gastroenterol Hepatol 23: 546–550, 2008
5. Nemoto T et al: Stomach and Intestine 45: 190–202, 2010
6. Monma K, et al: Stomach and Intestine 40: 1239–1254, 2005
7. 'Stomach and Intestine' Editing Committee: Atlas of the Stomach and Intestine 1, Igaku Shoin, pp 32–33, 2001
8. Nagasako K, et al. (eds):Atlas of Gastrointestinal Endoscopy, Bunkodo, p 60, 2001
9. Muto M, et al: J Clin Oncol 28: 1566–1572, 2010
10. Japan Society for Head and Neck Cancer (eds). General Rules for Clinical Studies on Head and Neck Cancer (4th edition), Kanehara Shuppan, 2005.
11. Japan Esophageal Society (eds). Japanese Classification of Esophageal Cancer (Revised 10th edition), Kanehara Shuppan, pp 40–42, 2008.
12. Monma K, et al: Stomach and Intestine 42: 673–682, 2007
13. Arima M, et al: Endoscopia Digestiva 17: 2076–2083, 2005
14. Inuyama Y (ed.) Tumors of the head and neck (Client 21), Nakayama Shoten, pp 367–368, 2000
15. Reichart PA, et al: Oral Oncol 41: 551–561, 2005
16. Takeda M et al: Cancers of the head and neck 33: 470–475, 2007
17. Parkin DM, et al: Int J Cancer 80: 827–841, 1999
18. Yokoyama A, et al: Cancer Sci 97: 905–911, 2006
19. Takubo K: Pathology of the Esophagus (2nd edition), Sogo Igakusha, pp18–23, 1996
20. Makuuchi H: Gastroenterology 4: 493–499, 1986
21. Inoue H, et al: Dig Endosc 9: 16–18, 1997
22. Makuuchi H: Stomach and Intestine 38: 317–330, 2003
23. Matsubara T, et al: J Clin Oncol 21: 4336–4341, 2003
24. Muto M, et al: Cancer 101: 1375–1381, 2004
25. Yoshimura N et al: Gastroenterol Endosc 51 (Suppl 1): 814, 2009
26. Goda K et al: Gastroenterol Endosc 18: 1427–1435, 2006
27. Monma K, et al: Stomach and Intestine 30: 337–345, 1995
28. Inoue H, et al: Dig Endosc 8: 134–138, 1996
29. Arima M, et al: Gastroenterol Endosc 40: 1125–1137, 1998
30. Devesa SS, et al: Cancer 83: 2049–2053, 1998
31. Hongo M, et al: Aliment Pharmacol Ther 20 (Suppl 8): 50–54, 2004
32. Sharma P, et al: Gastrointest Endosc 64: 167-175, 200632) Goda K, et al: Gastrointest Endosc 65: 36–46, 2007
33. Committee for Classification of Barrett's Esophageal Cancer, Japanese Society for Diseases of the Esophagus: Survey of Barrett's Esophageal Cancer. Japanese Society for Diseases of the Esophagus Committee Activity Reports (2002), pp 70–73, 2002
34. Makuuchi H: Jpn J Gastroenterol 97: 1233–1242, 2000

Part III

Atlas of NBI: Stomach and Duodenum

Diagnostic System

7

Kenshi Yao

The gastric mucosa is a glandular epithelium containing projections and indentations such as crypts, so various anatomical structures can be visualised using magnifying endoscopy with narrow-band imaging (M-NBI). If you do not understand what anatomical structure corresponds with the actual image that has been visualised, you cannot make a medical analysis, and the normal gastric fundic gland mucosa and pyloric gland mucosa present totally different magnified endoscopic images (microvascular pattern and microsurface pattern).

As far as possible, we have tried to make this chapter an objective atlas and to standardise the terminology describing M-NBI findings with anatomical terminology.

K. Yao
Department of Endoscopy, Fukuoka University Chikushi Hospital,
1-1-1 Zokumyoin, Chikushino 818-8502, Japan
e-mail: yao@fukuoka-u.ac.jp

M. Muto et al. (eds.), *Atlas of Endoscopy with Narrow Band Imaging*,
DOI 10.1007/978-4-431-54243-8_7

7.1 Anatomical Components of the Glandular Epithelium Examined Using M-NBI

Figure 7.1 shows an example of the superficial layers of the normal fundic glandular mucosa, showing the vertically extending crypt epithelium, the image visualised using projected narrow-band light (upper diagram) and the corresponding histological diagram (lower diagram) [1]. The subepithelial capillaries (SECs) are visualised as a dark brown polygonal capillary pattern and the marginal crypt epithelium as a semitransparent white border surrounding the crypt opening. The crypt opening (CO) is seen as a dark brown oval-shaped hole. The area between crypt and crypt is called the intervening part (IP).

Although not described in detail in this chapter, in the gastric antrum and in pathological mucosa such as a tumour or inflammatory changes, crypts running perpendicular to the mucosal surface are uncommon, so dark brown crypts are not visualised even when using M-NBI.

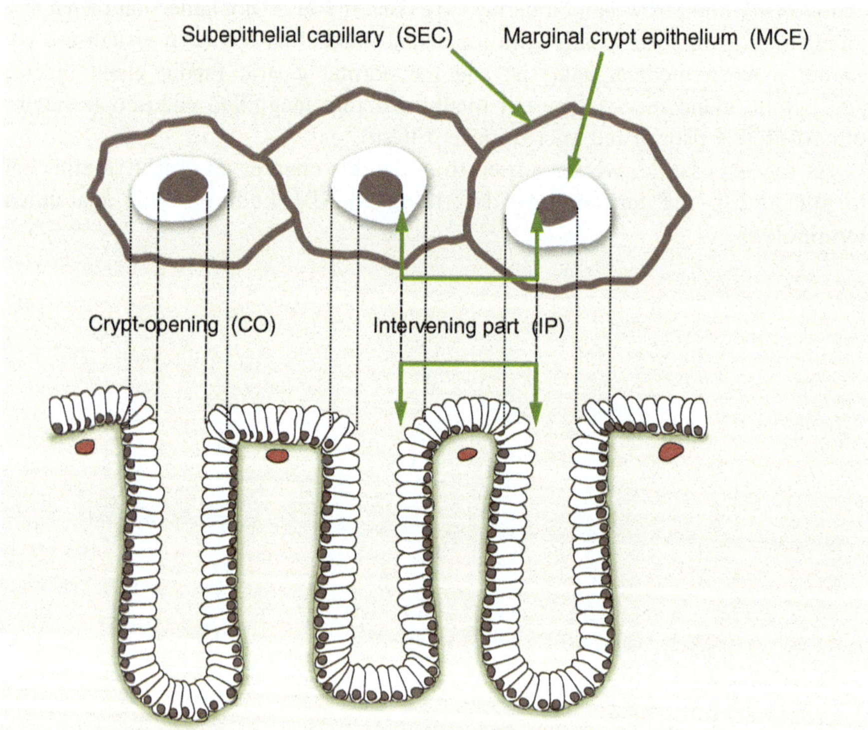

Fig. 7.1 Anatomical structures viewed in glandular epithelium (histological cross-sectional diagram and corresponding M-NBI image) (Reprinted from Yao [1])

7.2 Principles for Interpretation of M-NBI Findings

When analysing M-NBI findings, the author (1) separately and independently analyses the microvascular pattern (V) and the microsurface pattern (S) using the anatomical components indicated in Table 7.1 and then (2) interprets the V and S components with reference to consistent diagnostic criteria, which we have designated the VS classification system. The reason for this is there are limitations to a system of classification based on combinations of V and S. M-NBI endoscopic images of the normal gastric mucosa in the fundic and pyloric gland regions are completely different, and the addition of chronic gastritis makes the findings even more complicated.

Table 7.1 Anatomical components used in the VS (vessel plus surface) classification system for M-NBI

V: microvascular (MV) pattern
1. SECN: subepithelial capillary network
2. CV: collecting venule
3. MV: pathological microvessel
S: microsurface (MS) pattern
1. MCE: marginal crypt epithelium
2. CO: crypt opening
3. IP: intervening part

7.3 VS Classification System Applied to the Differential Diagnosis Between Cancer and Noncancer

As shown in Table 7.2 and Fig. 7.2, the microvascular pattern (V) is classified as either regular, irregular or absent. At the same time, the microsurface pattern (S) is classified as either regular, irregular or absent.

Next, referring to the diagnostic criteria in Table 7.3, we determine whether the lesion is cancer or noncancer. Specifically, when we examine a localised lesion under magnification, we determine if either of the following two conditions apply:

1. There is a clear demarcation line (DL) between the lesion and non-lesion area, and the subepithelial microvascular pattern (V) displays an irregular MV pattern.
2. There is a clear DL between the lesion and non-lesion area, and the mucosal microsurface pattern (S) is irregular, i.e. an irregular MS pattern.

The diagnosis is cancer if either (1) or (2) is present and noncancer if the findings are other than (1) and (2).

Although the above diagnostic criteria cannot diagnose all cancers, in a study by the authors [2] 97 % of cancers met these diagnostic criteria. Cancers that do not fit these criteria should be treated as special cases, diagnosed with reference to their individual characteristic findings or dealt with clinically by taking biopsies to establish the diagnosis.

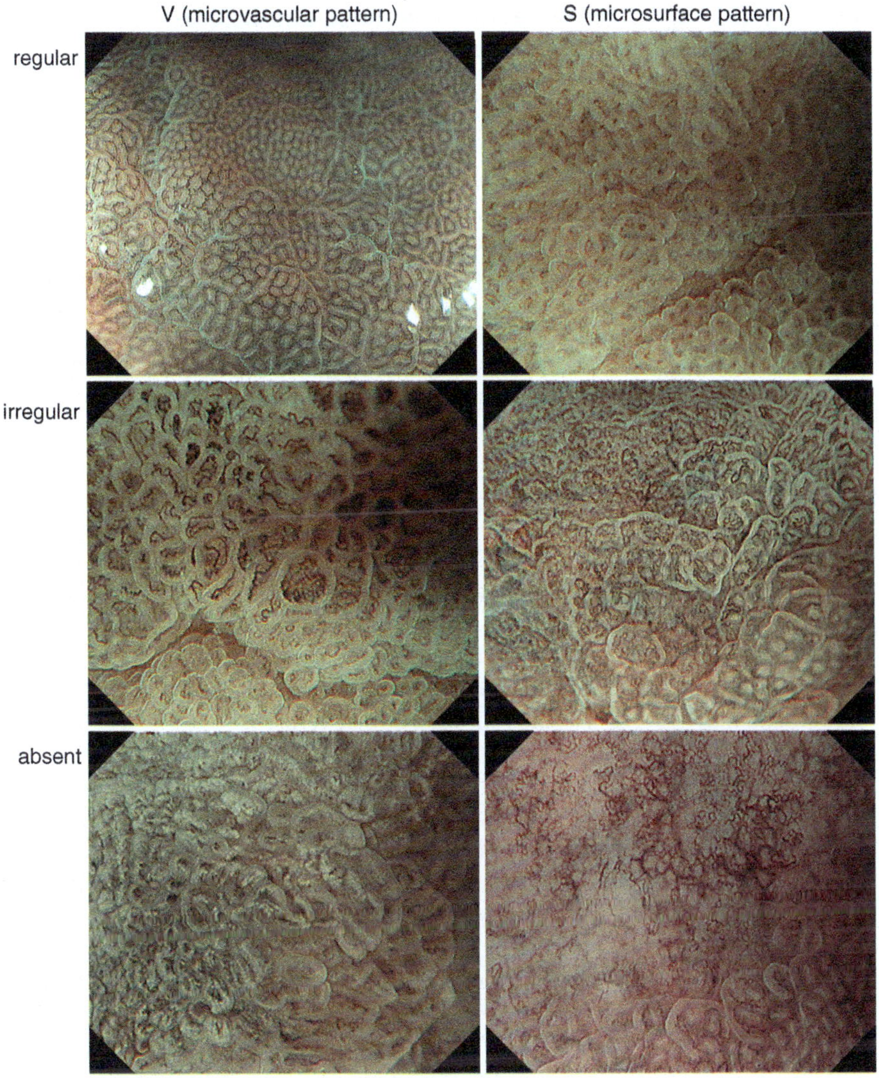

Fig. 7.2 VS classification

Table 7.2 Classification of gastric mucosa (differentiation between cancer and noncancer) using the VS classification based on the M-NBI findings

V: regular/irregular/absent MV pattern
S: regular/irregular/absent MS pattern

Table 7.3 HGD/EC diagnostic criteria according to M-NBI based on VS classification system

1. Irregular MV pattern with a demarcation line (DL), and/or
2. Irregular MS pattern with a demarcation line (DL)

HGD high-grade dysplasia, *EC* early cancer

7.4 Finding of Demarcation Line Between Lesion and Background Mucosa

7.4.1 Demarcation Line (DL)

A demarcation line (DL) is defined as a margin that can be identified by differences in the microvascular pattern (V) or microsurface pattern (S) between the lesion and non-lesion area. The presence or absence of a DL is an effective diagnostic marker for differentiation between gastritis and gastric cancer and for the detection of epithelial tumours. When examining a flat reddened lesion, if a DL cannot be discerned in the peripheral area, cancer can be excluded with a high degree of probability [3].

On the other hand, if a demarcation line is present, we examine the V and S components of the mucosa in detail, and if an irregular MV pattern and/or irregular MS pattern are observed, the diagnosis of cancer can be made. In other words, a demarcation line is an essential condition for a diagnosis of cancer, whereas an irregular MV pattern or irregular MS pattern is a sufficient condition.

7.4.2 Intraepithelial Microinvasion (IEMI)

Detailed examination of the marginal area of a cancer may reveal a cancer-specific VS, continuous with the cancer mucosa, in the intervening part of the MCE of the background mucosa. This has the following two patterns:

1. Cancer-specific irregular MV pattern under the noncancerous epithelium of the marginal area, termed subepithelial invasion
2. Destruction of the noncancerous epithelial structure, with replacement by a cancer-specific irregular MV pattern or irregular MS pattern, termed superficial invasion

7.5 Findings Within the Lesion

The general rule for VS classification of a lesion is that the V and S components should be analysed separately. In addition, when cancer has been diagnosed, a supplementary analysis should be made of the relationship between V and S.

7.5.1 Combined Morphology of V and S (VS Concordance)

In general, the normal and noncancerous (chronic gastritis, hyperplastic lesions, etc.) mucosa follows the anatomical principle that subepithelial capillaries and vessels are located in areas corresponding to the IP (VS concordance). However, in cancers with poor differentiation or deep invasion, this principle no longer applies, and findings where the relationship between MCE (S) and blood vessels (V) is not necessarily concordant (the IP (S) is destroyed or the orientation of the MCE (S) and blood vessels (V) do not match). The dissociation or divergence between the V and S components is termed VS discordance.

1. VS concordant
   Blood vessels are present in areas corresponding to the IP subepithelium, surrounded by the MCE.
2. VS discordant
   Blood vessels are not consistently present in areas corresponding to the IP subepithelium surrounded by the MCE, indicating dissociation between the distribution and direction of the epithelium and microvessels.
3. Not determined (ND)
   When the correlation between the epithelial structure and microvascular morphology is unclear, and it is not possible to determine the relationship between the two, it is recorded as 'not determined'.

7.6 Exceptions to the VS Classification System

In Chap. 2, we used standardised terminology and description methods based on the VS classification system. However, for some diseases such as MALT lymphoma and carcinoids, there is insufficient accumulated experience, so they should be regarded as exceptions and the VS classification system is not applied.

References

1. Yao K (ed.). Zoom gastroscopy, pp 57–69. 2013. Springer.
2. Yao K, et al. *Endoscopy* 2009; **41**: 462–467.
3. Yamada S, et al. Gastrointest Endosc 2014; 79: 55–63.

Atlas of Normal Appearance in the Stomach and the Duodenum

8

Kenshi Yao

K. Yao
Department of Endoscopy, Fukuoka University Chikushi Hospital,
1-1-1 Zokumyoin, Chikushino 818-8502, Japan
e-mail: yao@fukuoka-u.ac.jp

M. Muto et al. (eds.), *Atlas of Endoscopy with Narrow Band Imaging*,
DOI 10.1007/978-4-431-54243-8_8

8.1 Normal Fundic Glandular Mucosa

8.1.1 M-NBI Findings

1. Microvascular architecture (V): regular honeycomb-like subepithelial capillary network (SECN) pattern and regular collecting venule (CV) pattern
2. Microsurface structure (S): regular oval crypt opening (CO) pattern and circular marginal crypt epithelium (MCE) pattern
3. Microvascular architecture and microsurface structure (VS): concordant, gastric body type (epithelium within vessel pattern)

8.1.2 Explanation

8.1.2.1 Non-magnified WLI Appearance (Fig. 8.1a)

In the normal fundic gland mucosa free of *Helicobacter pylori* infection, the collecting venules (CVs) reported by Yagi et al. are visualized as a regular arrangement of collecting venules (RAC).

8.1.2.2 M-NBI Appearance (Maximal Magnifying Ratio) (Fig. 8.1b, c)

Microvascular architecture (V): Comprising the brown subepithelial capillaries (SECs) and the CVs visualized as cyan coloured, the shape of each individual SEC is polygonal (many are pentagonal), and these anastomose repeatedly with each other, forming a regular honeycomb-like subepithelial capillary network (SECN) pattern. These subepithelial capillary networks feed into the CVs. In the normal fundic glandular epithelium, these subepithelial capillary networks and collecting venules have a regular shape and arrangement.

Microsurface structure (S): The anatomical structures visualized are the brown crypt openings (COs) and the white belt-like structures of the marginal crypt epithelium (MCE). The crypt openings are in a circular or oval shape, and MCE surrounds crypt opening.

Part of Figures 8.1b has been magnified and shown as Fig. 8.1c. Figure 8.1c has been divided into the NBI images obtained with central wavelengths of 415 nm (Fig. 8.1d) and 540 nm (Fig. 8.1e). As shown in Fig. 8.1d, the narrow bandwidth (central wave length 415 nm) enables good visualization of the shape of the SECs, MCE, and COs. On the other hand, as shown in Fig. 8.1e, the CVs are clearly delineated using 540 nm NBI.

Correlation between microvascular architecture and microsurface structure (VS) (Fig. 8.1d): The subepithelial capillaries are located in the subepithelial area of intervening part, (VS concordant). Inside the polygonal capillaries are the circular or oval COs and the circular or oval MCE (epithelium within vessel pattern, gastric body type).

8.1.2.3 Histological Findings

Figure 8.1f shows a biopsy sample of normal fundic glandular mucosa. Compared to the pyloric glandular epithelium, the intervening part is narrow and the density of the glandular crypts are high. The glandular crypts run in a comparatively vertical direction.

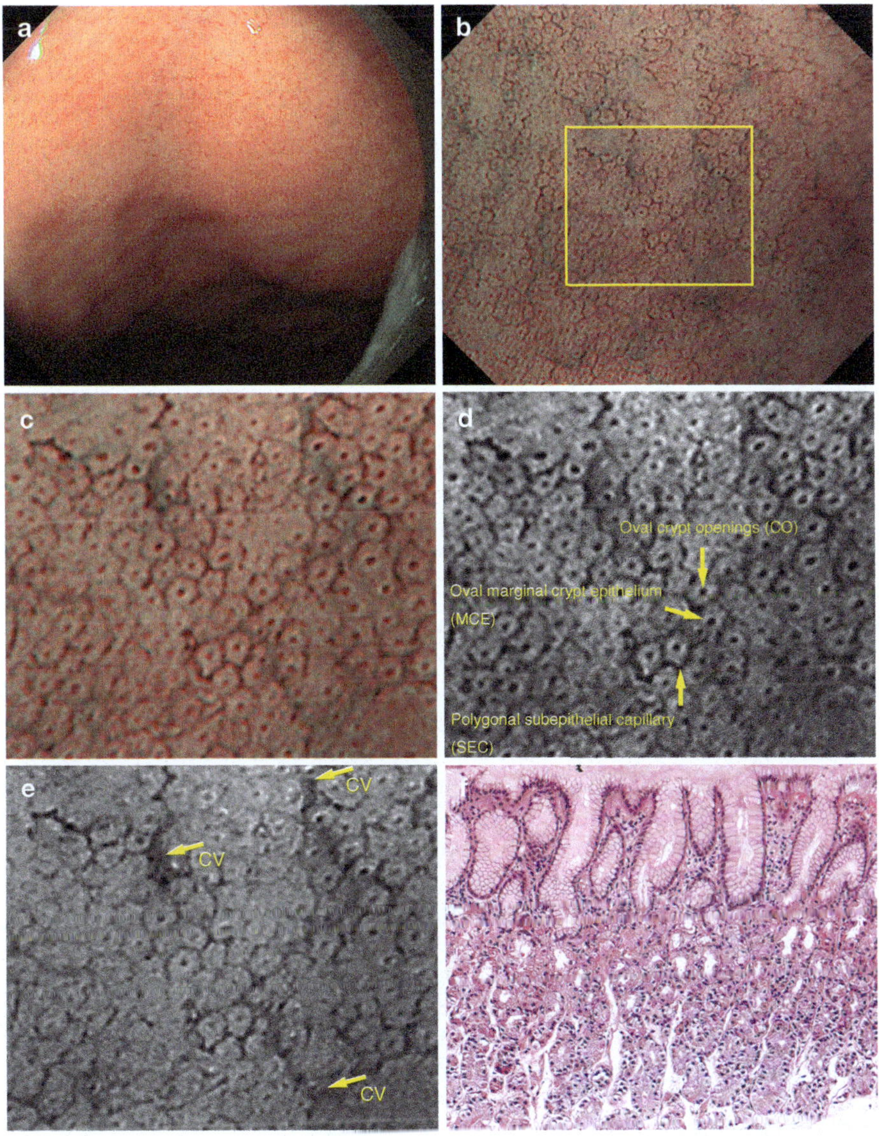

Fig. 8.1 Normal fundic glandular mucosa. (**a**) Non-magnified WLI appearance. (**b**) M-NBI appearance. (**c**) Enlarged M-NBI apperance. (**d**) M-NBI image optained with central wavelength of 415 nm. (**e**) M-NBI image optained with central wavelength of 540 nm. (**f**) Histological findings

8.2 Normal Pyloric Glandular Mucosa

8.2.1 M-NBI Findings

1. Microvascular architecture (V): regular coil-shaped subepithelial capillary network (SECN) pattern with absence of regular collecting venule (CV) pattern
2. Microsurface structure (S): regular curved marginal crypt epithelium (MCE) pattern
3. Microvascular architecture and microsurface structure (VS): concordant, gastric antral type (vessel within epithelium pattern)

8.2.2 Explanation

8.2.2.1 Non-magnified WLI Appearance (Fig. 8.2a)

In the normal pyloric glandular mucosa observed using non-magnified WLI, the collecting venules (CVs) are observed infrequently, and the mucosa has a uniform light-reddened appearance.

8.2.2.2 M-NBI Appearance (Maximal Magnifying Ratio) (Fig. 8.2b, c)

Microvascular architecture (V): The brown SECs are visualized, but unlike the fundic glandular mucosa, the cyan-coloured collecting venules (CVs) are visualized only infrequently. The morphology of the individual SECs is coil shaped and open looped (Fig. 8.2d). These form a regular coil-shaped SECN pattern. Although not shown in this atlas, the SECs are sometimes closed looped, forming a subepithelial reticular network.

Microsurface structure (S): This mainly comprises belt-like structures of MCE, and unlike the gastric fundic glandular mucosa, brown COs are only visualized infrequently. The morphology of the MCE is usually curved or polygonal, sometimes linear, with a regular distribution (Fig. 8.2e).

Correlation between microvascular architecture and microsurface structure (VS): The SECs are located beneath the intervening part (IP) (VS concordant). As shown in Figure 8.2e, capillaries are surrounded by a polygonal epithelium (vessel within epithelium pattern, gastric antral type).

8.2.2.3 Histological Findings

Figure 8.2f shows a biopsy sample of normal pyloric glandular mucosa. Compared to the fundic glandular epithelium, the IP is wide, and the density of the glandular crypts is low. Few glandular crypts run in a vertical direction.

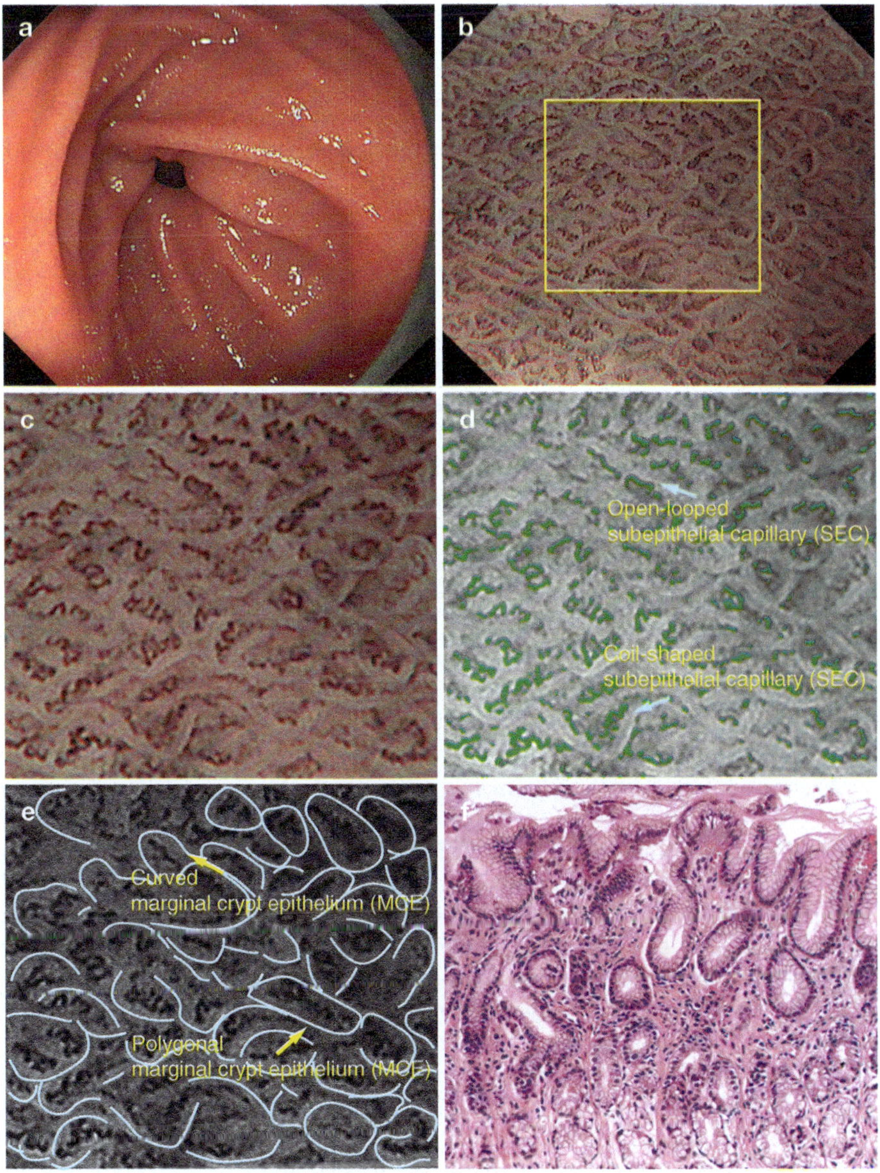

Fig. 8.2 Normal pyloric glandular mucosa. (**a**) Non-magnified WLI appearance. (**b**) M-NBI appearance. (**c**) Enlarged M-NBI appearance. (**d**) Gray scale image of M-NBI appearance. (**e**) Gray scale image of M-NBI appearance. (**f**) Histological findings

8.3 Normal Duodenal Mucosa

8.3.1 M-NBI Findings

1. Microvascular architecture (V): regular villous subepithelial capillary network (V-SECN)
2. Microsurface structure (S): regular curved or oval-shaped marginal villous epithelium (MVE)

8.3.2 Explanation

8.3.2.1 Non-magnified WLI Appearance (Fig. 8.3a)

In a normal duodenal mucosa, the valves of Kerckring (circular folds) run in equally and regularly spaced rings. Examination in detail reveals minute granular protuberances thought to be villous structures spread out on the surface.

8.3.2.2 M-NBI Appearance (Maximal Magnifying Ratio) (Fig. 8.3b, c)

Figure 8.2b shows the non-water-immersed appearance and Figure 8.2c the water-immersed appearance.

Microvascular architecture (V): In general, the V-SECN forms anastomoses, which can be observed lined up regularly directly beneath the villous epithelium. At times, they can be observed flowing into the villous venules (VV) (Fig. 8.3b light blue arrow) in the deep part.

Microsurface structure (S): This mainly comprises the MVE, mainly visualized as a white belt-like structure (Fig. 8.3d) (the opening of the crypts are deeper than the villi (Fig. 8.3f), so normally they are not visualized). The MVE morphology varies according to the direction from which it is visualized, appearing round to oval when viewed perpendicular to the mucosa surface and curved when observed obliquely. The villi bordering the MVE generally show a fingerlike or leaf-like and occasionally ridge-like morphology. Examination using the water immersion technique shows the villi swaying in the water flow, a morphological characteristic of normal villi (Fig. 8.3c).

Although reproducibility varies depending on the direction of observation, light blue crests (LBCs) can always be visualized in the periphery of the normal duodenal MVE (Fig. 8.3e).

Correlation between microvascular architecture and microsurface structure (VS): In the duodenum, loop-shaped capillaries are located inside the villi bordering the marginal villous epithelium (MVE) in a leash-like arrangement and can be clearly discerned forming anastomoses inside the villi (Figs. 8.3b, c).

8.3.2.3 Histological Findings

Figure 8.3f shows a biopsy sample of normal duodenal mucosa. The epithelium comprises long thin villi and crypts. The V-SECNs are distributed beneath the villous epithelium.

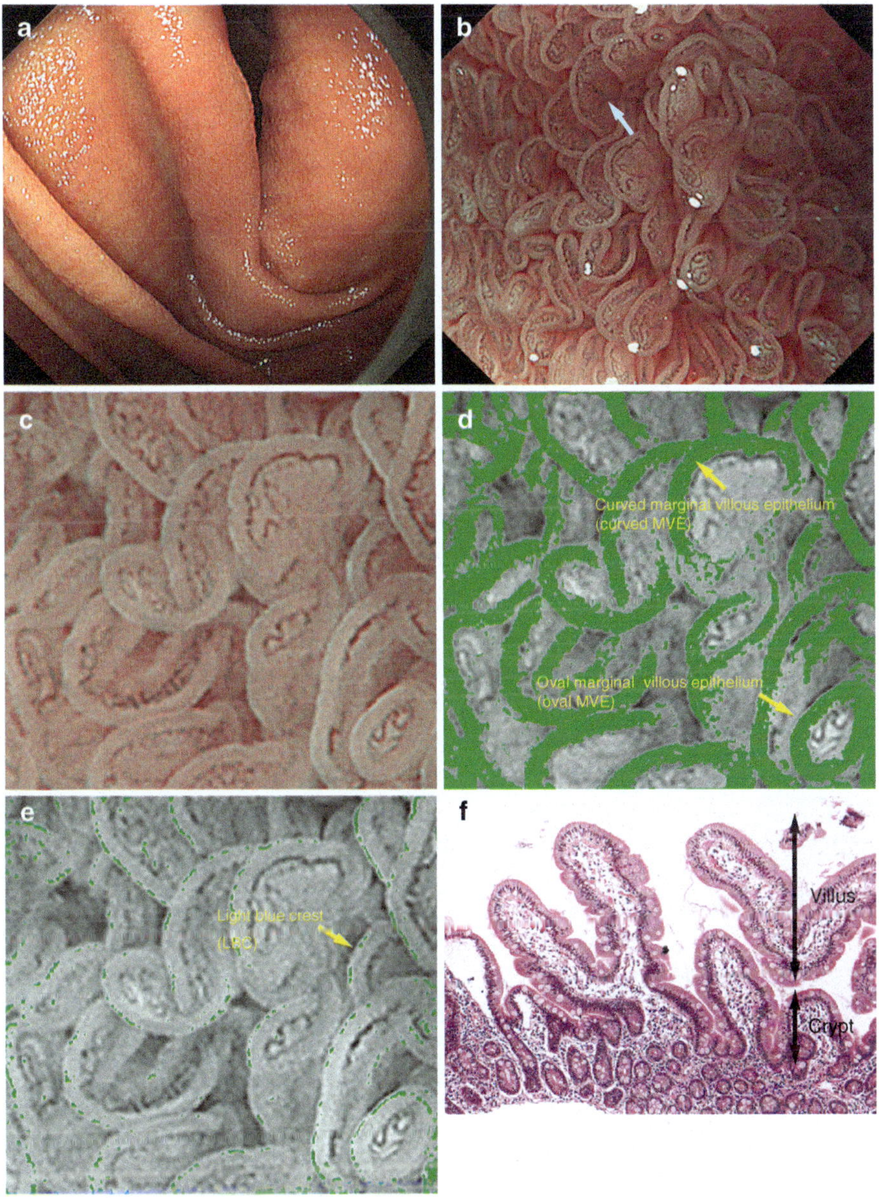

Fig. 8.3 Normal duodenal Mucosa. (**a**) Non-magnified WLI appearance. (**b**) M-NBI appearance (Non-water immersed). (**c**) Enlarged M-NBI appearance (Water immersed). (**d**) Morphology of marginal villons epithelium (MVE). (**e**) Extraction of light blue crest (LBC). (**f**) Histological findings

Atlas of Nonneoplastic Lesions in the Stomach

9

Kenshi Yao, Noriya Uedo, Hisashi Doyama, and Hirohisa Machida

K. Yao (✉)
Department of Endoscopy, Fukuoka University Chikushi Hospital,
1-1-1 Zokumyoin, Chikushino 818-8502, Japan
e-mail: yao@fukuoka-u.ac.jp

N. Uedo
Department of Gastrointestinal Oncology, Osaka Medical Center for Cancer and Cardiovascular Diseases, Osaka, Japan

H. Doyama
Department of Gastroenterology, Ishikawa Prefectural Central Hospital, Kanazawa, Japan

H. Machida
Machida Gastroenterical Hospital, Osaka, Japan

M. Muto et al. (eds.), *Atlas of Endoscopy with Narrow Band Imaging*,
DOI 10.1007/978-4-431-54243-8_9

9.1 Chronic Gastritis and Atrophic Gastritis

Endoscopic diagnosis of chronic gastritis associated with *Helicobacter pylori* (HP) infection using only conventional non-magnified endoscopy has suffered limitations and lacked reproducibility. In recent years, Yagi et al. [1] and Nakagawa et al. [2] have demonstrated that magnifying endoscopic examination of the fundic glandular mucosa can be used to diagnose, accurately and objectively, HP-negative normal mucosa, HP-associated chronic gastritis, and atrophic gastritis (Fig. 9.1a–f were reproduced from [3] with permission).

9.1.1 M-NBI Appearance

9.1.1.1 Type 1 (HP-Negative, Normal Fundic Glandular Mucosa, Fig. 9.1a)

1. Microvascular architecture (V): Brown polygonal (pentagonal or hexagonal) subepithelial capillaries (SECs) surround the periphery of the crypt openings (COs), forming a regular subepithelial capillary network (SECN) with a honeycomb-like appearance. These honeycomb-like SECNs flow into the collecting venules (CVs, Fig. 9.1a arrows) visualized as cyan colored.
2. Microsurface structure (S): Inside the polygonal subepithelial capillaries (SECs) can be found the white semitransparent round marginal crypt epithelium (MCE), inside which are the round COs. Their morphologies are uniform, with a regular arrangement.

9.1.1.2 Type 2 (Fundic Glandular Mucosa with Mild Active Gastritis, Mild Atrophy, Associated with HP Infection, Fig. 9.1b)

1. Microvascular architecture (V): A slightly dilated SECN is seen, although the distribution maintains a regular honeycomb-like pattern. The main difference from the normal mucosa is that no CVs can be visualized.
2. Microsurface structure (S): The round MCE and COs preserve the same structure as the normal mucosa.

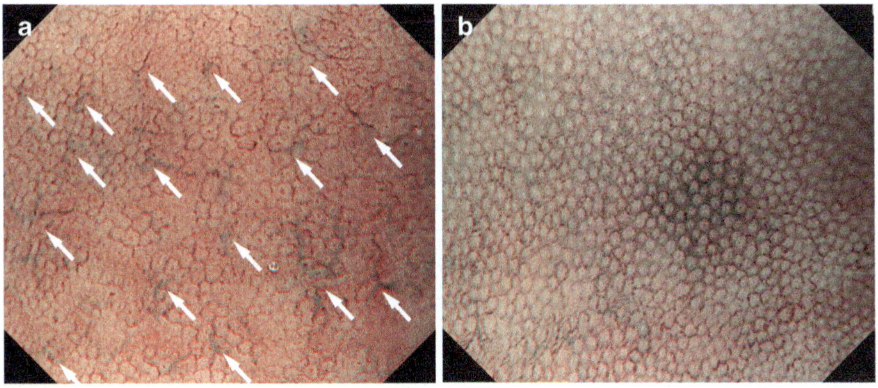

Fig. 9.1

9.1.1.3 Type 3 (Fundic Glandular Mucosa with Severe Strong Active Gastritis Associated with HP Infection, Fig. 9.1c)

1. Microvascular architecture (V): A dilated SECN is shown, with loss of the honeycomb-like pattern. CVs are also not visualized.
2. Microsurface structure (S): The MCE has lost its normal rounded structure and appears curved or oval shaped. Brown COs are not visualized.

9.1.1.4 Type 4 (Fundic Glandular Mucosa with Mild Active Gastritis and Marked Atrophic Gastritis, Fig. 9.1d)

1. Microvascular architecture (V): The normal honeycomb-like pattern is lost, and CVs (Fig. 9.1d arrows) are once again visualized. However, their morphology is irregular compared to normal CVs [2].
2. Microsurface structure (S): This is the absent MS pattern where no MCE or COs can be visualized.

9.1.2 Histological Findings

In the biopsy specimen (Fig. 9.1e) taken from the site shown in Fig. 9.1c, we see infiltration of large numbers of inflammatory cells into the fundic glandular mucosa. Compared to the normal mucosa, the crypt structure has altered, either dilated, inclined, or branched. Accompanying the extensive inflammatory cell infiltration, the intervening parts (IP) are also widened.

In the biopsy specimen (Fig. 9.1f) taken from the site shown in Fig. 9.1d, the number of infiltrating inflammatory cells is less, and the fundic glands have atrophied and disappeared. There is diffuse intestinal metaplasia. The mucosa is markedly thinned.

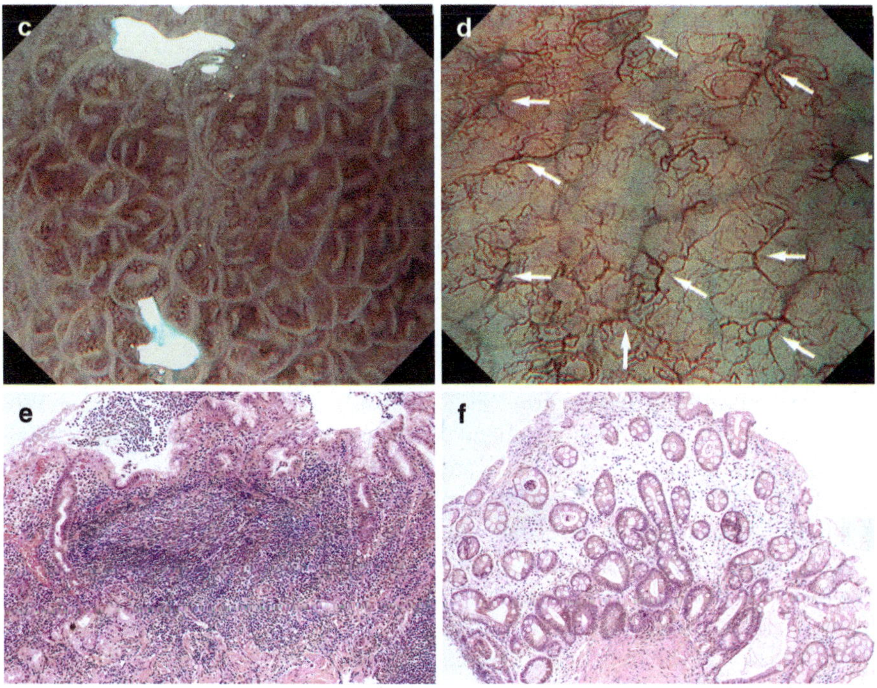

Fig. 9.1 (continued)

9.2 Intestinal Metaplasia (LBC+)

Intestinal metaplasia is associated with an increased risk of differentiated gastric carcinoma. The conventional non-magnified endoscopic findings of intestinal metaplasia which are of gray-white granular protuberances (specific intestinal dysplasia) are well known. Many cases of intestinal metaplasia are flat, however, so the sensitivity is low for this kind of finding alone, and the endoscopic diagnosis of intestinal metaplasia was considered difficult.

9.2.1 Explanation

Intestinal metaplasia is visualized as a whitish mucosa on non-magnified WLI appearance (Fig. 9.2a). Non-magnified NBI shows the non-metaplastic mucosa as brown and the intestinal metaplasia as areas with light blue crests (LBCs) (Fig. 9.2b).

M-NBI examination of the non-metaplastic mucosa reveals a broad subepithelial capillary network (SECN) in the intervening parts (IPs) (Fig. 9.2c upper part). In the area of intestinal metaplasia, the SECN has become dilated, tortuous blood vessels, and the marginal crypt epithelium (MCE) is broad and cloudy white (Fig. 9.2c lower part). This difference in the ratio of blood vessels to epithelium is believed to play a part in the color differences in this image. Apart from that, in areas of intestinal metaplasia, light blue lines are visible at the epithelial margins (surface). These are called light blue crests (LBCs), a useful finding for the detection of intestinal metaplasia in cases of *Helicobacter pylori* (*H. pylori*)-associated gastritis [4]. The inference is that this phenomenon involves strong reflection of short-wavelength narrow band light (415 nm) by the brush borders of the areas of intestinal metaplasia.

In fundic mucosa with *H. pylori*-associated inflammation or atrophy, the crypt openings (COs) may become round, or short or long lines, and with further progression of atrophy and intestinal metaplasia, the surface structure changes from a ridge-like to a papillary pattern. For this reason, areas of intestinal metaplasia in which LBCs are visualized have mainly crest-shaped to papillary surface structures, but in the gastric body, LBCs are mainly seen associated with a surface structure with COs (Fig. 9.2d). This differs from the circular COs observed in the *H. pylori*-positive fundic glandular mucosa, where a stellate morphology is common (Fig. 9.2d arrow). This should be recognized as a subtype of intestinal metaplasia.

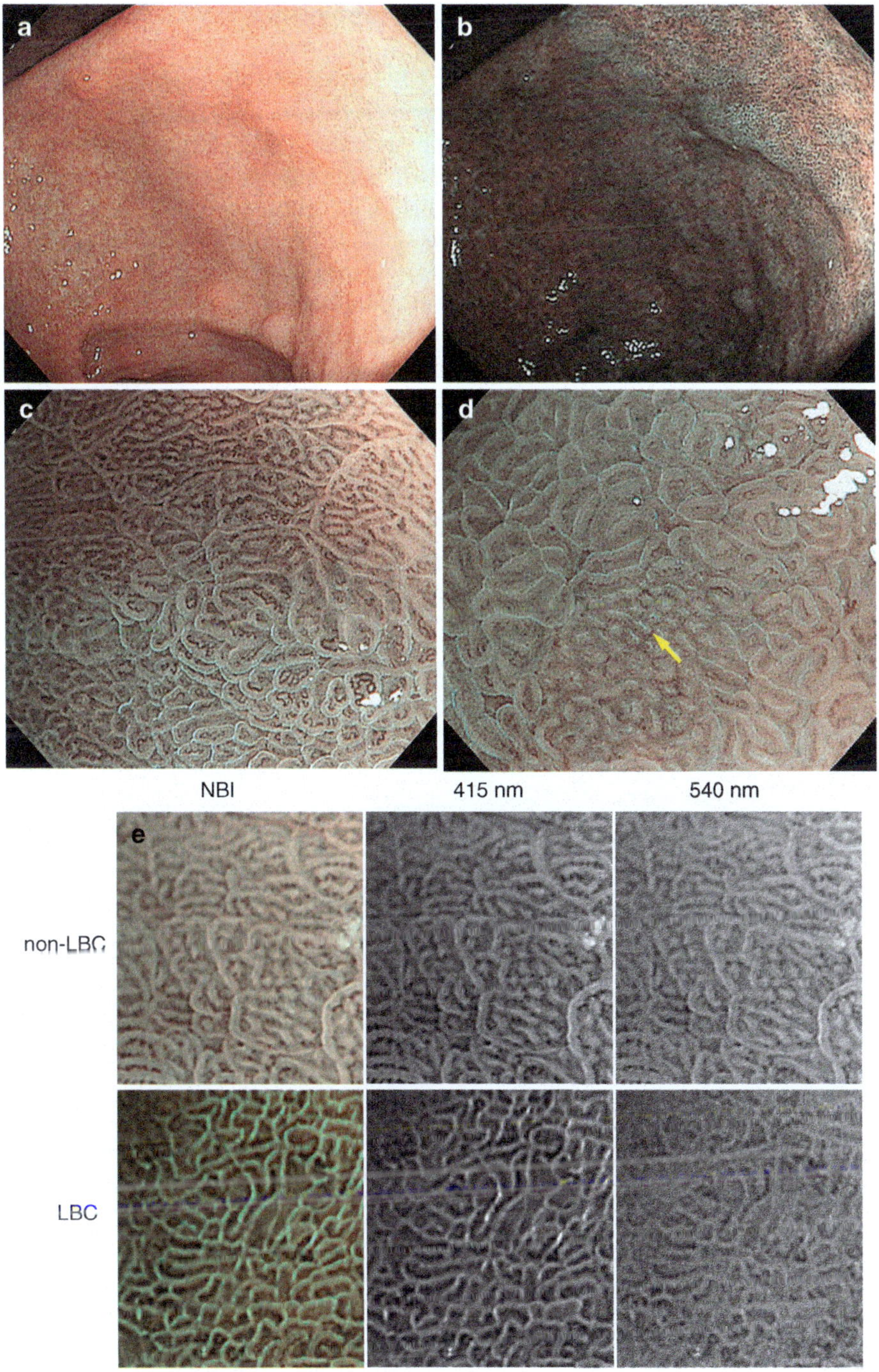

Fig. 9.2

9.2.2 Differentiation Using the NBI Appearance

One finding requiring differentiation from LBC is that of white lines on the MCE of the non-metaplastic mucosa. This phenomenon is thought to occur when examining the superficial layers of the crypt epithelium from the incident light direction due to overlapping backward scattering light. NBI applies color simulation to images obtained from projection of narrow band light with central wavelengths of 415 and 540 nm. In Fig. 9.2e the left column shows simulated color composite NBI images, the center column 415 nm grayscale images, and the right column 540 nm grayscale images. The non-LBCs in the surface crypt epithelium of the upper row of photographs are images from 415 nm reflected light allocated to green and blue simulated colors and 540 nm light allocated to red simulated color (seen as white in black and white images), so it is seen as white combining all of green, blue, and red, and they are arranged more thinly than LBCs (Fig. 9.2e). In comparison, in the lower row for LBCs, 415 nm light is more strongly reflected, so it appears light cyan with green and blue mixed, and the shape is large and slightly irregular (Fig. 9.2e). It is conjectured that the villous structure of the brush border of the intestinal metaplasia mucosal surface epithelium has these light characteristics.

9.3 Intestinal Metaplasia (WOS+)

9.3.1 M-NBI Findings

1. Microvascular architecture (V): absent MV pattern
2. Microsurface structure (S): regular MS pattern (WOS +, speckled)
3. Microvascular architecture and microsurface structure (VS): not determined

9.3.2 Explanation

The microvascular pattern is an important indicator for interpreting magnified endoscopic findings, but in some epithelial tumors and intestinal metaplastic mucosa, there is a white opaque substance (WOS) on the mucosal surface, so in some cases the subepithelial blood vessels in the IP cannot be visualized, as reported by the author and others [6, 7]. When the blood vessels (V) cannot be clearly seen, I record this as "absent MV pattern" and instead of V use the white opaque substance (WOS) as a marker of the microsurface structure pattern (S) and conduct a magnifying endoscopic examination.

In this section, I present an early stomach cancer with WOS (+) intestinal metaplasia present in the noncancerous background mucosa. Light blue crests (LBCs) are also an objective marker of intestinal metaplasia visualized using M-NBI. The two are optically different, in that LBCs can only be visualized using NBI, but that WOS can be visualized using either WLI or NBI.

9.3.2.1 WLI Appearance

A pale irregular depressed lesion can be seen on the anterior wall of the gastric antrum (Fig. 9.3a). This is a type 0-IIc early gastric cancer. The color of the noncancerous background on the oral side is also white (arrow). Magnified WLI (Fig. 9.3b) examination focusing on the area indicated by the arrow in Fig. 9.3a (background mucosa on the oral side of the cancer) is unable to visualize vessels due to the presence of WOS.

9.3.2.2 M-NBI Appearance

M-NBI examination delineates the WOS more clearly, and LBCs are visualized at the same time (Fig. 9.3c, d). However, WOS and LBCs do not always appear at the same time. Whereas LBCs are visualized lining the marginal crypt epithelium (MCE), WOS is normally located in the IPs. In other words, the two features are localized in different sites. When we look at another area in detail at maximum magnification (Fig.9.3e), we see only speckled WOS on the intervening part epithelium of the intestinal metaplasia but LBCs are not visualized.

9.3.2.3 Histological Findings

Histological examination of the noncancerous mucosa from the oral side of this endoscopic submucosal dissection (ESD) specimen reveals diffuse intestinal metaplasia containing goblet cells and Paneth cells (Fig. 9.3e). The gastric proper gland is atrophic and cannot be identified. In other words, these are the histological findings of metaplastic and atrophic gastritis.

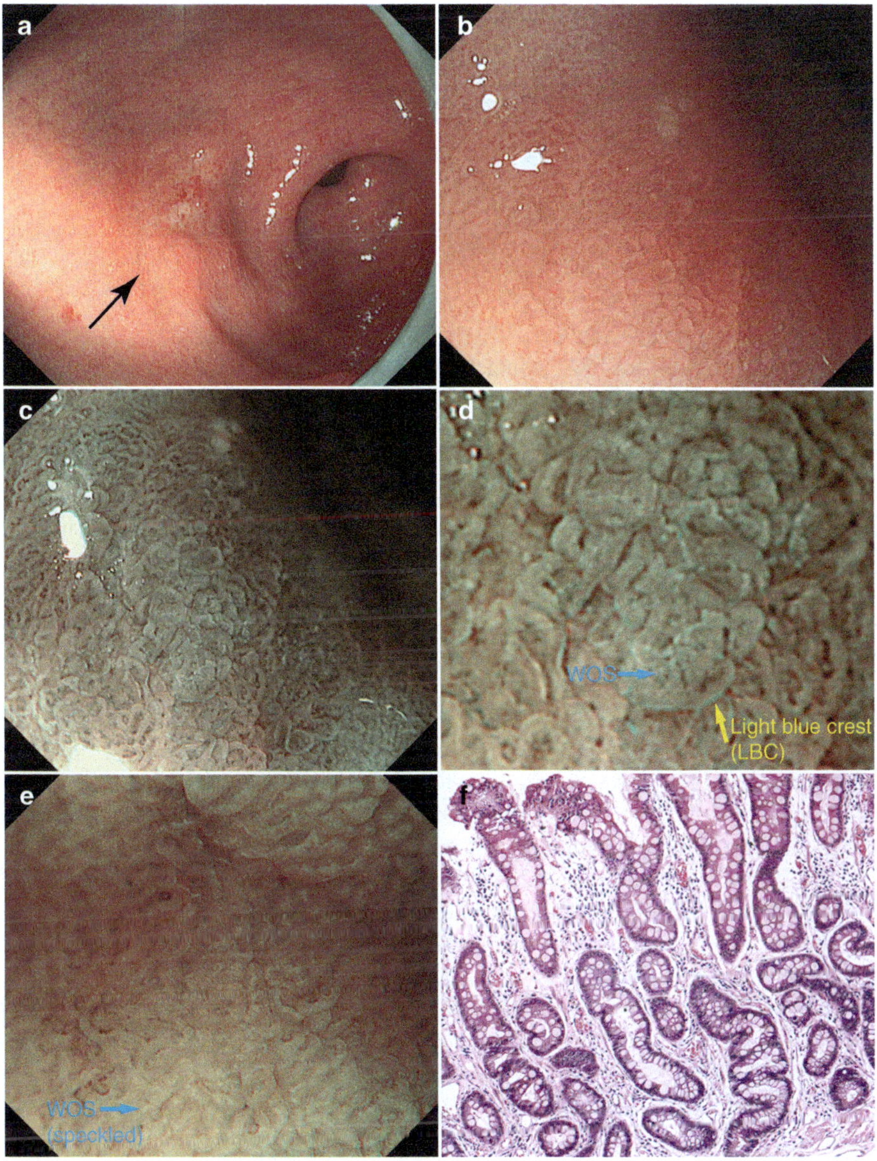

Fig. 9.3

9.4 Hyperplastic Polyp

9.4.1 M-NBI Findings

1. Margin (demarcation line: present or absent)
2. Lesion (VS classification: regular MV plus regular MS pattern)

9.4.2 Explanation

9.4.2.1 WLI Appearance

Hyperplastic polyps of the stomach are normally strongly reddened colored (Fig. 9.4a). When small they are semispherical, but as they grow larger, they change shape from semipedunculated to pedunculated, often associated with surface erosion. When dye is sprayed (Fig. 9.4b), the surface appears smooth and presents a regular gastric mucosal microsurface pattern.

M-WLI of the marginal area often reveals a clear demarcation line at the base of the protrusion, as shown in Fig. 9.4c. However, in some lesions, the surrounding V and S gradually change into a hyperplastic polyp morphology, and a clear demarcation line (DL) is not formed.

9.4.2.2 M-NBI appearance

S: The MCE shows a white, curved to linear morphology, forming a regular IP (Fig. 9.4d, e). Between the MCE can be seen dark slit-shaped crypt openings (COs). The individual sections of MCE have a consistent width and are large compared to the surrounding background mucosa, forming a widened brownish IP. The IPs (↔) have a constant width.

V: The IP subepithelium has a high vascular density, so the IPs overall are brown, and each microvascular pattern has low contrast making it difficult to classify. Blood vessels directly under the epithelium are mainly regular open-looped dilated microvessels.

VS concordance: This is a VS concordant finding, with microvessels located beneath the IP epithelium. The widened brownish IPs are characteristic. This is a gastric antral type (vessel within epithelium pattern) where the blood vessels are located in the IP subepithelium enclosed by the MCE.

9.4.2.3 Histological Findings

Histological examination of the biopsy reveals epithelium composed of foveolar epithelium with a rich clear cellular structure, associated with dilatation of the crypts (Fig. 9.4f). Within the wide IP spaces, we can see a rich proliferation of microvessels, with mild fibrosis and infiltration of inflammatory cells.

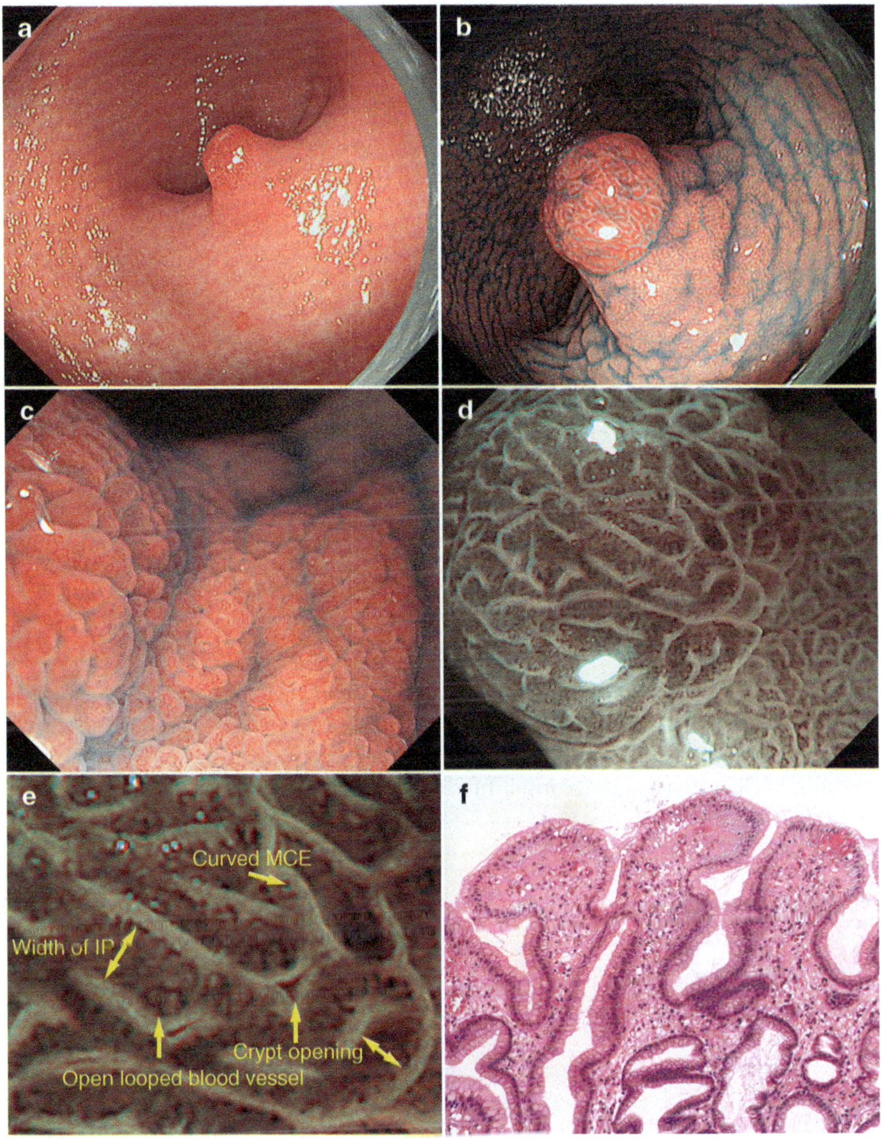
a
b
c
d
e
Curved MCE
Width of IP
Crypt opening
Open looped blood vessel
f

Fig. 9.4

9.5 Fundic Gland Polyp

9.5.1 M-NBI Findings

1. Marginal area (demarcation line: present or absent)
2. Lesion (VS classification: regular MV pattern plus regular MS pattern)

9.5.2 Explanation

9.5.2.1 WLI appearance

Fundic gland polyps, mainly found in the mucosa free of *H. pylori* infection in the fundic gland region (gastric body and fundus), are smooth-surfaced protruding lesions varying from the same color as their surrounds to light red. When a lesion is small, it varies from a superficial raised to a nonpedunculated protrusion (Fig.9.5a), but as it gets larger it becomes a semipedunculated protruding lesion (Fig. 9.5b), and the reddened coloration becomes stronger and fresher (Fig. 9.5b).

9.5.2.2 M-NBI Appearance

Background Mucosa

Figure 9.5c shows normal gastric fundic gland mucosa. This presents a regular honeycomb-like subepithelial capillary network (SECN) pattern with regular collecting venule (CV) pattern plus regular oval crypt opening (CO) pattern and circular MCE pattern (see "Normal fundic gland mucosa").

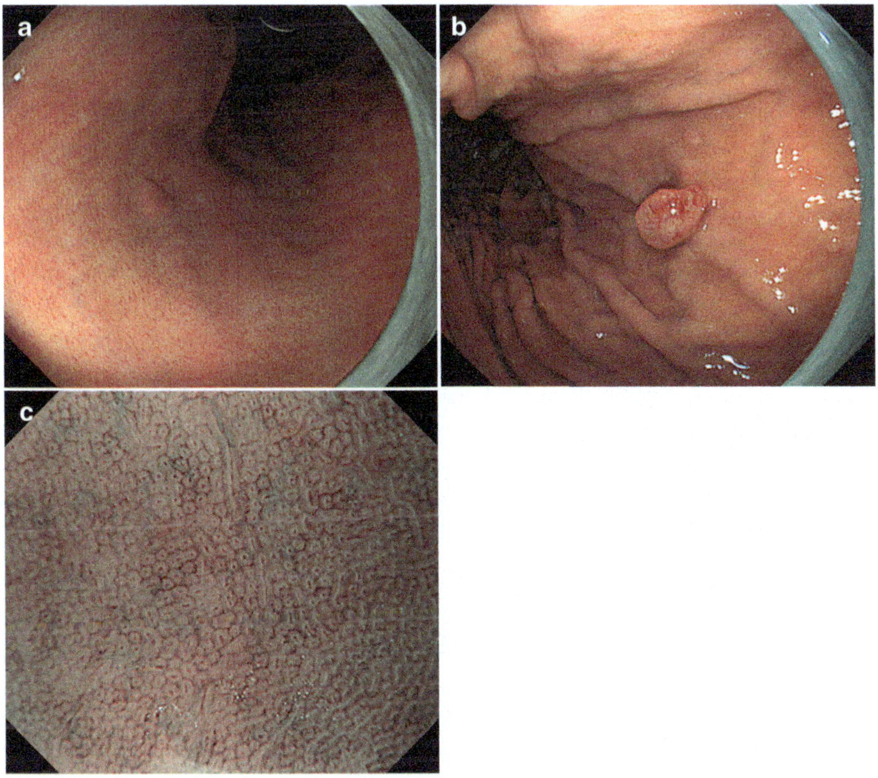

Fig. 9.5

Lesion

This small polyp has essentially the same microvascular architecture (V) and microsurface structure (S) as the surrounding background mucosa (Fig. 9.5d). When a lesion grows larger and semipedunculated, these features change slightly (Fig. 9.5e).

V: Each polygonal vessel in the honeycomb-like SECN becomes enlarged, and the blood vessel dilates and thickens. This is often associated with markedly dilated branching light cyan blood vessels with a morphology resembling CVs.

S: The marginal crypt epithelium (MCE) has a circular morphology, with an unchanged density, but it does become larger, and the COs also become oval and larger. It is characteristic that the intervening parts (IPs) become wider in association with these changes. Although not shown on the figures in this section, occasionally large COs are seen.

VS concordance: Essentially the same findings as the normal fundic gland mucosa. While a clear demarcation line (DL) is often delineated in the marginal area, in some cases there is a gradual change from background mucosa to the polyp VS.

9.5.2.3 Histological Findings

Figure 9.5f shows the histological findings of a biopsy specimen of the semipedunculated polyp shown in Figs. 9.5b and 9.5e. The surface spacing between crypts has become wider, and the IP is wide compared to the normal gastric fundic glandular mucosa. The lamina propria is slightly edematous, but no significant inflammatory cell infiltration is seen. Characteristic features are marked hyperplasia and cystic dilatation of the fundic glands.

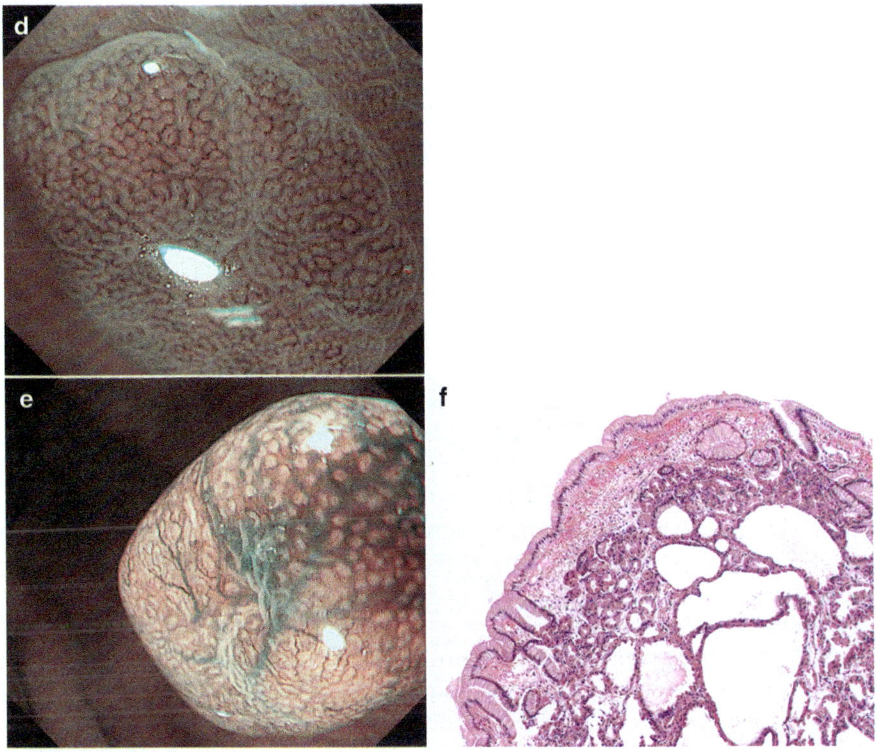

Fig. 9.5 (continued)

9.6 Localized Gastritis (Flat) Requiring Differentiation from Gastric Cancer

Helicobacter pylori infection causes inflammatory cell infiltration of the gastric mucosa after an extended period inducing mucosal changes such as atrophy and intestinal metaplasia, resulting in a variety of morphological changes to the gastric mucosa. Mucosal changes due to chronic gastritis can be diffuse or localized, and it is important to differentiate the latter from a small early gastric cancer.

9.6.1 Explanation

This patient underwent endoscopic submucosal dissection (ESD) for early gastric cancer of the anterior wall of the gastric angle 2 years ago.

9.6.1.1 WLI appearance

At a follow-up upper gastrointestinal tract endoscopy, a flat reddened lesion 7–8 mm in size was detected on the posterior wall of the upper gastric body (Fig. 9.6a).

9.6.1.2 M-NBI Appearance

M-NBI shows the surface microstructure (S) of the surrounding mucosa to range from ridge-like to papillary, whereas in some parts of the lesion, microvessels form an irregular network structure (Fig. 9.6b). Examination of the periphery of the lesion at maximal magnifying ratio reveals reticular to slightly dilated subepithelial capillaries (SECs) surrounded by distinct marginal crypt epithelium (MCE) in the surrounding gastritic mucosa (Fig. 9.6c upper part). The blood vessels of the lesion (Fig. 9.6c lower part) form an irregular network comprising slightly distended SECs interwoven together. Findings characteristic of tumor vessels, such as irregular dilatation and tortuosity, are infrequent in these narrow vessels, and unlike a cancer their shape resembled some of the blood vessels in the surrounding gastritic mucosa. A distinct demarcation line (DL) between the surface structure of the lesion and the surrounding mucosa can be seen at the left side of this image (Fig. 9.6b), whereas on the right side (Fig. 9.6c) the change is gradual and the margin unclear.

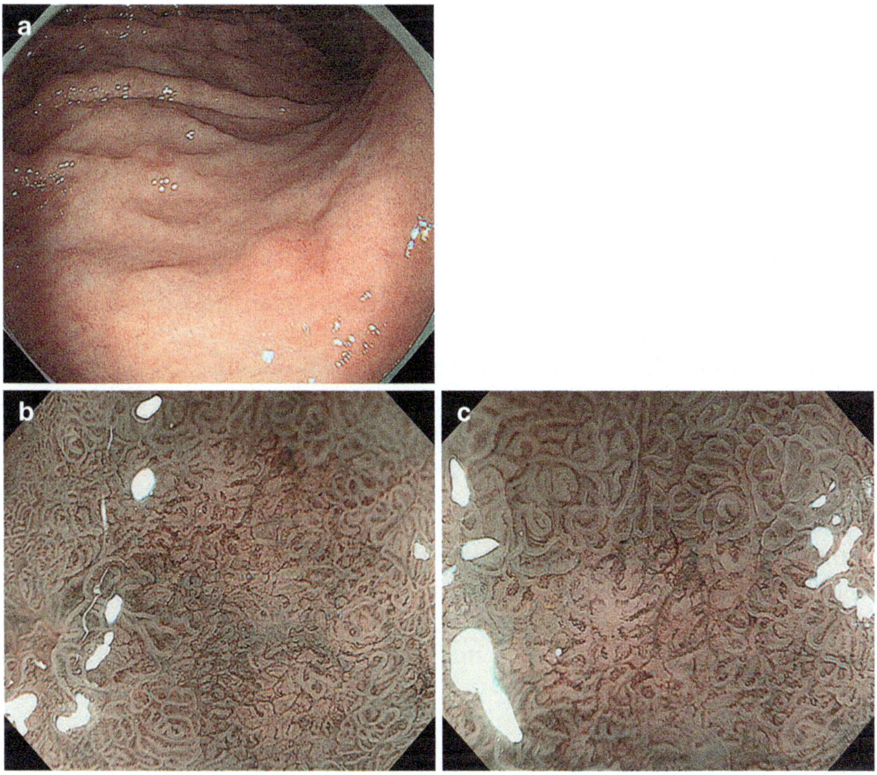

Fig. 9.6

9.6.1.3 Histological Findings

Although nonneoplastic changes were suspected on the basis of the above findings, a target biopsy was taken from this area to eliminate the possibility of tumor. Histopathological examination revealed only inflammation, with no findings suggesting a neoplasia (Fig. 9.6d).

9.6.2 Diagnostic Pointers for NBI

9.6.2.1 Typical Appearance of Nonneoplastic Localized Gastritis (Fig. 9.6e)

A cluster of fine SECs form a regular vascular network. The individual vessels forming the network structure are basically uniform in morphology and size, and crypt openings (COs), surrounded by the distinct marginal crypt epithelium (MCE), are regularly arranged within the network (Regular MV pattern plus regular MS pattern with a demarcation line).

9.6.2.2 Typical Appearance of Differentiated Cancer (Fig. 9.6f)

Dilated irregular tumor blood vessels form a network structure. The MCE is indistinct, and the individual vessels forming the network structure are nonuniform in diameter, morphology, and size (Irregular MV pattern plus absent MS pattern with a demarcation line).

9.6.2.3 When Taking a Biopsy

Differentiation between cancer and noncancer is easy when a lesion presents a typical appearance as shown in Fig. 9.6e, f, but if even one slightly atypical element is present as demonstrated in Fig. 9.6b, c, a biopsy should be taken without hesitation, not relying solely on the visual findings.

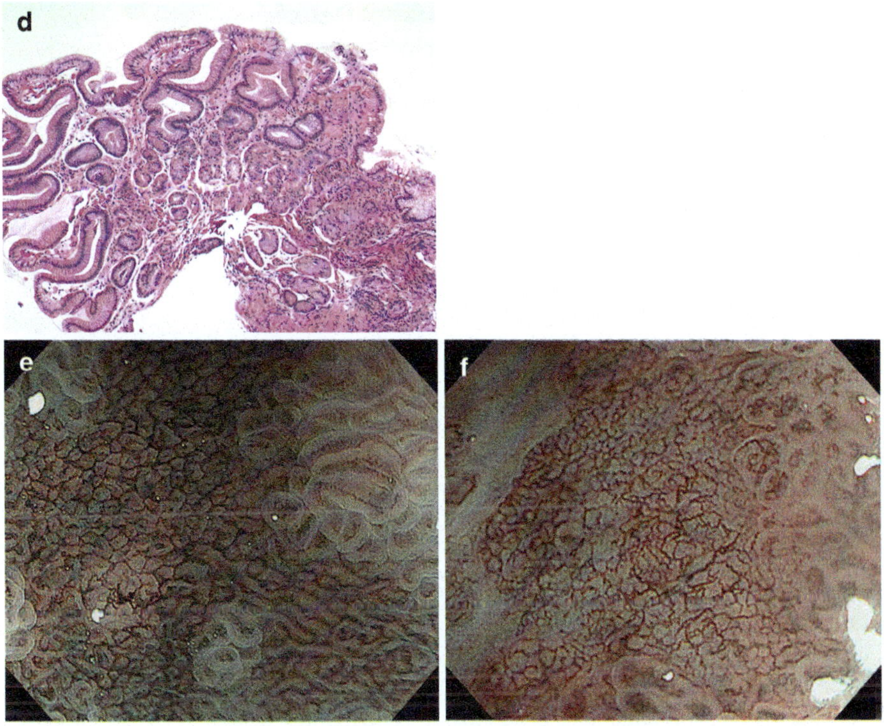

Fig. 9.6 (continued)

9.7 Localized Gastritis (Depressed) Requiring Differentiation from Gastric Cancer

9.7.1 M-NBI Findings

1. Marginal area (demarcation line: absent)
2. Lesion (VS classification: regular MV pattern plus absent MS pattern)

9.7.2 Explanation

9.7.2.1 WLI Appearance

We can see a reddened depressed lesion 3 mm in diameter toward the anterior wall of the greater curvature of the lower gastric body (Fig. 9.7a). Non-magnified WLI appearance reveals an irregular demarcation line (DL) in one area, making differentiation from a small type 0-IIc lesion difficult.

9.7.2.2 M-NBI Appearance

M-NBI examination at low magnification showed clear differences between the surface structure of the depression and the background mucosa, and proliferation of capillaries within the depression (Fig. 9.7b). However, at this magnification, evaluation of the microsurface structure (S) and microvascular structure (V) is not possible, so differential diagnosis of the lesion is difficult.

M-NBI examination at the maximal magnifying ratio (Fig. 9.7c, d) reveals scant oval marginal crypt epithelium (MCE) almost at the center of the depression, but in general MCE cannot be visualized, and the finding was of an absent MS pattern. Although the proliferation of microvessels in the depression shows an asymmetrical distribution and nonuniform morphology. But, no inequality of diameter or nonuniformity in size is seen, and the directionality is also relatively consistent. Furthermore, many blood vessels (Fig. 9.7d arrow) can be seen extending from the depressed area straight out into the surrounding mucosa maintaining the same direction, yielding the finding of a regular MV pattern.

No MCE could be detected in almost the entire lesion, so VS concordance could not be assessed.

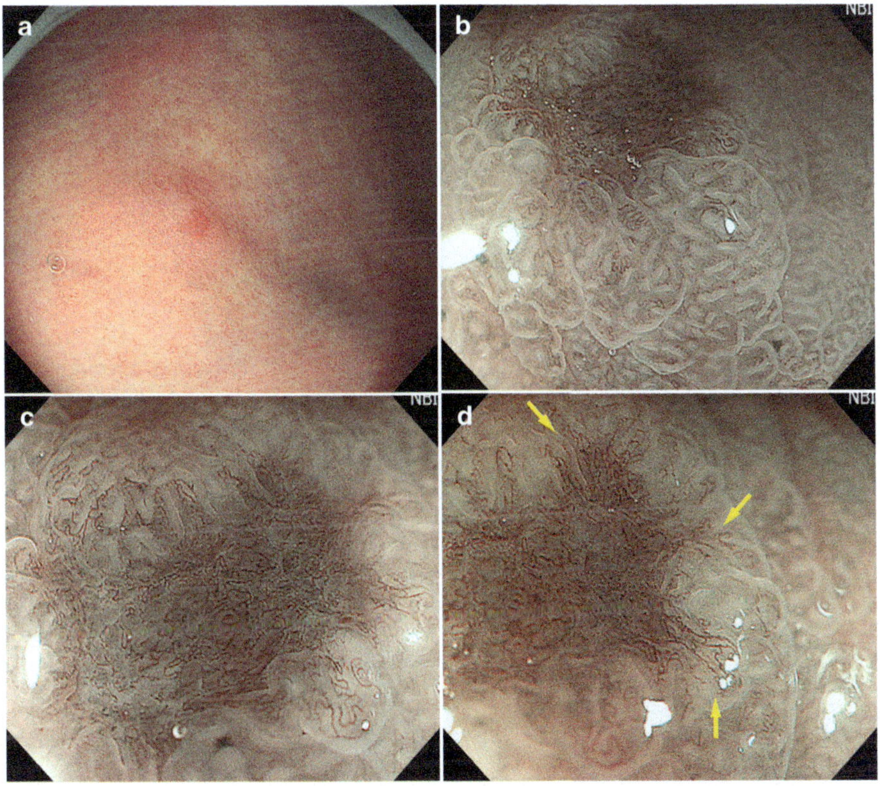

Fig. 9.7

From the above findings, the diagnosis was made of noncancer and localized gastritis. Figure 9.7e shows the M-WLI appearance of the same area as shown in Fig. 9.7c, in which it is difficult to discern any microvessels.

9.7.2.3 Histological Findings

Histological examination of the biopsy specimen revealed chronic gastritis (Fig.9.7f).

9.7.3 Diagnostic Pointers for NBI

Microvessels are easily delineated using M-NBI. In this lesion, some asymmetrical distribution and morphological variability is seen in the microvessels, but there is no nonuniformity of diameter or size, and directionality is relatively consistent.

No DL could be delineated using V, and characteristic of gastritis microvessels were seen extending from the depressed area straight out into the surrounding mucosa maintaining the same direction, gradually merging into surrounding capillaries.

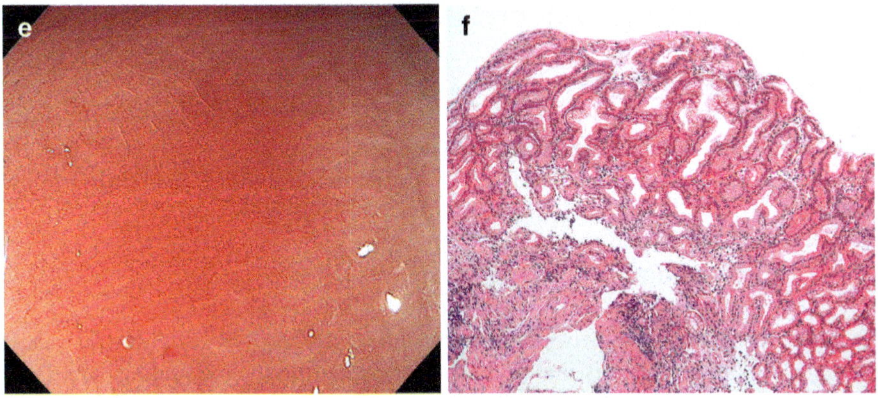

Fig. 9.7 (continued)

9.8 Gastric Ulcer Scar

9.8.1 M-NBI Findings

1. Marginal area (demarcation line: absent)
2. Lesion (VS classification: regular MV pattern plus absent MS pattern)

9.8.2 Explanation

In order to differentiate between a gastric ulcer scar and an early gastric cancer associated with a scar, it is important to know what the typical findings are. Even with M-NBI imaging, unless mucosal convergence is present, the findings of white scars (S2 stage) are almost the same as the surrounding chronic gastritis. Accordingly, in this section I will discuss red scars (S1 stage).

9.8.2.1 WLI Appearance

Non-magnified WLI appearance reveals an ulcer scar with central-reddened coloration on the posterior wall of the upper gastric body (Fig. 9.8a). M-WLI (low magnification) is unable to delineate a distinct demarcation line between the reddened area and the surrounding background mucosa (Fig. 9.8b).

9.8.2.2 M-NBI Appearance (Maximal Magnifying Ratio, Fig. 9.8c–e)

Background mucosa (Fig. 9.8c), convergent folds

V: The subepithelial capillaries (SECs) are open or closed looped, with a symmetrical distribution and regular arrangement.

S: The marginal crypt epithelium (MCE) has a mainly curved to oval morphology and is lined by light blue crests (LBCs). The intervening parts (IPs) have a consistent width and regular arrangement.

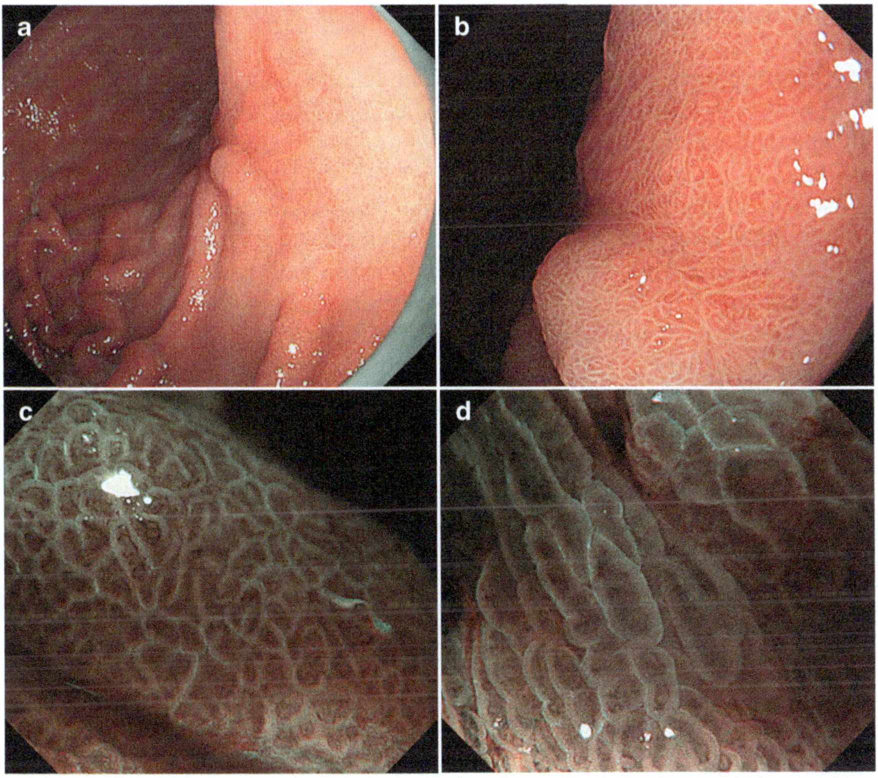

Fig. 9.8

Lesion part (Fig. 9.8d, e), regenerative epithelium

V: The subepithelial microvessels are open or closed looped, with a high vascular density, so frequently the morphology of individual blood vessels cannot be discerned, and the IPs appear brown.
S: The MCE is mainly curved, oval, or highly elliptical, forming IPs that vary from oval to highly elliptical. The epithelium exhibits a consistent directionality toward the ulcer scar, with a regular arrangement. No LBCs are seen.
VS concordance: This is a VS concordant finding with microvessels distributed beneath the IP epithelium. Characteristic findings are blood vessels distributed in concordance with the highly elliptical IPs and brown areas of high absorbency of narrow band light.

9.8.2.3 Histological Findings

This biopsy sample was taken from the area of regenerative epithelium shown in Fig. 9.8e. Epithelial cell cytoplasm in the section between the arrows are somewhat basophilic, indicating this is regenerative epithelium with no intestinal metaplasia. In the wide stroma of the IPs, we can see infiltration by chronic inflammatory cells and proliferation of dilated microvessels. On the other hand, the mucosa apart than regenerative epithelium shows intestinal metaplasia.

9.8.3 Diagnostic Pointers for NBI

The biggest difference between regenerative epithelium in an ulcer scar and a tumor is the absence of a demarcation line between the reddened regenerative epithelium and the background mucosa in the former.

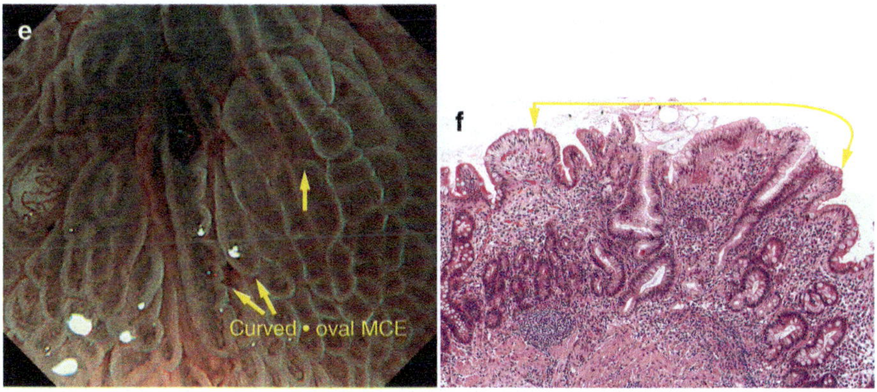

Fig. 9.8 (continued)

9.9 Gastric Xanthoma

9.9.1 M-NBI Findings

1. Marginal area (demarcation line: absent)
2. Lesion (VS classification: regular MV pattern plus absent MS pattern, LBC +)

9.9.2 Explanation

A gastric xanthoma is a benign lesion commonly seen in the mucosa with *H. pylori* gastritis. Generally, these lesions are flat to superficial elevated and yellow in coloration. In this section we present the typical findings of a gastric xanthoma, for the rare occasions that differentiation is required from an intramucosal flat undifferentiated early gastric cancer.

9.9.2.1 WLI appearance

Non-magnified WLI appearance reveals a reddened type 0-IIa early gastric cancer (yellow arrow) on the posterior wall of the gastric antrum, on the oral side of which we can see a flat yellow-white xanthoma (blue arrow) (Fig. 9.9a).

9.9.2.2 M-NBI Appearance (Fig. 9.9a–e)

Weak Magnification (Fig. 9.9b)

The background mucosa V comprises small-looped subepithelial capillaries (SECs), and the S curved to polygonal marginal crypt epithelium (MCE) lined by LBCs, forming a regular MV pattern plus regular MS pattern (LBC+). These regular patterns continue up to the xanthoma and the absence of a distinct demarcation line (DL) differs greatly from an epithelial neoplastic lesion.

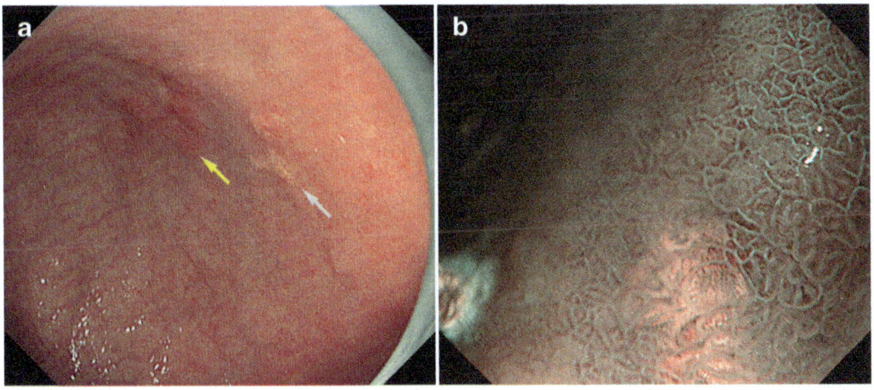

Fig. 9.9

Maximal Magnifying Ratio (Fig. 9.9c–e)
The microvascular pattern and microsurface pattern of the lesion are identical to the surrounding mucosa, and we can identify it as a subepithelial lesion. Compared to the intramucosal undifferentiated cancer (signet ring cell carcinoma), it is characteristic that neither the blood vessels of the covering epithelium nor the MCE are extended. Magnification of part of Figs. 9.9d and 9.9e allows us to confirm that the morphology of the surrounding SECs and MCE is well preserved. Unlike the situation when WOS is present, capillaries directly under the epithelium can be visualized.

9.9.2.3 Histological Findings

This lesion was resected at ESD together with the early cancer (Fig. 9.9f). We can see an aggregation of histiocytes with a foamy and basophilic cytoplasm in the lamina propria. Focusing on the surface layers, histiocytes are located beneath the SECs (arrowed), which remain unchanged, so we can understand why the morphology of the SECs and MCE are well preserved when delineated using M-NBI. Histologically, this lesion can be distinguished from the signet ring cell carcinoma because the nuclei are not peripherally located within the cell.

9.9.3 Diagnostic Pointers for NBI

Gastric xanthomas differ from undifferentiated cancers in that even within the lesion, the SEC and MCE morphologies are the same as the background mucosa. Naturally, a DL can also not be seen.

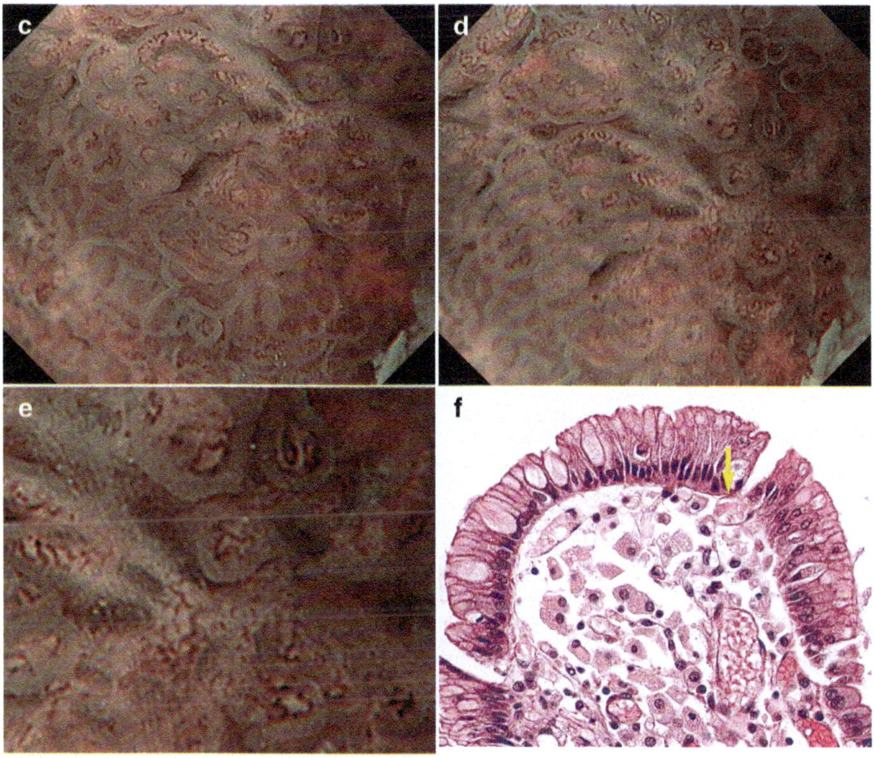

Fig. 9.9 (continued)

9.10 Angiodysplasia

Angiodysplasia is a condition where blood vessels within the submucosa and mucosa dilate and proliferate; it is also known as angioectasia. One, or a small number of blood vessels, becomes distended and appears in a limited location separate from the usual mucosal capillary network, forming an oval reddened patch with a distinct margin [8].

Angiodysplasia may require treatment if it causes bleeding resulting in anemia, but this is uncommon.

9.10.1 M-NBI Findings

1. Marginal area (demarcation line: absent)
2. Lesion part (VS classification: regular MV pattern plus regular MS pattern)

9.10.2 Explanation

9.10.2.1 WLI Appearance

Non-magnifying WLI endoscopic examination reveals a flat or slightly protruding reddened lesion. Closer examination shows capillaries radiating out toward the periphery from the lesion, which we can see is formed by an aggregation of microvessels. In an actual case, we see a localized reddened patch under non-magnified examination (Fig. 9.10a), and with M-WLI capillaries can be seen radiating out toward the periphery (Fig. 9.10b).

9.10.2.2 M-NBI Appearance

Non-magnifying NBI examination shows that the diameter of the blood vessel comprising the lesion is considerably greater than the few capillaries visualized in the surface layers of the surrounding mucosa. Although the vascular diameters are greater, even using M-NBI we cannot detect any irregular features, such as nonuniform diameter or morphology (Fig. 9.10c). Confirmation of these characteristic findings allows us to make a firm diagnosis.

9.10.2.3 Histological Findings

Histological examination reveals dilatation of capillaries, venules, and veins in the lamina propria and submucosa.

9.10.3 Diagnostic Pointers for NBI

Although extremely rare, some early cancers will present a strong red coloration similar to angiodysplasia when examined using non-magnifying WLI. Cancers have a demarcation line (DL), irregular MV pattern, or irregular MS pattern. An understanding of the characteristics of angiodysplasia, a benign vascular lesion, presented in this section will be helpful in making the differential diagnosis.

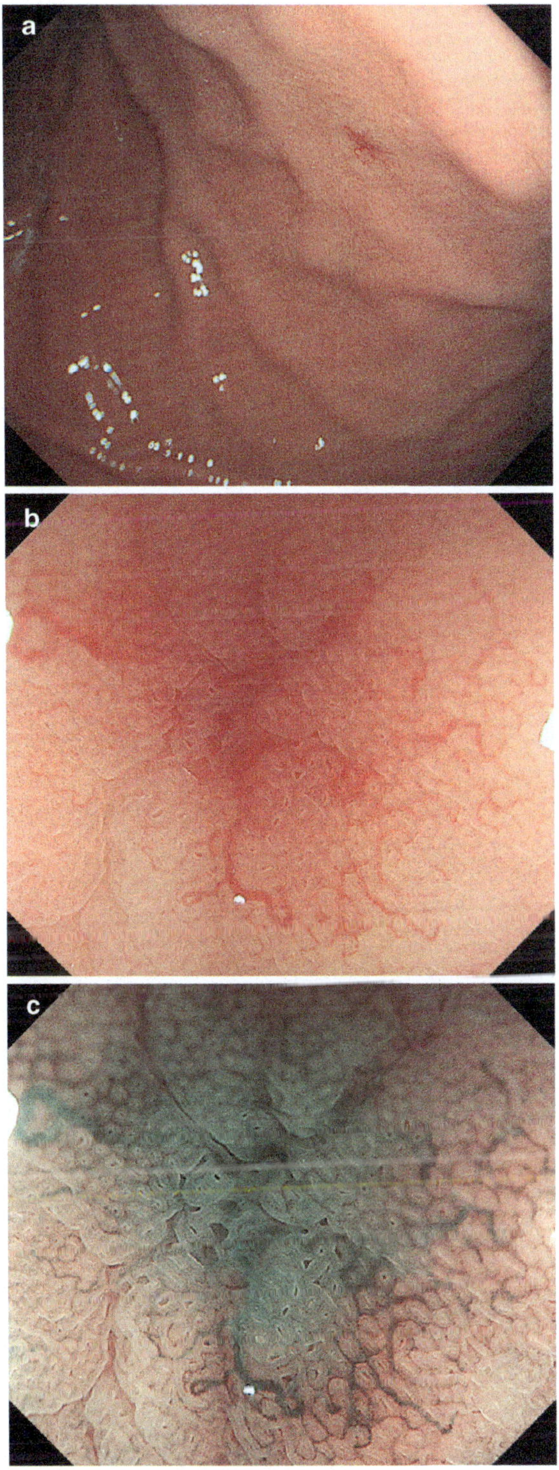

Fig. 9.10

References

1. Yagi K, et al.: *Endoscopy* 2002; **34:** 376–381
2. Nakagawa S, et al.: *Gastrointest Endosc* 2003; **58:** 71–95
3. Yao K. *Helicobacter Research* 2010; **14:** 224–227.
4. Uedo N, et al. *Endoscopy* 2006; **38:** 819–824.
5. Uedo N. *Endoscopy* 2008; **40:** 881. (Response to letter)
6. Yao K. *Gastrointest Endosc* 2008; **68:** 574–579.
7. Yao K. *Gastrointest Endosc* 2009; **70:** 402–403
8. Sakai Y, et al. *Stomach and Intestine* 2000; **35:** 763–769.

Atlas of Neoplastic Lesions in the Stomach

10

Kenshi Yao, Hisashi Doyama, Noriya Uedo, Takashi Nagahama, and Shoko Ono

K. Yao (✉)
Department of Endoscopy, Fukuoka University Chikushi Hospital, 1-1-1 Zokumyoin, Chikushino 818-8502, Japan
e-mail: yao@fukuoka-u.ac.jp

H. Doyama
Department of Gastroenterology, Ishikawa Prefectural Central Hospital, Kanazawa, Japan

N. Uedo
Department of Gastrointestinal Oncology, Osaka Medical Center for Cancer and Cardiovascular Diseases, Osaka, Japan

T. Nagahama
Department of Gastroenterology, Fukuoka University Chikushi Hospital, Chikushino, Japan

S. Ono
Division of Endoscopy, Hokkaido University Hospital, Sapporo, Japan

M. Muto et al. (eds.), *Atlas of Endoscopy with Narrow Band Imaging*,
DOI 10.1007/978-4-431-54243-8_10

10.1 Gastric Adenoma (Elevated)

10.1.1 Case 1

10.1.1.1 M-NBI Findings

1. Marginal area (demarcation line: present)
2. Lesion (VS classification: regular MV pattern plus regular MS pattern, LBC +)

10.1.1.2 Explanation

Non-magnifying WLI endoscopic examination reveals a smooth-surfaced pale superficial elevated lesion (arrow, Fig. 10.1a) on the posterior wall of the gastric antrum. M-NBI examination using the maximal magnifying ratio delineates a distinct demarcation line (DL) (arrow, Fig. 10.1b) where the surrounding regular MV pattern plus regular MS pattern disappears. Although the microvascular pattern of the lesion is not clearly visualized, the individual blood vessels have a polygonal morphology and form a regular network. The regular arrangement of oval to curved marginal crypt epithelium (MCE) comprises a regular MS pattern. The crypt openings (COs) enclosed by the MCE are neatly lined with light blue crests (LBCs). The VS pattern is the gastric body type with MCE located with polygonal vessels.

Figure 10.1c shows the histological findings of the ESD specimen (arrow indicates the margin). The tumor on the left side shows atypical glands with mild-to-moderate grade atypia, the finding of a tubular adenoma. Immunostaining of the tumor epithelium was positive for CD10 (figure not shown). The nontumor background mucosa comprises crypt epithelium free of intestinal metaplasia.

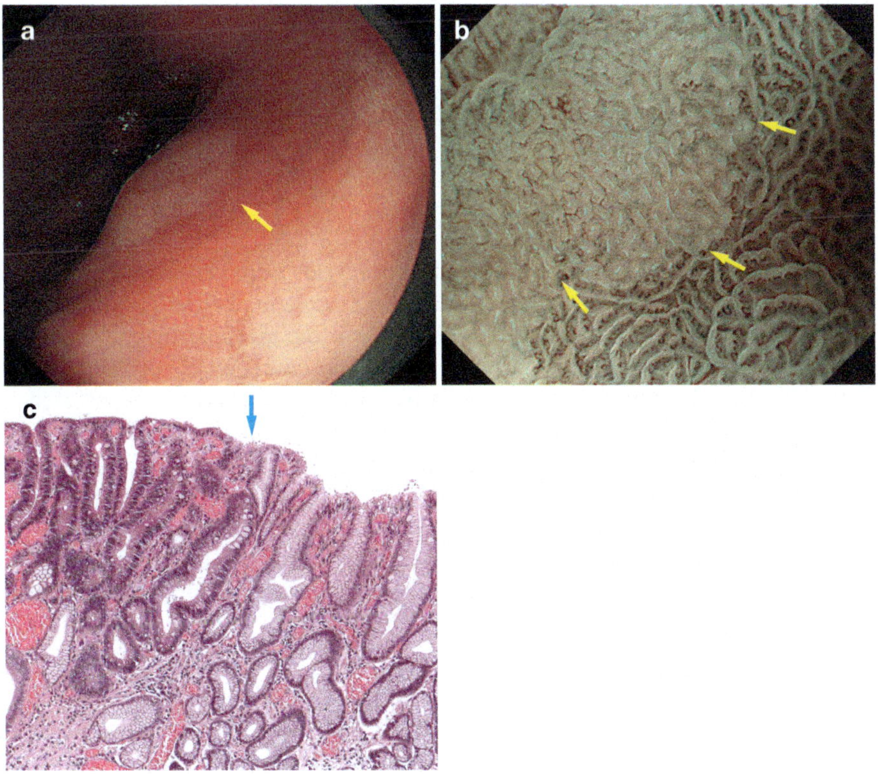

Fig. 10.1

10.1.2 Case 2

10.1.2.1 M-NBI Findings

1. Marginal area (demarcation line: present)
2. Lesion (VS classification: absent MV pattern plus regular MS pattern, WOS +, speckled)

10.1.2.2 Explanation

Non-magnifying WLI endoscopic examination reveals a smooth-surfaced pale flat elevated lesion (arrow, Fig. 10.2a) on the lesser curvature of the gastric antrum. M-NBI examination of the center of the lesion at the maximal magnifying ratio (Fig. 10.2b) reveals the presence of white opaque substance (WOS), and since blood vessels of the subepithelial vessels cannot be visualized at all, this was assessed as an absent MV pattern. Using WOS as a marker of the microsurface pattern, WOS is distributed corresponding to the regular intervening parts (IPs), with a morphology varying from reticulate to maze-like, so this was assessed as a regular MS pattern. Although not shown in the figures, this lesion has a distinct demarcation line (DL).

Histological examination of the ESD specimen yielded the diagnosis of tubular adenoma with moderate atypia with a low degree of differentiation into goblet cells (Fig. 10.2c).

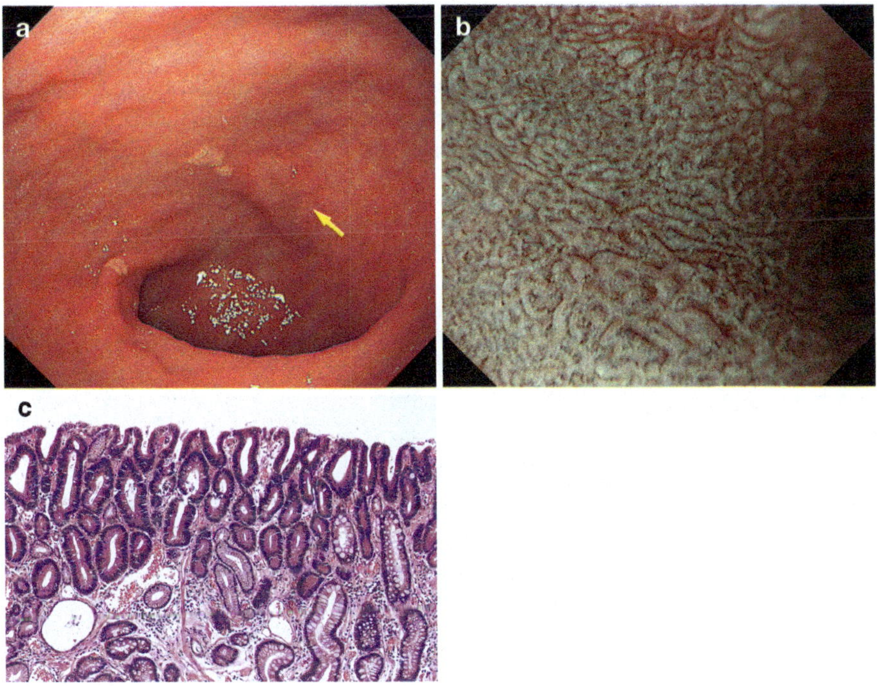

Fig. 10.2

10.2 Gastric Adenoma (Depressed Type)

Depressed gastric adenomas are comparatively rare. Irregular margin and reddened coloration are considered effective in detecting gastric cancers using non-magnifying WLI, but often a definitive diagnosis cannot be reached with non-magnifying WLI and biopsy alone, and endoscopic treatment in the form of "total biopsy" is often required.

10.2.1 M-NBI Findings

1. Marginal area (demarcation line: present)
2. Lesion (VS classification: regular MV pattern plus regular MS pattern)

10.2.2 Explanation

10.2.2.1 Non-magnifying WLI Appearance

We can see a reddened depressed lesion 9×6 mm in the vicinity of the post-ESD ulcer scar on the posterior wall of the gastric antrum (Fig. 10.3a, b). An irregular demarcation line (DL) could be delineated using non-magnifying WLI, so this lesion could not be differentiated from a type IIc cancer.

10.2.2.2 M-NBI Appearance

M-NBI at a low magnifying ratio revealed a distinct demarcation line (DL) due to differences in the surface structure between the marginal area of the lesion and the background mucosa (Fig. 10.3c). However, at this magnification we cannot discern the microvascular pattern or microsurface pattern, making a qualitative analysis difficult.

M-NBI at the maximal magnifying ratio (Fig. 10.3d, e) reveals a round- to oval-shaped marginal crypt epithelium (MCE), with a uniform width, within the lesion. The size of the individual intervening parts (IPs), enclosed by MCE, is slightly smaller than in the background mucosa, and despite the slight nonuniformity in size, the directionality, distribution, and arrangement are relatively uniform. The vessels in the IPs of the lesion are slightly smaller and denser compared to the background mucosa, but their morphology is relatively uniform. Their distribution is symmetrical and their arrangement regular. Vessels are located beneath the epithelium of the IPs enclosed by MCE, so there is no VS discordance. From these findings, the diagnosis of a gastric adenoma was made.

10.2.2.3 Histological Findings

Histological examination of this ESD specimen demonstrated a tubular adenoma with mild to moderately atypical tumor glands and a regularly arranged stroma (Fig. 10.3f).

10.2.3 Diagnostic Pointers for NBI

The characteristics of this adenoma visualized in detail using M-NBI at the maximal magnifying ratio are as follows:

1. The presence of a distinct DL.
2. A regular MS pattern is seen, although the IPs are slightly small with mildly nonuniform size.
3. A regular MV pattern is seen, although the vessels are slightly small and dense.

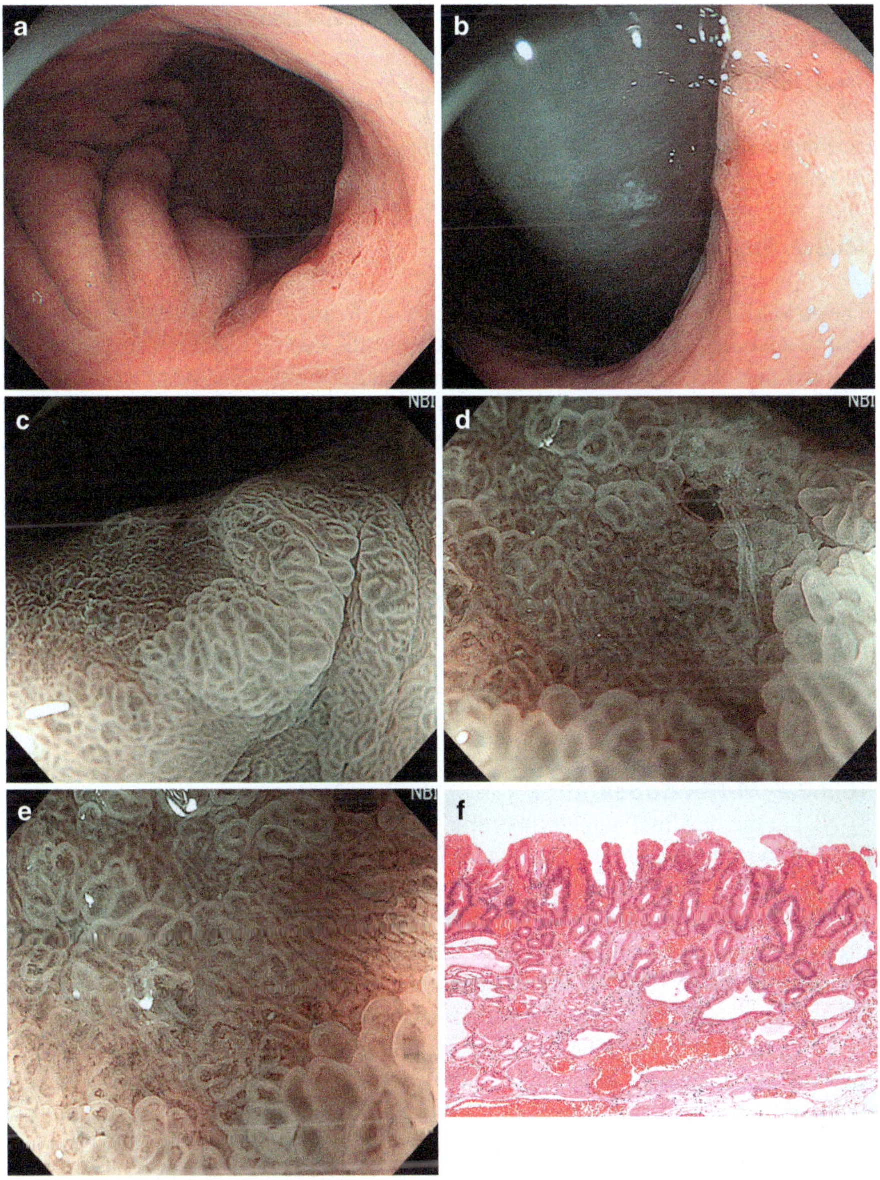

Fig. 10.3

10.3 Very Well-Differentiated Adenocarcinoma

10.3.1 M-NBI Findings

1. Marginal area (demarcation line: present)
2. Lesion (VS classification: irregular MV pattern plus irregular MS pattern, LBC +)

10.3.2 Explanation

The pathohistological definition and clinical significance of a very well-differentiated gastric adenocarcinoma remain unclear. Clinically, even if cancer is suspected and a biopsy performed, it can be difficult to make the definitive diagnosis of cancer due to the mild degree of cellular atypia. In this section, we present a very well-differentiated intestinal-type adenocarcinoma diagnosed using an M-NBI gastroscope, even though histological examination of a biopsy specimen was unable to differentiate between adenocarcinoma and intestinal metaplasia (Fig. 10.4a reprinted by permission of [1]).

10.3.2.1 Non-magnifying WLI Appearance

We can see a reddened shallow depressed lesion on the small curvature of the gastric fundus (Fig. 10.4a). Indigo carmine dye spraying renders the slightly irregular border more distinct, and the surface of the depression has a microgranular to unstructured appearance (Fig. 10.4b).

10.3.2.2 M-NBI Appearance

M-NBI at the maximal magnifying ratio (Fig. 10.4c) reveals a distinct demarcation line (DL, arrows) where the surrounding regular MV pattern plus regular MS pattern disappears. Detailed examination shows that, compared with the orderly marginal crypt epithelium (MCE) in the surrounds, the MCE in the lesion interior has a strongly varied morphology, from curved to sawtooth shaped. Magnification of the center of the tumor (Fig. 10.4d) reveals the morphology of the MCE to be sawtooth shaped, like pounding waves (jagged), and the intervening parts (IPs) enclosed by the MCE to have an irregular (rough) morphology with nonuniform sizes, so this is assessed as an irregular MS pattern. Other characteristics of this lesion are that the width of the MCE is not uniform for each section, or between sections. Bright cyan reflections, or light blue crests (LBCs), are seen lining the MCE (Fig. 10.4d, arrow). Little nonuniformity is seen in the sizes of the loop-shaped microvessels, but their morphology varies strongly, assessed as an irregular MV pattern (Fig. 10.4c).

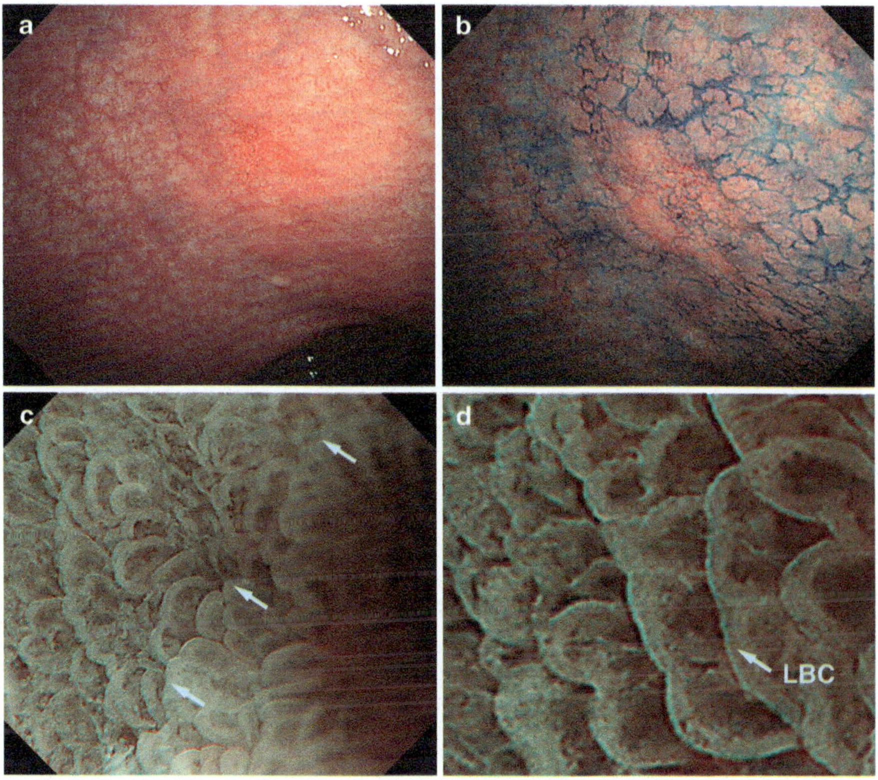

Fig. 10.4

10.3.2.3 Histological Findings

Figure 10.4e shows the hematoxylin-stained neoplastic section of the ESD specimen. Although the histological appearance resembles complete intestinal metaplasia, and there is little cellular atypia, the diagnosis of very well-differentiated gland cancer was made on the basis of the structural atypia.

Anti-CD10 immunostaining (Fig. 10.4f) showed that this tumor was CD10 positive, positive for MUC2 mucin staining, and negative for MUC5AC and MUC6, expressing only the intestinal mucin phenotype.

10.3.3 Diagnostic Pointers for NBI

The main characteristics of this lesion are the irregular MCE morphology and the presence of LBCs. It is important to have plentiful experience of benign lesions such as depressed areas of intestinal metaplasia and have a good understanding of the typical noncancerous appearance.

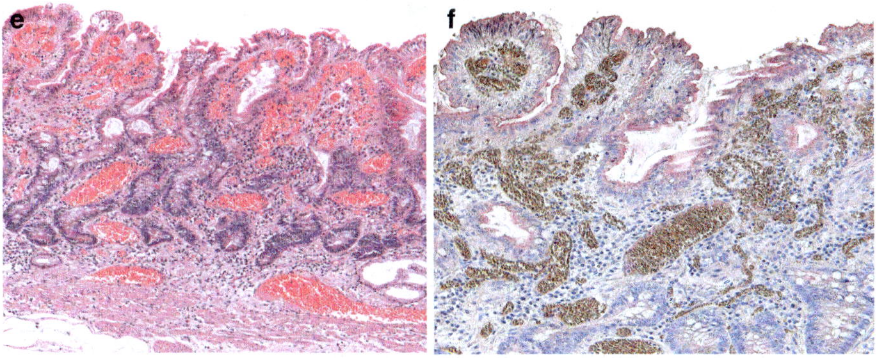

Fig. 10.4 (continued)

10.4 Early Gastric Cancer (Differentiated): Type I

10.4.1 M-NBI Findings

1. Marginal area (demarcation line: present)
2. Lesion (VS classification: irregular MV pattern plus irregular MS pattern)

10.4.2 Explanation

The M-NBI gastroscopic appearances of type 0-I early gastric cancers are varied. In this section, we present this type 0-I early stage gastric cancer presenting a histologically irregular papillary morphology as a case study in the interpretation of magnified endoscopic findings.

10.4.2.1 Non-magnifying WLI Appearance

We can see a reddened, markedly elevated semipedunculated lesion on the lesser curvature of the gastric antrum (Fig. 10.5a). The lesion bleeds easily and displays a microgranular surface when sprayed with indigo carmine (Fig. 10.5b).

10.4.2.2 M-NBI Appearance

The marginal crypt epithelium (MCE) presents an irregular saw-toothed morphology, consistent with the irregular papillary histological appearance (Fig. 10.5c). In one part of the tumor, we can see irregular microvessels beneath the epithelium of the intervening part (IP) enclosed by circular MCE (Fig. 10.5d), presenting the so-called vessel within epithelial circle (VEC) pattern [2]. The IPs are nonuniform in morphology and irregular in size. Accordingly, it is easy to assess this as an irregular MS pattern.

Although the microvascular pattern is rich in variety, as shown in Fig. 10.5e, with polygonal loop-shaped vessels repeatedly and irregularly anastomosing with each other forming an irregular MV pattern, there is no VS discordance.

10.4.2.3 Histological Findings

As shown in Fig. 10.6f, histological examination of the ESD specimen shows that this tumor contains a mixture of a papillary adenocarcinoma and a tubular adenocarcinoma with marked structural and cellular atypia. This explains the variegated magnified endoscopic findings, as the histological structure is not uniform.

10.4.3 Diagnostic Pointers for NBI

Type 0-I cancers can present a variety of appearances, so a detailed analysis of the microvascular pattern and microsurface structure, and accurate evaluation of any irregularities, is important in differentiating between malignant and benign lesions.

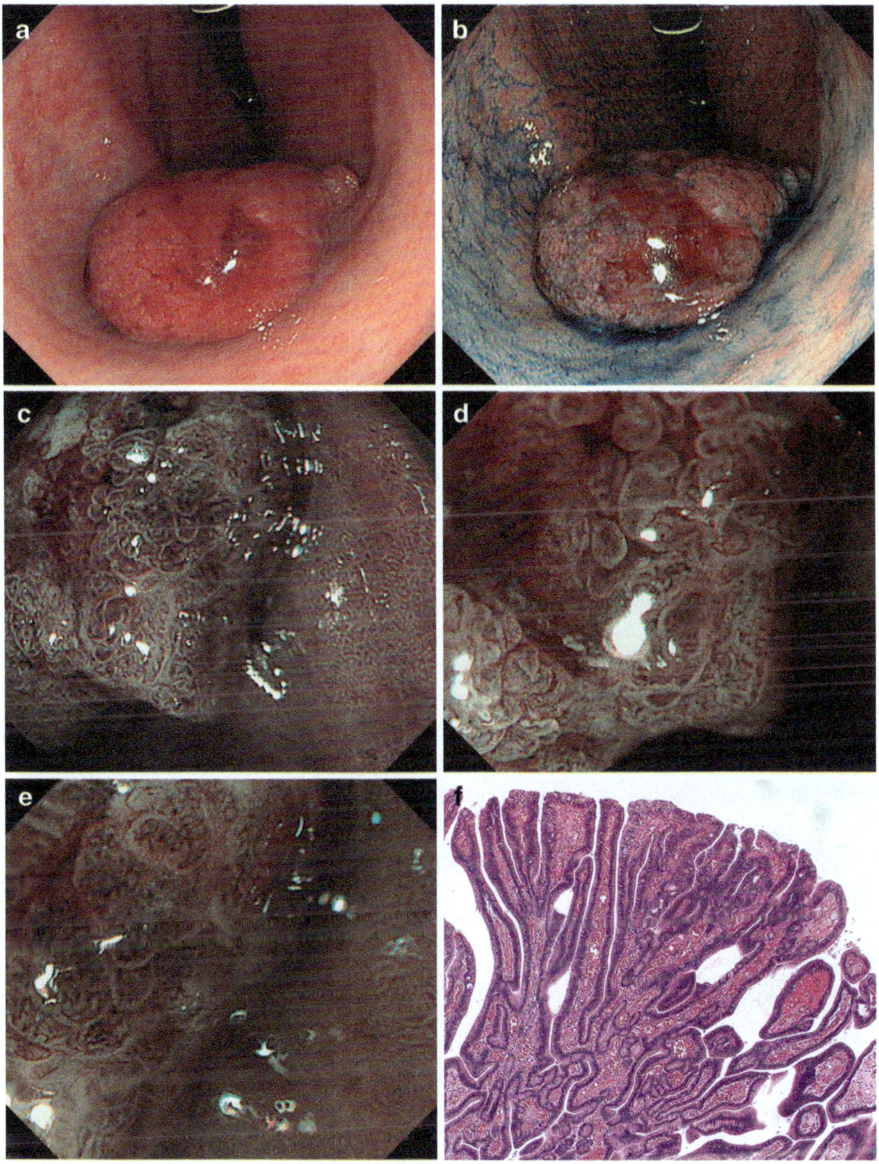

Fig. 10.5

10.5 Early Gastric Cancer (Differentiated): Type IIa (1)

10.5.1 M-NBI Findings

1. Marginal area (demarcation line: present)
2. Lesion (VS classification: irregular/absent MV pattern plus irregular MS pattern, WOS +)

10.5.2 Explanation

The M-NBI appearances of superficial elevated type (0-IIa) early gastric cancers also vary considerably. In this and the next section, we present two representative examples of the interpretation of the endoscopic findings.

10.5.2.1 Non-magnifying WLI Appearance

We can see a low reddened superficial elevated-type lesion on the lesser curvature of the gastric antrum (Fig. 10.6a). The red coloration is mottled in appearance, and the lesion bleeds easily. Spraying with indigo carmine does not clearly visualize the surface microstructure, rendering it almost without structure (Fig. 10.6b).

10.5.2.2 M-NBI Appearance (Maximal Magnifying Ratio; Fig. 10.6c–e)

Background mucosa (Fig. 10.6c, e outside arrows)

The small, curved to round, relatively uniform marginal crypt epithelium (MCE), lined by light blue crests (LBCs), forms a regular MS pattern. The capillaries beneath the epithelium of the intervening part (IP) show a mainly uniform small open-looped morphology and form a regular MV pattern. A distinct demarcation line (Fig. 10.6c, e arrows) can be delineated in areas where the regular VS pattern is lost.

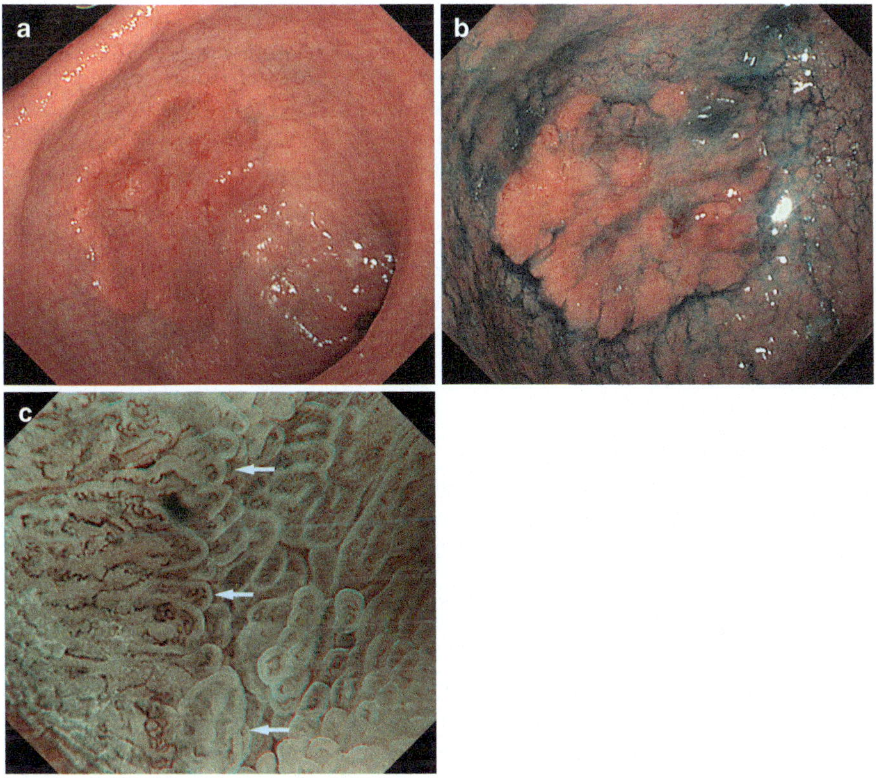

Fig. 10.6

Lesion

V: The individual microvessels have a nonuniform morphology, exhibiting a variety of shapes and sizes, including dilated tortuous irregular microvessels (Fig. 10.6c) and loop-shaped microvessels with distorted shapes (Fig. 10.6d). Their distribution is asymmetrical, and we can recognize this as a typical irregular MV pattern. In part of the lesion, the presence of white opaque substance (WOS) produces an absent MV pattern (Fig. 10.6c, e).

S: In this lesion, curved MCE can be visualized in part of the lesion, although not clearly (Fig. 10.6c, d). WOS, a marker of the microsurface structure, is used in the assessment of the S component. As shown in Fig. 10.6e, the WOS, varying from extremely small dots to a speckled pattern, has an uneven distribution and irregular arrangement, so we assess this as an irregular MS pattern.

10.5.2.3 Histological Findings

Fig. 10.6f shows the histological findings of the tumor marginal area. This is a tubular adenocarcinoma with marked structural and cellular atypia. In the noncancerous background mucosa, we can see diffuse intestinal metaplasia.

10.5.3 Diagnostic Pointers for NBI

A detailed analysis of the microvascular pattern and microsurface structure at the maximal magnifying ratio, and accurate evaluation of any irregularities, is important in differentiating between cancerous and noncancerous lesions.

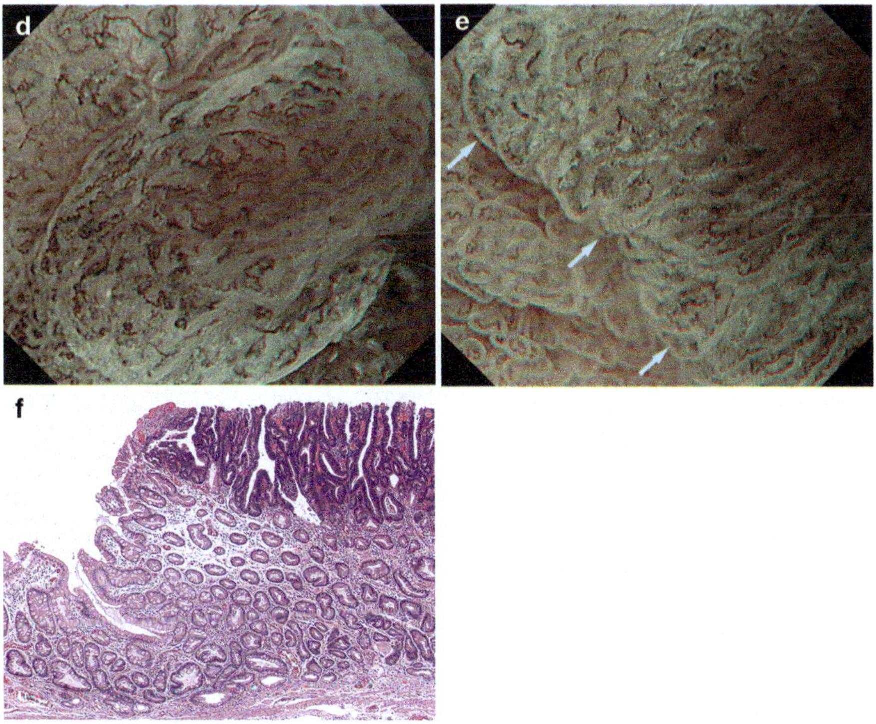

Fig. 10.6 (continued)

10.6 Early Gastric Cancer (Differentiated): Type IIa (2)

10.6.1 M-NBI Findings

1. Marginal area (demarcation line: present)
2. Lesion (VS classification: irregular MV pattern plus regular MS pattern)

10.6.2 Explanation

10.6.2.1 Non-magnifying WLI Appearance

We can see a low reddened superficial elevated-type (IIa) lesion on the posterior wall of the gastric antrum (Fig. 10.7a). The surface has a fine reddened tinge. Spraying with indigo carmine reveals fine granularity of the surface (Fig. 10.7b).

10.6.2.2 M-NBI Appearance (Fig. 10.7c–e)

S: Examination of the marginal area under low magnification (Fig. 10.7c) reveals a regular arrangement of round marginal crypt epithelium (MCE) inside the demarcation line (DL, arrowed). This is a regular MS pattern, comprising curved to rounded, small, relatively uniform MCE. Examination using the maximal magnifying ratio (Fig. 10.7d, e) delineates the MCE as a neat circular structure, more regular than the MCE of the background mucosa. The intervening parts (IPs) are larger than those in the surrounding background mucosa.

V: When the blood vessels are observed at maximal magnifying ratio (Fig. 10.7d, e), nonuniformly shaped loop-shaped blood vessels are observed in the IP sub-epithelia, so an irregular MV pattern can be determined. From the finding of these blood vessels, cancer can be diagnosed.

VS concordance: This is the vessel within the epithelial circle (VEC) pattern, the magnified endoscopy finding characteristic of papillary adenocarcinoma. No VS concordance can be identified in such a VEC pattern [2].

10.6.2.3 Histological Findings

Figure 10.7f shows the histological findings of the ESD specimen (appearance of the area displaying the VEC pattern) [2]. The rounded epithelium is formed by pure papillary adenocarcinoma, and the atypical epithelium with a narrow stroma forms long papillary structures. The left-right symmetrical MCE of the papillary adenocarcinoma and the microvessels distributed mainly in the narrow stroma correspond to the distinct VEC pattern observed using M-NBI endoscopy.

10.6.3 Diagnostic Pointers for NBI

The VEC pattern is all. The potential pitfall in this case is that we cannot make the diagnosis based only on the rounded epithelium. Conversely, the rounded epithelium is a cause for extra caution. If you see this feature, identify an irregular MV pattern using the maximal magnifying ratio, and then if a VEC pattern is detected, papillary adenocarcinoma is easy to diagnose [2].

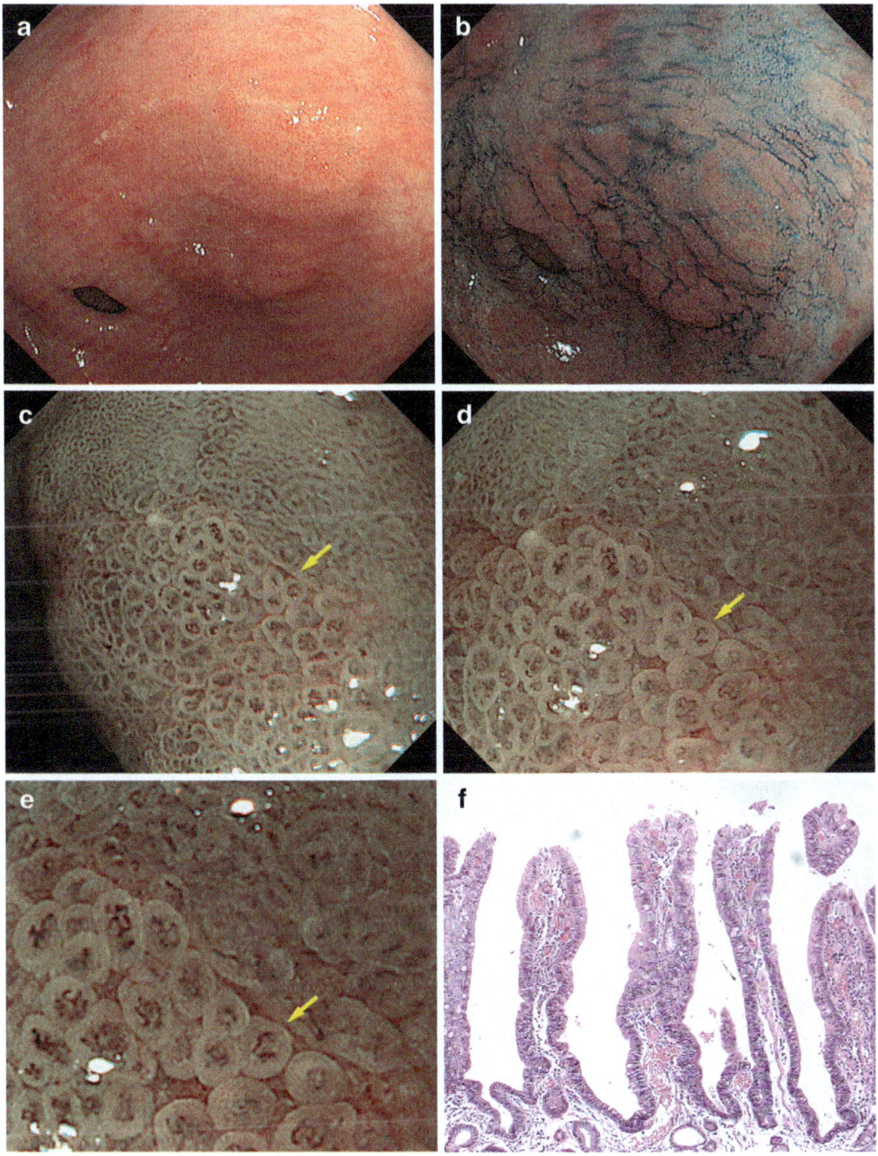

Fig. 10.7

10.7 Early Gastric Cancer (Differentiated): Type IIa (3)

In recent years, clinical trials have been conducted in efforts to expand the applications of methods such as ESD to excise larger UL (−)-differentiated M cancers. However, the margins of large lesions are sometimes indistinct, so more accurate margin delineation is required.

10.7.1 M-NBI Findings

1. Marginal area (demarcation line: present)
2. Lesion (VS classification: irregular MV pattern plus absent MS pattern)

10.7.2 Explanation

In this case, a routine endoscopy for a health checkup detected a 0-IIa lesion on the anterior wall of the lower gastric body. Biopsies yielded adenocarcinoma, so I was consulted whether endoscopic treatment was appropriate. On the initial endoscopic images, a granular elevated lesion was visualized, but the lesion could not be identified in its entirety, making it impossible to determine the line of resection (Fig. 10.8a).

10.7.2.1 Non-magnifying WLI Appearance

At the second endoscopic examination, the lesion was identified as a cluster of low protrusions on the anterior wall of the lower gastric body (Fig. 10.8b). Spraying 0.04 % indigo carmine made clearer the morphology of the protrusions (Fig. 10.8c). Careful observation revealed that the mucosa of the greater curvature side of the cluster of protrusions was slightly paler and appeared to form a margin (yellow arrowheads).

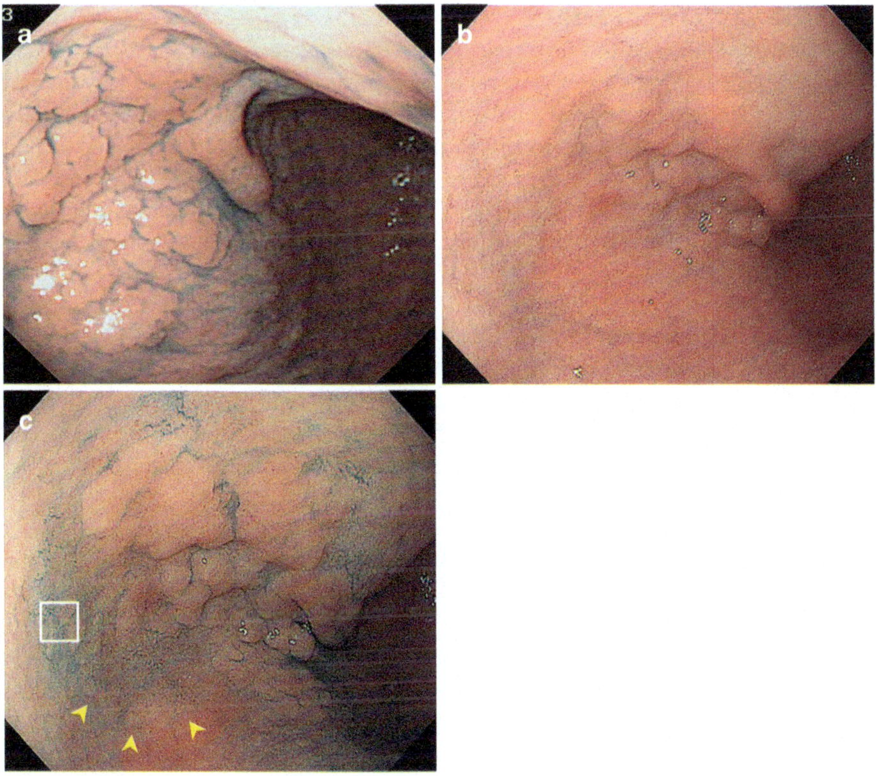

Fig. 10.8

10.7.2.2 M-NBI Appearance

M-NBI examination of this area (inside the white square in Fig. 10.8c) at an intermediate magnifying ratio reveals a regular microsurface pattern of the surrounding mucosa and a regular subepithelial capillary network (SECN) in the intervening parts (IPs). However, the microsurface pattern of the pale flat mucosa within the lesion has disappeared, with irregular microvessels forming a small network. This forms a clear demarcation line (DL) (Fig. 10.8d). The surgical margins were determined on the basis of these findings, and the lesion was excised using the ESD method (Fig. 10.8e).

10.7.2.3 Histological Findings

Histological examination confirmed that the lesion was completely excised in one piece. The surrounding gastric mucosa (Fig. 10.8f, right side) shows a papillary structure for the surface of the crypt epithelium, whereas the tumor (Fig. 10.8f, left side) has a flat surface with the cancer forming small glandular structures.

10.7.3 Diagnostic Pointers for NBI

Under magnification, the field of view is narrow, so we should first detect any abnormal areas using non-magnifying endoscopy and chromoendoscopy, then focus on the areas of interest. If we examine only the cancer, we may unknowingly overlook the horizontal spread of the lesion, so we should carefully examine the surrounding noncancerous mucosa and detect subtle changes in color or elevation. When comparing cancers with noncancerous mucosa clearly affected by chronic gastritis, a useful method is to identify the demarcation line between them, then observe the marginal area using M-NBI. Even when performing an M-NBI examination, the initial non-magnifying and chromoendoscopic findings are of fundamental importance.

If we commence the examination at the maximal magnifying ratio from the start, it is difficult to make an overall assessment or delineate the lesion margins. It is best to gradually increase the magnification as we evaluate the state of the mucosa using the microsurface pattern and delineate the DL, all the while comparing the findings with the non-magnifying and chromoendoscopic findings. Evaluation of the microvascular pattern requires the maximal magnifying ratio.

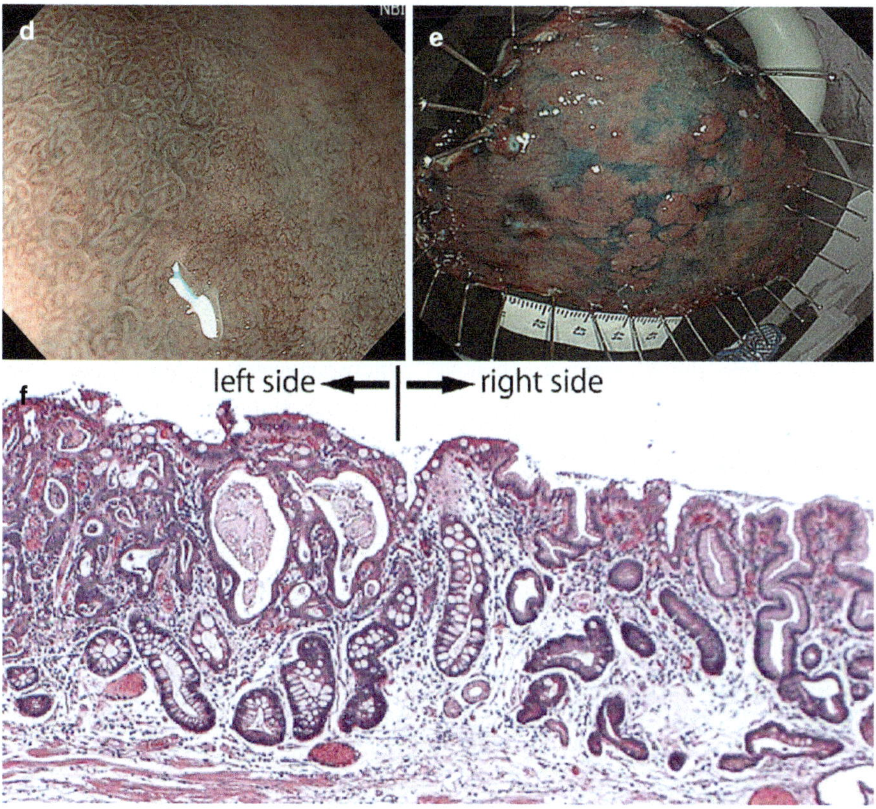

Fig. 10.8 (continued)

10.8 Early Gastric Cancer (Differentiated): Type IIa (4)

Important factors in distinguishing between elevated adenocarcinoma and adenoma endoscopically are said to include size, coloration, surface characteristics, and the presence of depressed elements. However, differentiation is difficult in many cases, and we anticipate that our ability to diagnose these lesions will improve with M-NBI [3].

10.8.1 M-NBI Findings

1. Marginal area (demarcation line: present)
2. Lesion (VS classification: irregular MV pattern plus irregular MS pattern)

10.8.2 Explanation

10.8.2.1 Non-magnifying WLI Appearance

We can see a slightly pale, superficial elevated lesion, 15×9 mm in size, with a distinct demarcation line (DL) on the posterior wall of the lower gastric body (Fig. 10.9a).

10.8.2.2 M-NBI Appearance

Figure 10.9b shows the M-NBI findings of the anal side of the lesion at low magnification. At first glance, we get the impression that the microsurface pattern is regular, and there is minimal microvessel proliferation. However, at this magnification ratio, of course, we should not try to evaluate the microvascular or microsurface patterns.

Examination of the oral side (Fig. 10.9c) and anal side (Fig. 10.9d) of the lesion using M-NBI at the maximal magnifying ratio yields a completely different evaluation of the microvascular pattern and the microsurface pattern. On the oral side of the lesion (Fig. 10.9c), the marginal crypt epithelium (MCE) has a uniform width and a morphology varying from oval to curved, with a symmetrical distribution and regular arrangement. The intervening parts (IPs) are larger than those in the background mucosa, with only slight variation in size. The microvessels have a uniform open-looped morphology, with no irregularity seen in distribution or arrangement. There is no VS discordance. No characteristic findings of cancer are detected in any of these parameters, so a degree of atypia corresponding to tubular adenoma was diagnosed. On the anal side of the lesion (Fig. 10.9d), however, the MCE is curved and nonuniform in size and width, with no directionality and with no continuity between sections of the epithelium. Furthermore, the microvessels are nonuniform in diameter and size, with an irregular distribution and a variety of morphologies, including irregular branching and anastomosing with each other. Lacking regularity, their distribution and directionality are dissociated from the IPs and MCE, being VS discordant. From the above, the anal side of the lesion shows the definite findings of a differentiated gastric cancer.

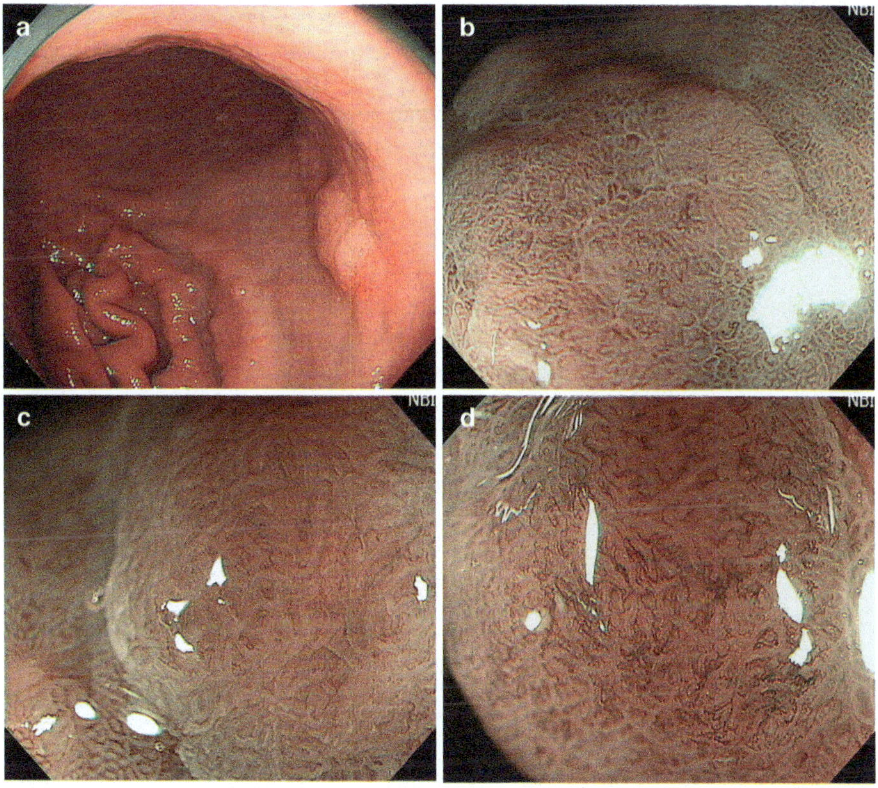

Fig. 10.9

10.8.2.3 Histological Findings

Histological examination of the ESD specimen shows that the oral side lesion has elements differentiated into an adenoma (Fig. 10.9e), whereas the anal side is clearly a well-differentiated tubular adenoma confined to the mucosa (Fig. 10.9f). The transition between the two is unclear, and the overall diagnosis is cancer.

10.8.3 Diagnostic Pointers for NBI

Using the maximal magnifying ratio, we are able for the first time to accurately see the difference in the degree of differentiation between the oral and anal side of this lesion. In this case, we are able to diagnose differentiated cancer based on the findings of the anal side.

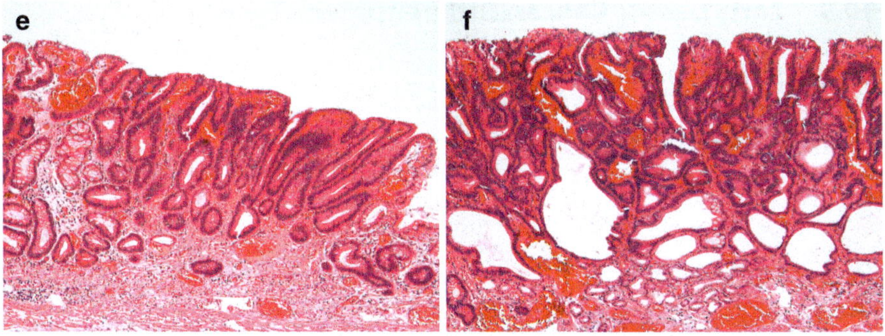

Fig. 10.9 (continued)

10.9 Early Gastric Cancer (Differentiated): Type IIb

10.9.1 M-NBI Findings

1. Marginal area (demarcation line: present)
2. Lesion (VS classification: irregular MV pattern plus absent MS pattern)

10.9.2 Explanation

The M-NBI gastroscopic appearances of superficial flat type (0-IIb) early gastric cancers also vary considerably. In this section we present a representative example of the interpretation of the endoscopic findings.

10.9.2.1 Non-magnifying WLI Appearance

On the posterior wall of the upper gastric body, we can see an area where the blood vessels of the background mucosa can no longer be visualized (Fig. 10.10a, blue arrows). The lesion surface is lightly reddened. Indigo carmine spraying reveals a flat localized lesion matching the area where the surrounding microgranular mucosal structure is lost (Fig. 10.10b). There is almost no height difference with the surrounding area.

10.9.2.2 M-NBI Appearance (Maximal Magnifying Ratio; Water Immersion Technique)

Background mucosa (Fig. 10.10c, d)

This is a regular MS pattern comprising small, relatively uniform marginal crypt epithelium (MCE) with a curved to round morphology. The margins of the MCE are lined by light blue crests (LBC). The capillaries beneath the intervening part (IP) of the epithelium are mainly uniform, small open or closed loops, forming a regular MV pattern. In the area that has lost the regular VS components, we can see a distinct demarcation line (DL) (Fig. 10.10c, d, blue arrows).

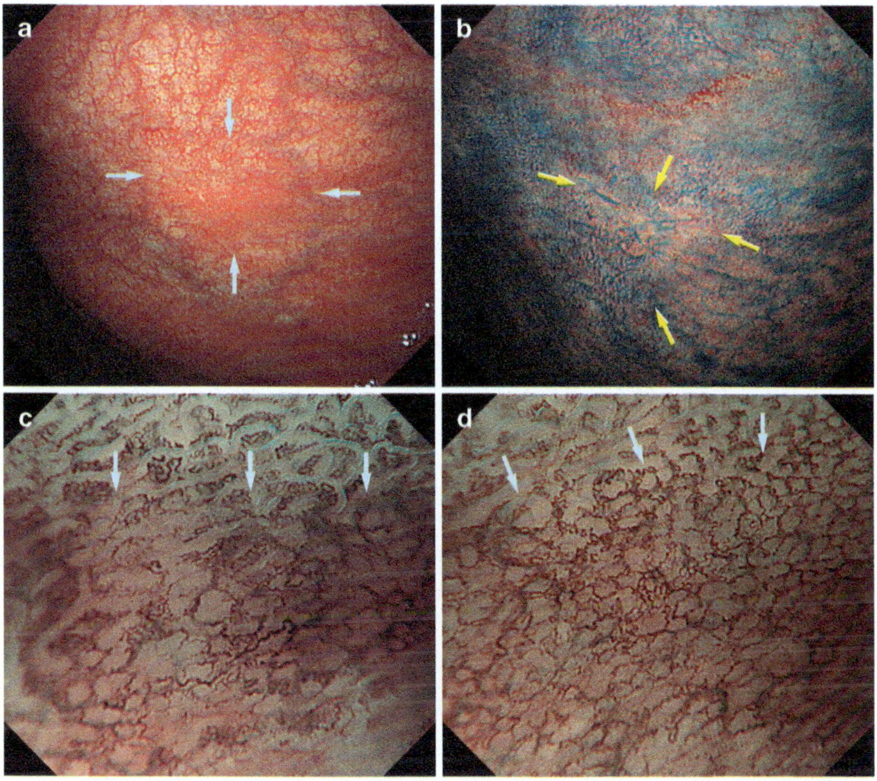

Fig. 10.10

Lesion

V: As shown in Fig. 10.10c, at the lesion margins we can see irregular, dilated, tortuous microvessels. There is marked nonuniformity of the diameter between individual vessels. As Fig. 10.10d shows, at first glance the tumor vessels appear to form a simple network, but as enlarged in Fig. 10.10e, we see irregular microvessels of various sizes and morphologies, from small round closed-looped vessels (blue arrow) to large irregular polygonal vessels (yellow arrow), far from a simple network. Only at the maximal magnifying ratio can these details be visualized. From these findings, we assess this as an irregular MV pattern.

S: In this lesion, the MCE cannot be clearly visualized as a consistent white semitransparent banded pattern, so this was assessed as an absent MS pattern (Fig. 10.10c–e).

10.9.2.3 Histological Findings

Figure 10.10f shows the ESD specimen. The arrow indicates the histological margin, with no height difference detected between the cancerous mucosa on the left and the noncancerous mucosa on the right. This tumor is a tubular adenocarcinoma with glandular lumen formation. However only a small number of crypts can be seen on the cancer epithelial surface. We consider that this histological structure is the reason why the MCE of this tumor is not visualized.

10.9.3 Diagnostic Pointers for NBI

Formation of a microvascular network cannot be used as a marker for differentiating between cancer and noncancer. As seen in this case, the individual microvessels have an irregular polygonal morphology and their lack of morphological uniformity is the evidence for an irregular MV pattern.

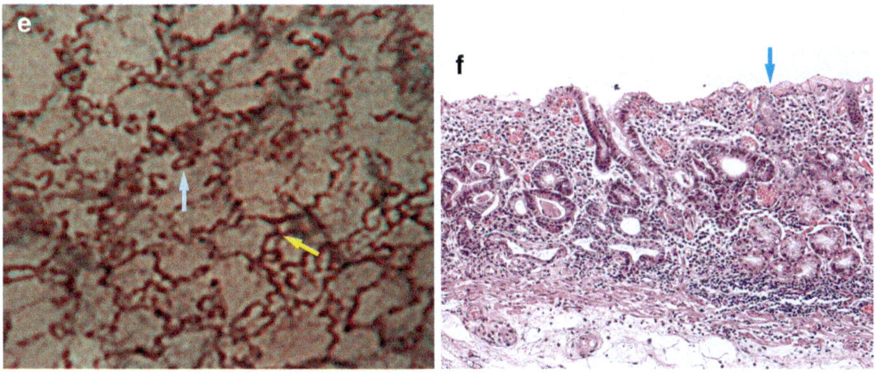

Fig. 10.10 (continued)

10.10 Early Gastric Cancer (Differentiated): Type IIc (1)

10.10.1 M-NBI Findings

1. Marginal area (demarcation line: present)
2. Lesion (VS classification: irregular MV pattern plus irregular MS pattern)

10.10.2 Explanation

The M-NBI gastroscopic appearances of superficial depressed type (0-IIc) early gastric cancers also vary considerably.

10.10.2.1 Non-magnifying WLI Appearance

We can see a reddened depressed lesion on the greater curvature of the gastric antrum (Fig. 10.11a). Following indigo carmine dye spraying, the margins of the depression are clearly delineated, and from the irregular margins of the inner protrusion, we can understand that this is a typical superficial depressed early cancer (Fig. 10.11b).

10.10.2.2 M-NBI Appearance (Water Immersion Technique)

The surrounding background mucosa displays regular curved marginal crypt epithelium (MCE), showing a regular MS pattern with light blue crests (LBCs) in one part. When we examine in the direction from the surrounds toward the depression (Fig. 10.11c), the regular epithelial structure disappears, forming a demarcation line (DL) corresponding to the margin of the depression. Focusing on the lesion interior (Fig. 10.11d), we see an irregular MV pattern comprising irregular loop-shaped microvessels of varied morphologies forming irregular anastomoses beneath the epithelium. The irregular MS pattern comprises an irregularly arranged MCE with a rich variety of rather saw-toothed and curved morphologies.

In a separate marginal area (Fig. 10.11e), we can see a section (yellow arrows) where an irregular MV pattern can be viewed beneath a regular MCE in the surrounding noncancer background mucosa. This was assessed as representing intraepithelial microinvasion (IEMI, subepithelial invasion).

10.10.2.3 Histological Findings

Figure 10.11e shows the ESD specimen, a section corresponding to the marginal area (Fig. 10.11f). As indicated by the arrow, this image shows intraepithelial microinvasion (IEMI, subepithelial invasion) by the tubular adenocarcinoma beneath the noncancerous mucosa at the marginal area.

10.10.3 Diagnostic Pointers for NBI

Identification of the irregular MV pattern and irregular MS pattern is easy in this case. When you are able to interpret the finding of intraepithelial microinvasion (IEMI) in the marginal area, you will be able to diagnose cancer with more confidence.

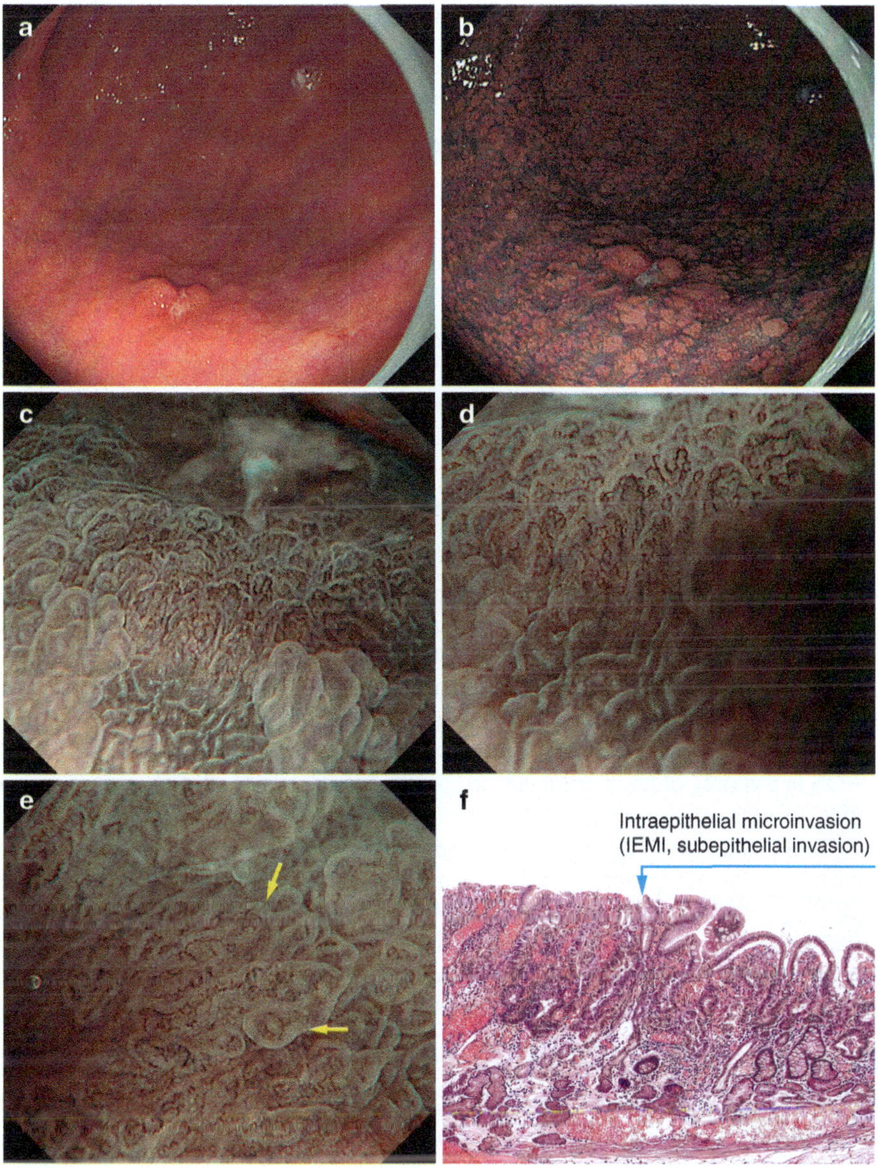
a
b
c
d
e
f
Intraepithelial microinvasion
(IEMI, subepithelial invasion)

Fig. 10.11

10.11 Early Gastric Cancer (Differentiated): Type IIc (2)

10.11.1 M-NBI Findings

1. Marginal area (demarcation line: present)
2. Lesion (VS classification: absent MV pattern plus irregular MS pattern)

10.11.2 Explanation

10.11.2.1 Non-magnifying WLI Appearance

On the anterior wall of the gastric antrum, we can see a pale depressed lesion (Fig. 10.12a). Following indigo carmine dye spraying (Fig. 10.12b), the margins of the depression are clearly delineated, forming a slightly irregular demarcation line (DL).

10.11.2.2 M-NBI Appearance

The noncancerous background mucosa shows a regular MV pattern, with small loop-shaped vessels in a regular arrangement, although in some areas the presence of speckled white opaque substance (WOS) makes it impossible to visualize the vasculature (Fig. 10.12c, d). The regular MS pattern comprises marginal crypt epithelium (MCE) with a curved to polygonal morphology in a regular arrangement (WOS +, speckled). At the tumor margin a distinct demarcation line (DL) can be delineated where the regular MV pattern plus regular MS pattern disappears. Within the demarcation line a proliferation of irregular blood vessels can be seen. The presence of WOS in a variety of sizes, from dots to speckled, prevents visualization of vessels in almost all other areas (Fig. 10.12e), so this was assessed as an absent MV pattern.

On the other hand, as the MCE was not clearly visualized, WOS was used as the marker for the MS pattern, assessed as an irregular MS pattern. In Fig. 10.12e we see a separate marginal area, where the regular speckled WOS of the noncancerous background mucosa (intestinal metaplasia) to the right of the arrow contrasts with the irregular and varied morphology of the fine WOS of the cancerous mucosa to the left of the arrow.

10.11.2.3 Histological Findings

Figure 10.12f shows the ESD specimen. This is a tubular adenocarcinoma with a high degree of structural atypia and cellular atypia. Diffuse intestinal metaplasia is seen in the noncancerous mucosa.

10.11.3 Diagnostic Pointers for NBI

When WOS is present and the microvascular pattern beneath the intervening part (IP) of the epithelium cannot be visualized, this is assessed as an absent MV pattern, and instead the microsurface structure is interpreted using the morphology of the MCE and WOS [4].

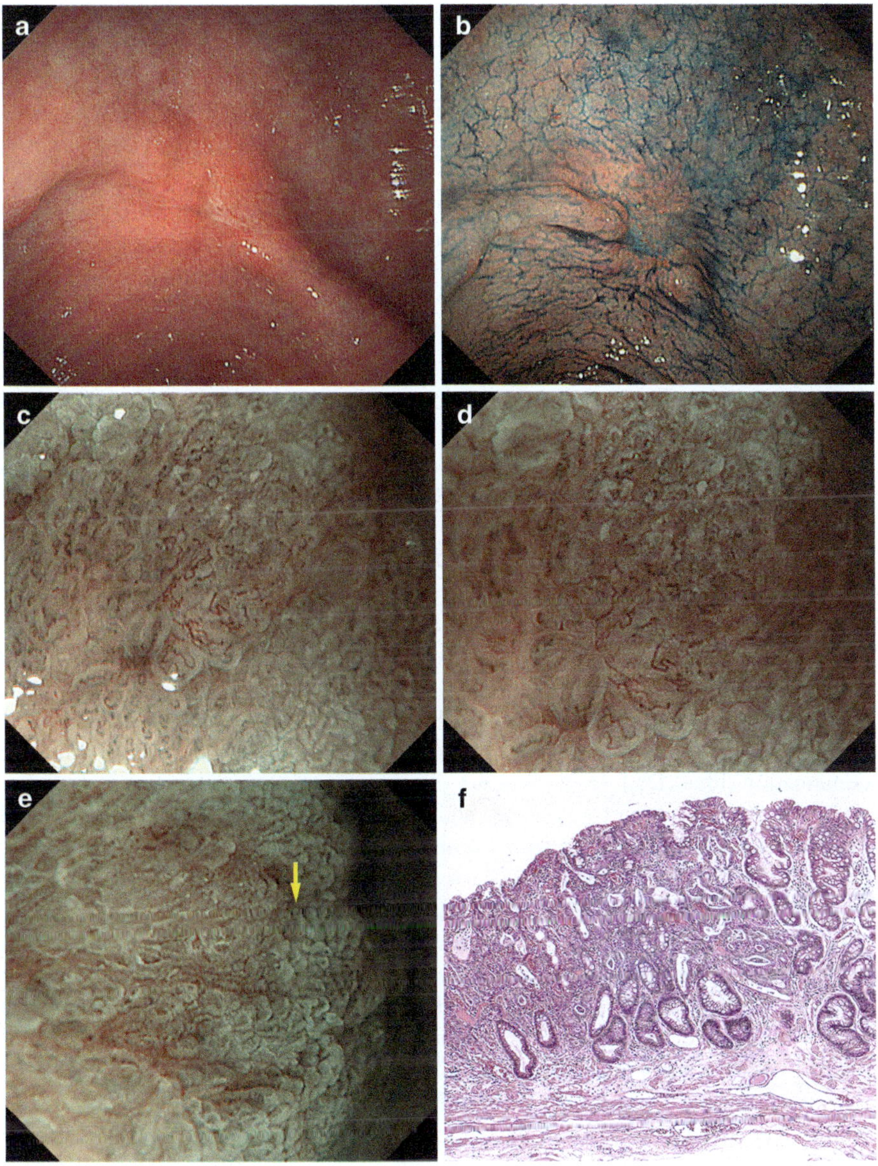

Fig. 10.12

10.12 Early Gastric Cancer (Differentiated): Type IIc (3)

Histological types of gastric cancer are broadly classified into differentiated cancers that form glandular structures and undifferentiated cancers that do not. Differentiated cancers can be further subclassified into those that form an obvious tubular structure, and those that present a papillary structure.

Advanced cancers often contain a mixture of different histological components, but some early gastric cancers also contain a variety of histological types and structures. These may be reflected in the histological findings, as in this case.

10.12.1 Explanation

The referring physician detected a type 0-IIc lesion on the posterior wall of the lower gastric body. Biopsies yielded the diagnosis of an adenocarcinomatous lesion, so the patient was referred here for endoscopic treatment.

10.12.1.1 Non-magnifying WLI Appearance

Non-magnifying WLI examination revealed a reddened depressed lesion on the posterior wall of the lower gastric body (Fig. 10.13a).

10.12.1.2 M-NBI Appearance

M-NBI examination of the reddened shallow depressed surface of the center of the lesion reveals irregular microvessels forming a fine reticular structure and a clear demarcation line (DL) (Fig. 10.13b). The vessels show an irregular reticular morphology with nonuniform shapes and sizes. Examination of the anal side of the depressed area under low magnification shows a vessel within epithelial circle (VEC) pattern, indicative of a papillary structure [2]. A distinct DL can be delineated on the anal side between the papillary structure and the surrounding mucosa (Fig. 10.13c, arrows). Focusing on the DL at the maximal magnifying ratio (Fig. 10.13d, arrows), we see crypt openings (COs) with uniform aperture widths in the surrounding mucosa. The microvessels in the intervening parts (IPs) are slightly dilated in places but maintain a regular subepithelial network. Based on the regular microsurface pattern but the irregular microvascular pattern within the lesion, this was diagnosed as a cancerous lesion. This region corresponds with the slightly whitish flat mucosa on the periphery of the reddened depression seen using non-magnifying WLI (Fig. 10.13a, arrowed).

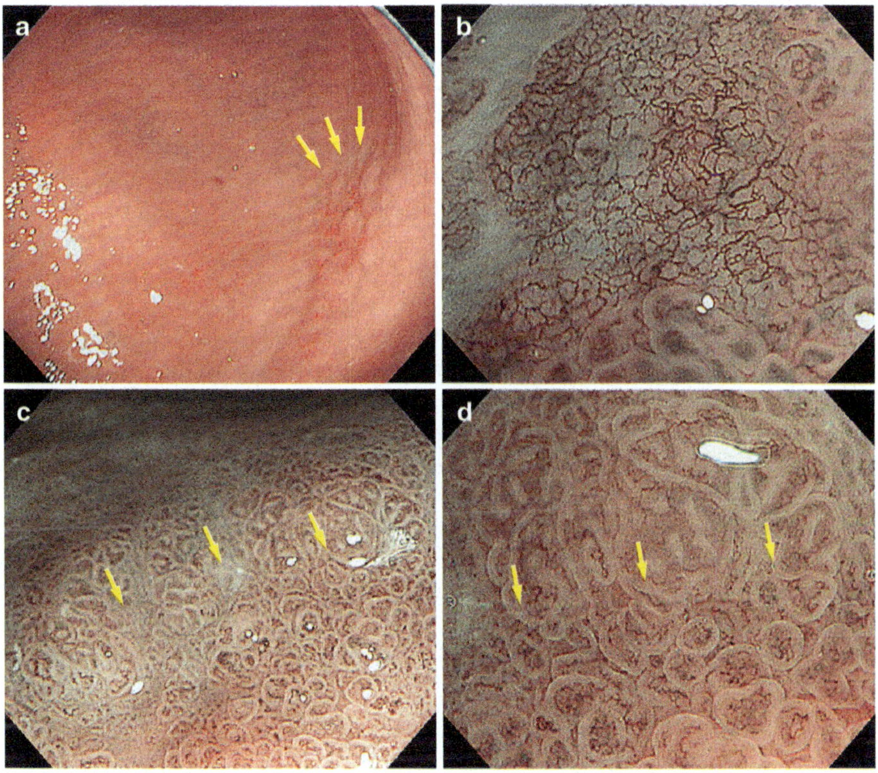

Fig. 10.13

10.12.1.3 Histological Findings

Based on the DL delineated using M-NBI, this lesion was resected at ESD. Histological examination of the resected specimen showed that the central depressed area was comparatively flat and formed small tubular glands (Fig. 10.13e), whereas the flat surrounding area presented a papillary epithelial morphology (Fig. 10.13f) which is corresponding to VEC pattern in Fig. 10.13c, d).

10.12.2 Diagnostic Pointers for NBI

When different histological types and structures exist within a lesion, when visualized endoscopically the demarcation line may be mistaken for the tumor margin. Under magnification, the field of view is limited, so evaluations should be made while comparing the findings with the non-magnifying and chromoendoscopic findings. It is also important to recognize the microsurface and microvascular patterns of the definitely normal surrounding mucosa and compare these with the tumor.

When the degree of atrophy and intestinal metaplasia are strong in the surrounding mucosa, the background mucosa also shows a papillary microsurface pattern, so the DL is often indistinct for a tumor with a VEC microsurface pattern. The DL should then be delineated on the basis of irregular morphology and nonuniformity of size in the microsurface pattern and the presence of irregular microvascular pattern.

Fig. 10.13 (continued)

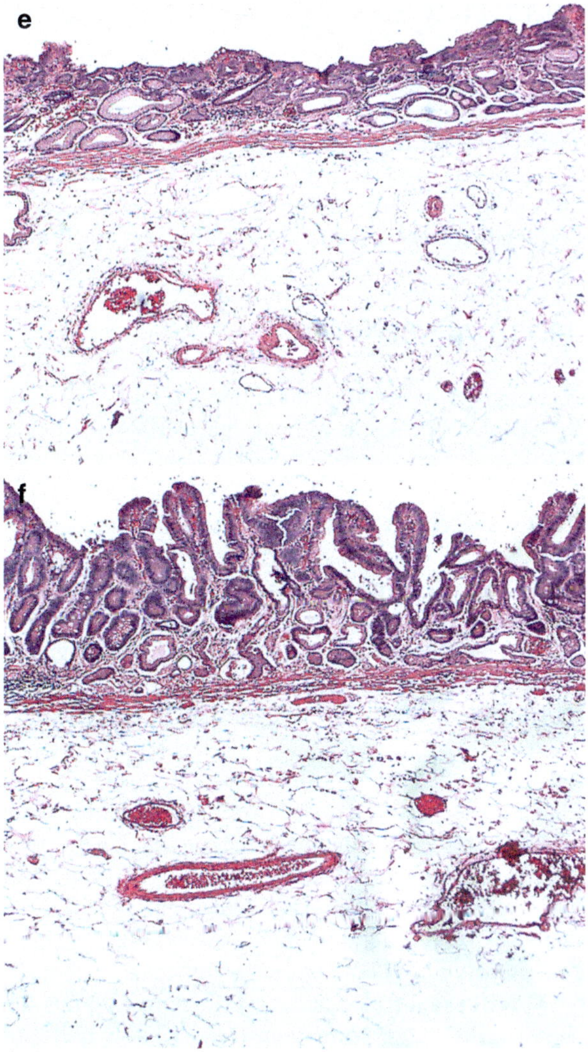

10.13 Early Gastric Cancer (Differentiated): Type IIc (4)

The differential diagnosis of depressed lesions lacking the characteristics of gastric cancer, such as irregular margins or spiny depression, is difficult using non-magnifying WLI endoscopy, and biopsies are often relied upon to provide the diagnosis. M-NBI observation has improved the diagnostic ability for depressed lesion such as this one, but we should be aware that an adequate diagnosis is not possible with magnified observation at anything less than the maximal magnifying ratio.

10.13.1 M-NBI Findings

1. Marginal area (demarcation line: present)
2. Lesion (VS classification: irregular MV pattern plus irregular MS pattern)

10.13.2 Explanation

10.13.2.1 Non-magnifying WLI Appearance

We can see a slightly indented, somewhat reddened lesion, 9 × 3 mm in size, near the gastric angle, on the lesser curvature of the lower gastric body. Using non-magnified WLI, we can discern few features suggestive of gastric cancer, and the margin is indistinct in part (Fig. 10.14a, arrows indicate lesion).

10.13.2.2 M-NBI Appearance

Under close NBI observation applying slight air suction, even without magnification we can see a distinct demarcation line (DL) corresponding to the margin of the depressed area (Fig. 10.14b). With M-NBI examination at low magnification, the microsurface pattern appears regular, and in part of the anal side of the lesion, we can visualize proliferating microvessels (Fig. 10.14c). However, detailed evaluation of these features is not possible at this magnification.

M-NBI examination at the maximal magnifying ratio (Fig. 10.14d, e) shows that the marginal crypt epithelium (MCE) has a uniform width but an asymmetrical distribution and a rounded, oval, polygonal or curved variegated morphology. The intervening parts (IPs) are nonuniform in size. Individual microvessels have nonuniform diameters and sizes, with an irregular distribution and varied morphology, including branching and anastomosing with each other. Their arrangement and directionality are irregular. From these findings, we made the diagnosis of differentiated gastric cancer. The arrow in Fig. 10.14e indicates the DL, delineated using the microsurface and microvascular patterns. In the noncancerous background mucosa outside the DL, we can see light blue crests (LBCs) lining the MCE. LBCs are rarely visualized within cancers themselves, and disappearance of the LBCs also helps to delineate the DL.

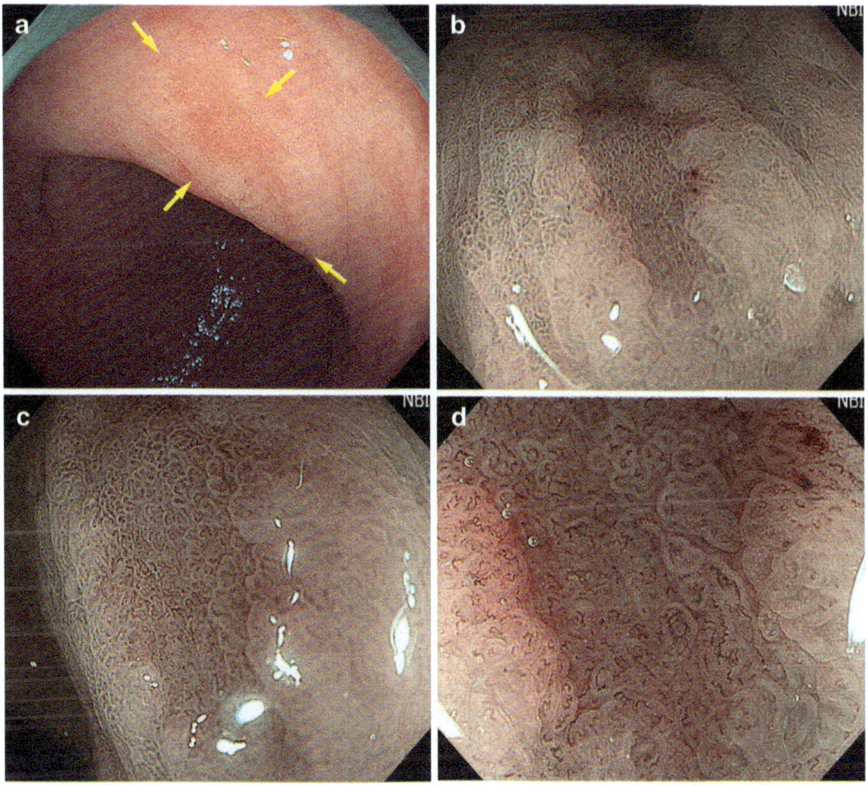

Fig. 10.14

10.13.2.3 Histological Findings

The ESD specimen in Fig. 10.14f corresponds to the endoscopic findings in Fig. 10.14e, with the histological finding of a well differentiated tubular adenocarcinoma.

10.13.3 Diagnostic Pointers for NBI

Examination at the maximal magnifying ratio reveals for the first time the irregular MV pattern plus irregular MS pattern and allows us to easily diagnose this lesion as a differentiated gastric cancer.

Close observation of lesions near the lesser curvature of the gastric angle is often difficult, and detailed observation at the maximal magnifying ratio is impossible unless the air inside the stomach is sufficiently suctioned.

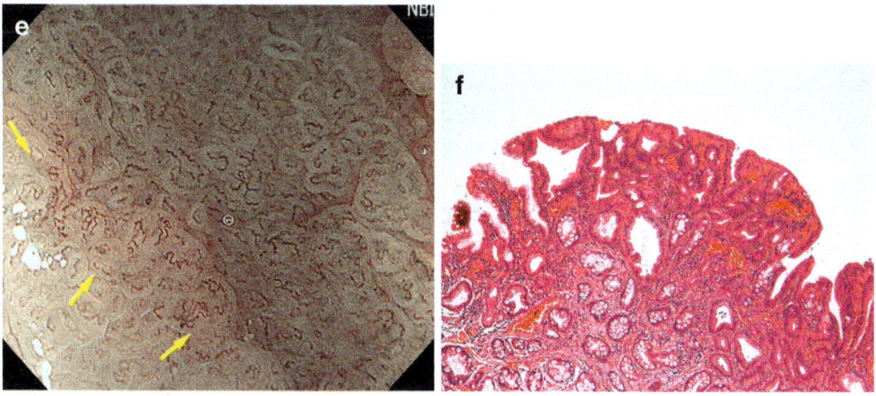

Fig. 10.14 (continued)

10.14 Early Gastric Cancer (Differentiated): Type IIc (UL +)

Superficial depressed (type 0-IIc) early gastric cancers are frequently associated with peptic ulceration. Conversely, when a gastric ulcer is detected endoscopically, we should always be aware of the possible existence of a cancer. In this section, we present a case in which non-magnifying WLI was only able to detect a gastric ulcer scar, but using M-NBI the diagnosis of gastric cancer could be made.

10.14.1 M-NBI Findings

1. Marginal area (demarcation line: present)
2. Lesion (VS classification: irregular MV pattern plus irregular MS pattern)

10.14.2 Explanation

10.14.2.1 Non-magnifying WLI Appearance

We can see mucosal convergence on the posterior wall of the gastric angle (Fig. 10.15a). Even dye spraying with indigo carmine (Fig. 10.15b) failed to reveal any findings suggestive of malignancy such as tapering of the fold tips.

10.14.2.2 M-NBI Appearance (Water Immersion)

The surrounding background mucosa displays a regular rounded marginal crypt epithelium (MCE) and loop-shaped subepithelial capillaries (SECs) (Fig. 10.15c). In a fairly narrow range on the anal side of the scar center, the regular VS pattern has disappeared in the area indicated by the arrows, forming a demarcation line (DL) (Fig. 10.15c–e). Inside of the demarcation line, we see an irregular MV pattern comprising irregular loop-shaped microvessels with a varied morphology. The irregular curved MCE, disappearing in one area, forms an irregular to absent MS pattern.

From the above findings, we diagnosed a type 0-IIc early gastric cancer (UL+) localized to a narrow area, associated with an ulcer scar.

10.14.2.3 Histological Findings

Histological examination of the ESD specimen (Fig. 10.15f) reveals a tubular adenocarcinoma localized to and growing replacing the surface layer. There are also some noncancerous glands present. Non-magnifying WLI and chromoendoscopy are limited in their ability to detect gastric cancers that display a histological structure like the one in this case.

10.14.3 Diagnostic Pointers for NBI

When we detect an ulcer scar using non-magnifying WLI, we routinely take a biopsy from the center of the lesion. Using M-NBI at low magnification, we search for and delineate the DL. We then raise the magnifying ratio and biopsy only lesions with an irregular MV pattern or irregular MS pattern internally. We would like to suggest this as a useful strategy.

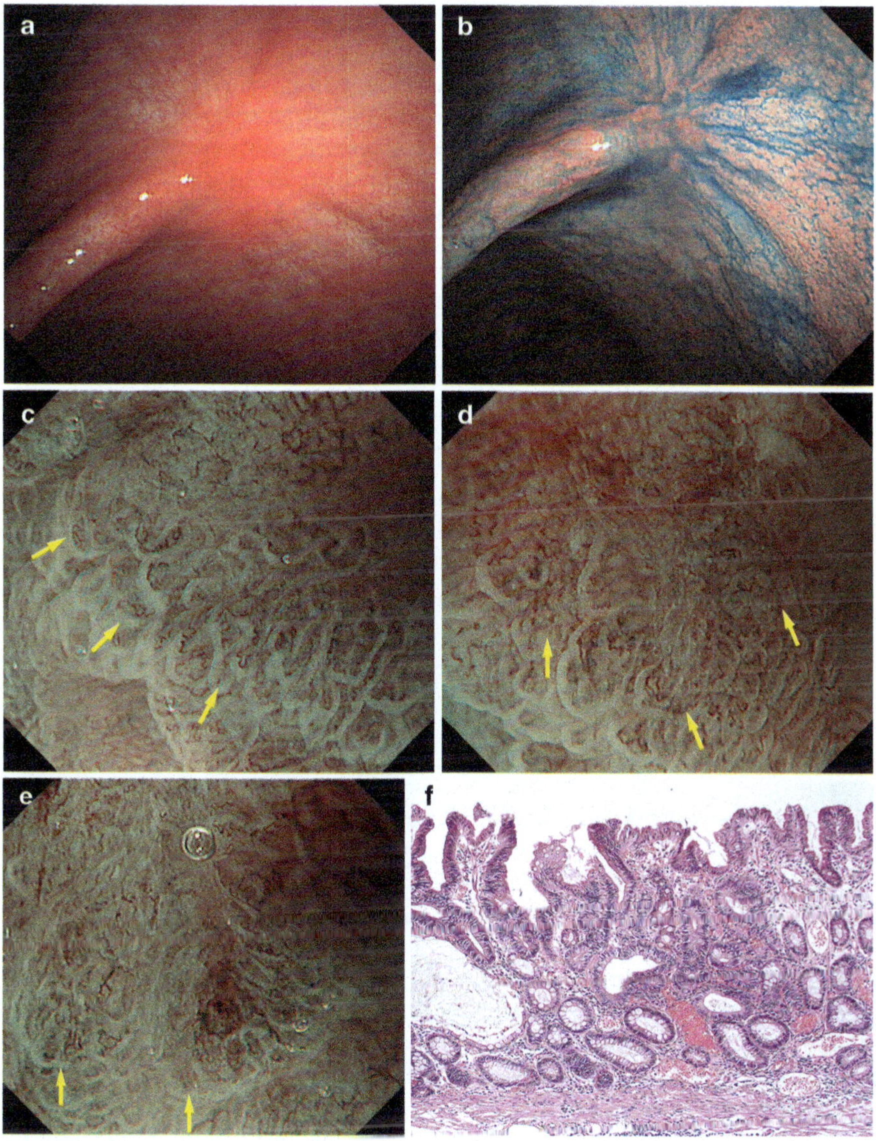

Fig. 10.15

10.15 Early Gastric Cancer (Undifferentiated): Type IIc (1)

Undifferentiated cancer cells develop from the gastric gland neck and proliferate within the lamina propria mucosae, destroying the gland neck. Accordingly, when the number of cancer cells within the lamina propria is extremely low, the cancer epithelial surface is covered by noncancer epithelium. Proliferation of cancer cells is associated with atrophy of the mucosa and erosion of the epithelium, and as the cancer proliferate, it becomes exposed on the surface epithelium [5]. Although M-NBI using the VS classification is said to be of limited value in diagnosing undifferentiated cancers from the microsurface pattern and microvascular pattern [6], it is possible to speculate about changes in the intramucosal histological architecture.

10.15.1 M-NBI Findings

We can see a 17-mm pale depressed lesion (Fig. 10.16a) with central reddened granularity on the greater curvature of the lower gastric body. Dye spraying revealed a type 0-IIc undifferentiated cancer with steep margins to the depressed area. Other than post-biopsy regenerative granules in the central area, within the depression we see the same gastric area pattern as the background mucosa (Fig. 10.16b). The surface epithelium is covered by noncancerous epithelium, and we can infer an intramucosal histological structure in which the cancer cells have thinly infiltrated the middle layer of the lamina propria.

10.15.2 Magnified Area A (Fig. 10.16a, b)

1. Marginal area (demarcation line: present)
2. Lesion (VS classification: regular MV pattern plus absent MS pattern)

10.15.2.1 M-NBI Appearance (Fig. 10.16c)

Microvascular pattern (V): The morphology of each blood vessel in the background mucosa is a uniform-sized closed loop, anastomosing with each other to form a network. The distribution is symmetrical, the arrangement regular, and the density uniform, so this is assessed as a regular microvascular (MV) pattern. Within the depressed inner region, we also see a regular MV pattern resembling the background mucosa, so from the microvascular pattern, we cannot delineate a demarcation line (DL) between the tumor and the background mucosa.

Microsurface pattern (S): The marginal crypt epithelium (MCE) of the background mucosa is regularly arranged and distributed. It forms a DL corresponding to the depressed area. Although MCE can be discerned in part of the depression, it is either indistinct or absent, so this was assessed as an absent MS pattern.

10.15.2.2 Histological Findings

Elements of poorly differentiated adenocarcinoma and signet-ring cell carcinoma have infiltrated the middle layers of the lamina propria, covered by noncancerous mucosa with a flattened or blunted surface epithelium (Fig. 10.16d).

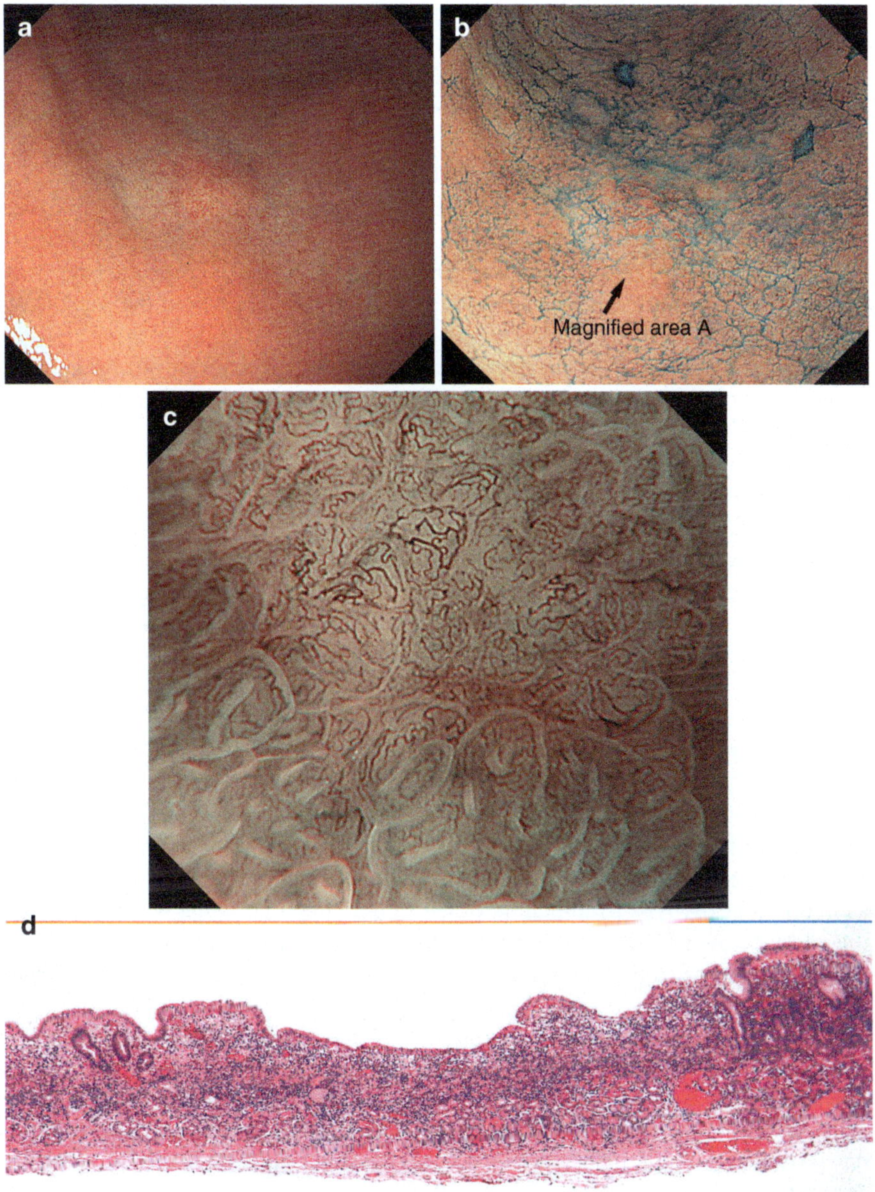

Fig. 10.16

10.15.3 Magnified Area B (Fig. 10.16e, f)

1. Marginal area (demarcation line: absent)
2. Lesion (VS classification: regular MV pattern plus regular MS pattern)

10.15.3.1 M-NBI Appearance (Fig. 10.16g)

Microvascular pattern (V): The individual vessels in the background mucosa have a uniform-sized closed- or open-looped morphology, with a symmetrical distribution, regular arrangement, and uniform density, assessed as a regular microvascular (MV) pattern. A similar regular MV pattern is seen within the depression, and a DL cannot be detected.

Microsurface pattern (S): Curved MCE can be seen within both the background mucosa and the depression, so this was assessed as a regular MS pattern. A DL cannot be discerned at the margin of the depressed area.

10.15.3.2 Histological Findings

At the infiltration border observed under magnification, the surface layer epithelium with a regular tubular structure like the background epithelium has regular arrangement, and the poorly differentiated adenocarcinoma and signet-ring cell carcinoma have infiltrated only the middle part of the mucosal lamina propria without destruction of surface part (Fig. 10.16h).

10.15.4 Diagnostic Pointers for NBI

The histological features common to magnified areas A and B are relatively thin infiltration of undifferentiated cancer into the middle layers of the lamina propria and coverage by noncancerous epithelium. With pathohistological structures such as in this case, M-NBI examination of the tumor shows a regular MS pattern, and the presence of cancer cannot even be detected. We recommend the 4-point biopsy taken from the surrounding mucosa to delineate the margins of undifferentiated cancers.

The pathohistological structural differences between magnified areas A and B are due to differences in the morphology and structure of the covering noncancerous epithelium. The surface epithelium of magnified area A is flattened or blunted, seen using M-NBI as an absent MS pattern in which the MCE was not visualized. While the surface epithelium of magnified area B shows the same morphology as that of the background mucosa, seen using M-NBI as regular as pattern.

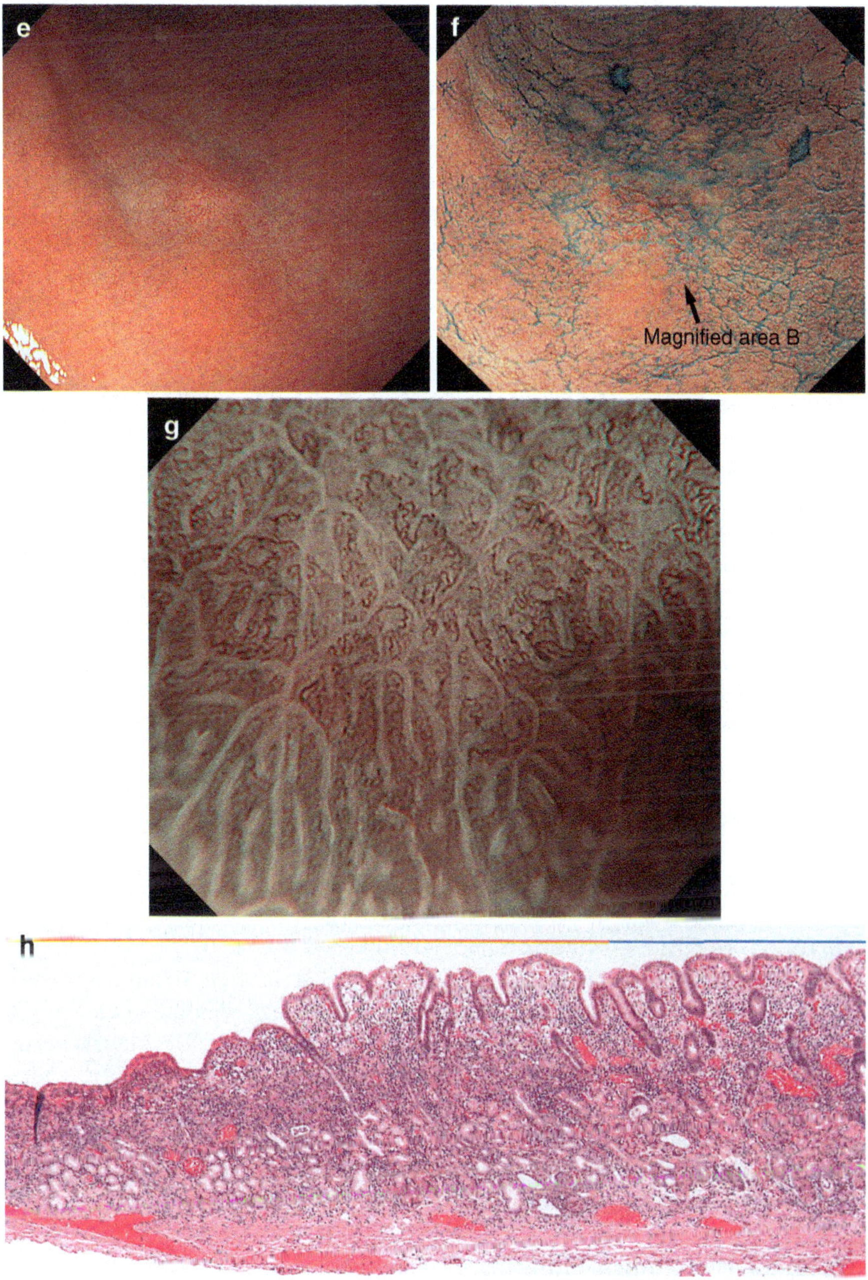

Fig. 10.16 (continued)

10.16 Early Gastric Cancer (Undifferentiated): Type IIc (2)

The clinical presentation of gastric cancers varies not only through the histological variability of the cancer cells themselves, but also the temporal factors related to growth and infiltration. The M-NBI findings of undifferentiated cancers are variable, from a regular microvascular pattern (V) and a regular microsurface pattern (S), similar to that seen in chronic gastritis, to an extremely irregular VS. This is thought to reflect various factors, such as the thickness and location of intramucosal cancer cells, the presence of infiltrating inflammatory cells or a desmoplastic reaction, and histological architecture of the background mucosa.

10.16.1 Non-magnifying of the Surface Epithelium WLI Findings

On the greater curvature of the gastric fundus, we can see a pale irregular depressed lesion with a number of reddened granules inside, 35 mm in size, associated with a barely discernible convergence of folds (Fig. 10.17a, e). Dye spraying reveals that the depression has steep and distinct margins and regenerative reddish granularities extending from the vicinity of the convergent folds on the anal side of the depression, whereas the oral side of the lesion comprises similar low granules (Fig. 10.17b, f). From these findings, this lesion is considered to be a type 0-IIc undifferentiated cancer (UL+) with thick proliferation of cancer cells as far as the mucosal surface, with repeated erosion and regeneration of the surface epithelium.

10.16.2 Magnified Area A (Fig. 10.17a, b)

Lesion (VS classification: regular MV pattern plus absent MS pattern)

10.16.2.1 M-NBI Examination (Fig. 10.17c)

Microvascular pattern (V): The individual vessels have a relatively smooth open-looped or in part small closed-looped morphology with little variability in diameter, anastomosing with each other to form a network. The vessels have a symmetrical distribution, regular arrangement, and uniform density, with a regular arrangement of collecting venules visualized in the background, so this was assessed as a regular MV pattern.

Microsurface pattern (S): The marginal crypt epithelium (MCE) is completely absent, so this was assessed as an absent MS pattern.

10.16.2.2 Histological Findings

Poorly differentiated adenocarcinoma and signet-ring cell carcinoma densely occupy the surface part of the mucosa, taking up one-third of its thickness, with no deeper invasion. The superficial epithelium is flattened, and the MCE structure has disappeared (Fig. 10.17d).

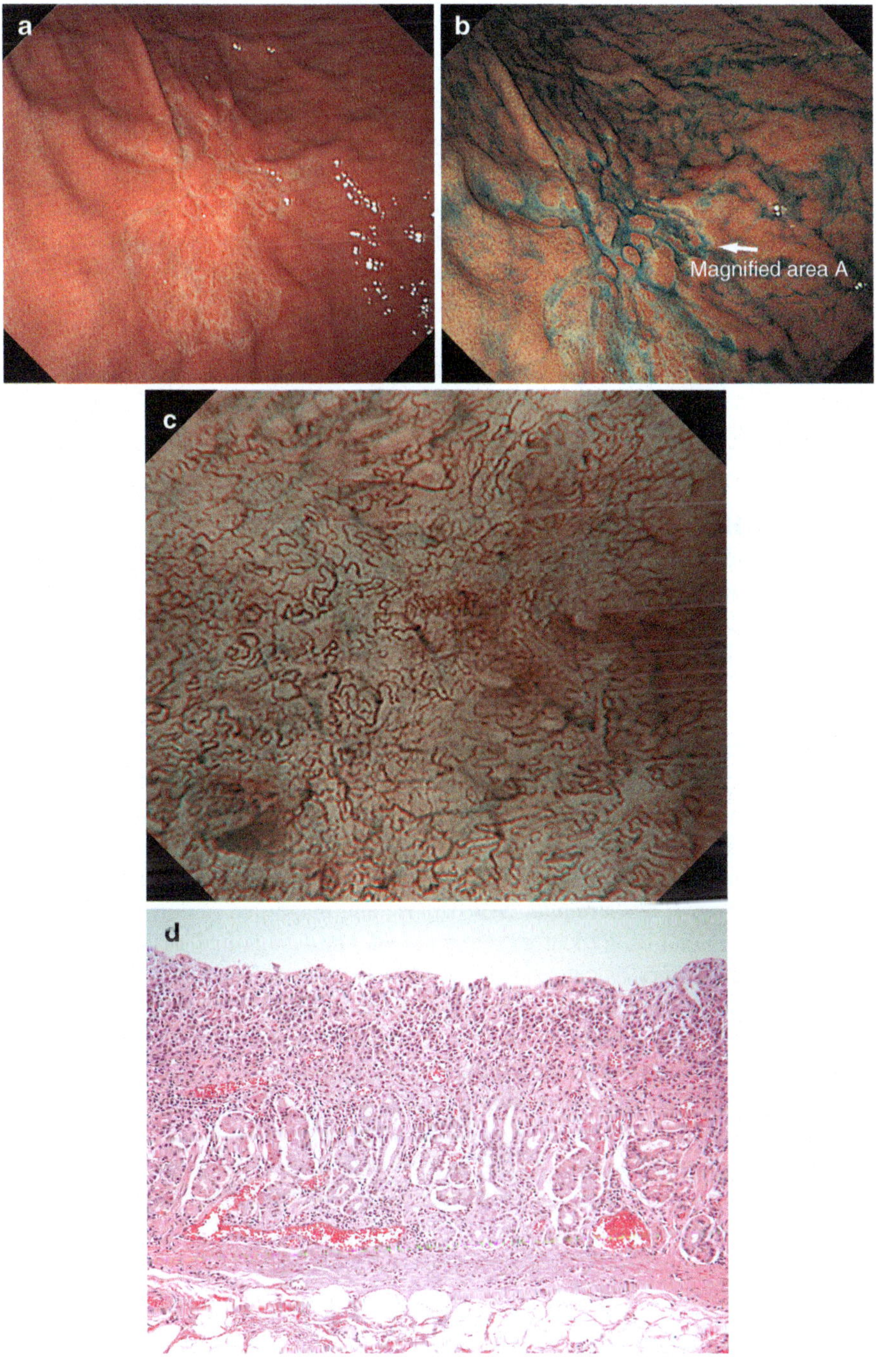

Fig. 10.17

10.16.3 Magnified Area B (Fig. 10.17e, f)

1. Marginal area (demarcation line: present)
2. Lesion (VS classification: irregular MV pattern plus absent MS pattern)

10.16.3.1 M-NBI Examination (Fig. 10.17g)

Microvascular pattern (V): The individual vessels within the depression are irregularly dilated, with a curved morphology, marked tortuosity, and nonuniform diameters, forming open-looped or in part small closed-looped shapes. Breaks and interruptions are common, and anastomoses uncommon. The distribution is asymmetrical, and the arrangement is irregular, with marked difference in density, so this was assessed as an irregular MV pattern.

Microsurface pattern (S): Based on the complete disappearance of the MCE, this was assessed as an absent MS pattern.

10.16.3.2 Histological Findings

In the magnified area, poorly differentiated adenocarcinoma and signet-ring cell carcinoma densely occupy the mucosal surface layer with deeper invasion. The crypts have disappeared (Fig. 10.17h). This is associated with a desmoplastic reaction inside the cancerous lesion.

10.16.4 Diagnostic Pointers for NBI

The common features in the magnifying endoscopic findings for magnified areas A and B are an absent MS pattern, dense proliferation of undifferentiated cancer in the superficial layers, an absent crypt structure, and a flattened surface. However, magnified region A has a regular MV pattern, and magnified region B an irregular MV pattern. Pathohistological examination of both magnified regions A and B reveals dense clusters of cancer cells in the mucosal surface layer. Although the epithelium is flattened, magnified region A has a thinner layer of intramucosal cancer compared to magnified region B, and in magnified region B a marked desmoplastic reaction can be seen within the cancerous lesion.

The magnified endoscopic findings in region A is similar to those of atrophic gastritis, making differentiation from cancer extremely difficult. On the other hand, as seen in magnified region B, as the intramucosal cancer layer increases in thickness, extending solidly as far as the surface layer, NBI-magnified examination will reveal a distinct irregular MV pattern.

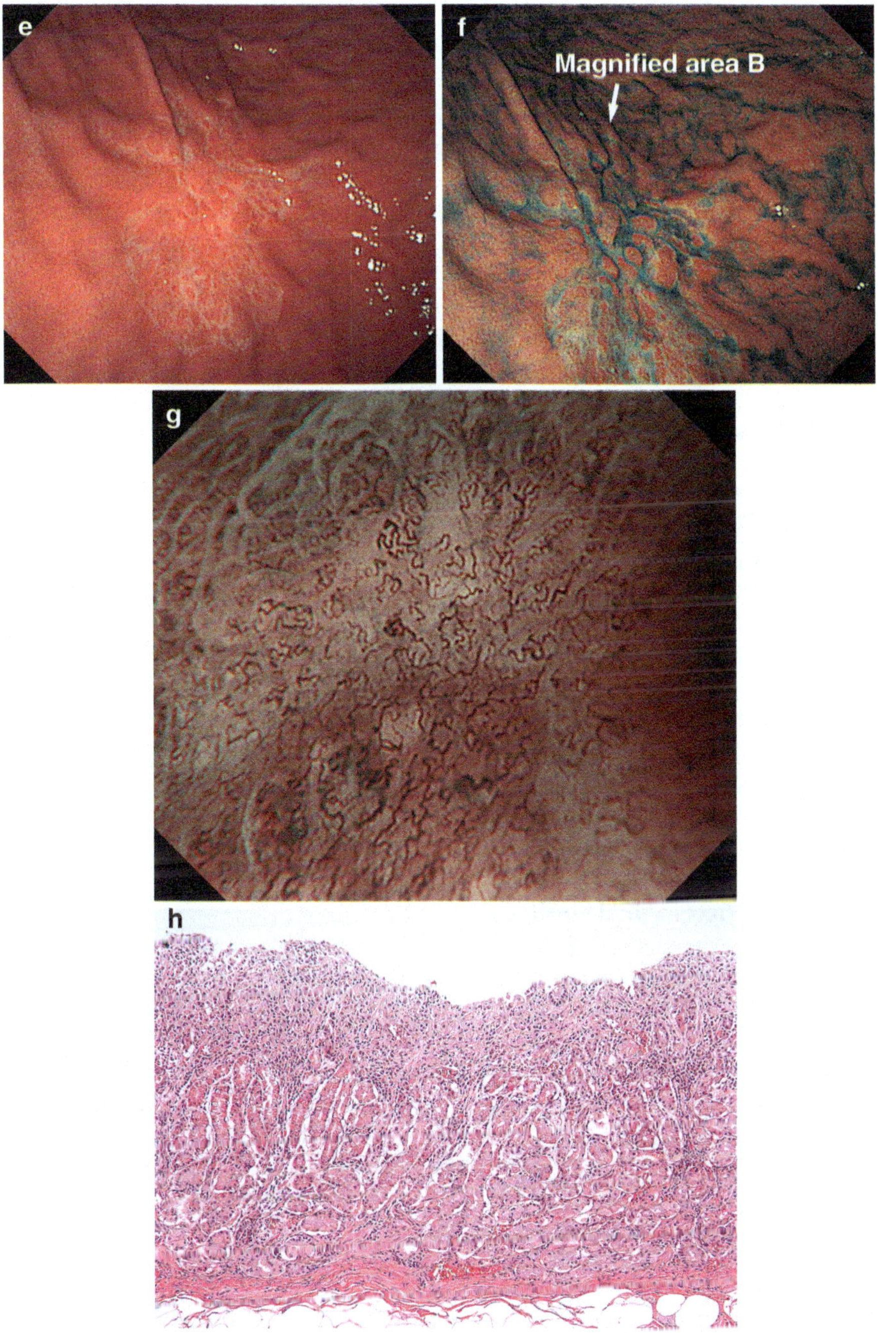

Fig. 10.17 (continued)

10.17 MALT Lymphoma [7]

MALT lymphomas, along with diffuse large cell lymphomas, are nonepithelial tumor occurring frequently in the digestive tract, particularly the stomach. The non-magnifying WLI endoscopic findings can be extremely varied, including erosions, ulceration, and gastric changes as well as elevated lesions including submucosal tumors (SMTs). The typical histological findings are of proliferation of small atypical B-cell lymphoid centrocyte-like cells, glandular destruction, and the lymphoepithelial lesion (LEL) infiltrative picture.

At the localized stage, *Helicobacter pylori* eradication therapy is the treatment of first choice, with good long-term results reported.

10.17.1 Explanation

10.17.1.1 Non-magnifying WLI Appearance

Non-magnifying WLI examination reveals a lesion on the posterior wall of the lower gastric body, with prominent surface irregularities almost the same color as the surrounding mucosa and small erosions scattered around its interior (Fig. 10.18a).

10.17.1.2 M-NBI Appearance

M-NBI examination shows that in one area, the microsurface pattern has completely disappeared, whereas collecting venules and microvessels can be visualized (Fig. 10.18b). In the marginal area (Fig. 10.18c), the remaining marginal crypt epithelium (MCE) is enlarged and distorted, and the intervening parts (IPs) are open and whitish. The subepithelial capillary network (SECN) is stretched, comprising loop-shaped or tortuous irregular vessels.

10.17.1.3 Histological Findings

Histological examination of the biopsy specimen shows dense lymphocyte and plasma cell infiltration and an LEL, yielding the diagnosis of MALT lymphoma (Fig. 10.18d).

10.17.1.4 After Eradication Therapy

Repeat endoscopy 1 month after eradication therapy (Fig. 10.18e) revealed irregularly arranged oval MCE and marked reduction in size of the unstructured area (Fig. 10.18f).

10.17.2 Diagnostic Pointers for NBI

The characteristic M-NBI findings of MALT lymphoma are a mixture of unstructured areas and remnant MCE, and dilation, distortion, and destruction of the remnant MCE may be visualized. Microvessels follow irregular courses, with little nonuniformity in diameter, and branch relatively infrequently. Collecting venules are visualized in one area.

Spot biopsy of unstructured areas is useful for the diagnosis and posttreatment evaluation.

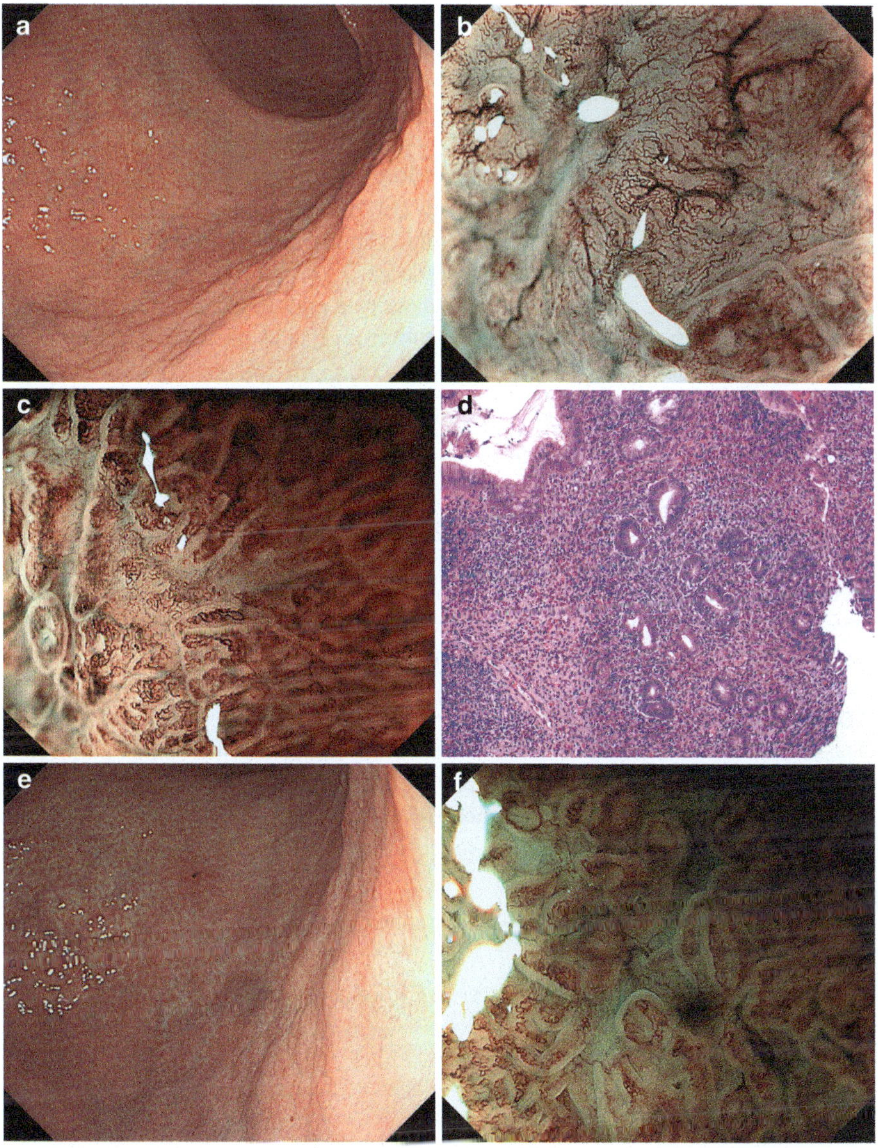

Fig. 10.18

10.18 Gastric Carcinoid Neoplasia, Type A Gastritis

For many years, atrophic gastritis has been broadly classified into fundic gland mucosal atrophy type (atrophic gastritis type A) and pyloric gland mucosal atrophy type (atrophic gastritis type B). In type A gastritis, due to autoimmune and other mechanisms, the fundic glands become diffusely atrophic, causing hypertrophy and neoplasia of the enterochromaffin-like cells (ECL cells) present in the fundic region associated with persistent hypergastrinemia, a state predisposing to endocrine cell micronests and carcinoids in the gastric mucosa.

In this section, we will focus on the magnifying endoscopic diagnosis of type A gastritis, and gastric carcinoid tumors arising from type A gastritis, and provide an overview of the relevant findings.

10.18.1 Explanation

10.18.1.1 Non-magnifying WLI Appearance

We can see a smooth-surfaced reddened elevated lesion on the posterior wall of the gastric body (Fig. 10.19a). Close examination following dye spraying (Fig. 10.19b) reveals marked dilatation of the surface blood vessels, and the sides of the protuberance are steeper than a typical submucosal tumor.

10.18.1.2 M-NBI Appearance

The surface is mainly composed of uniform width coarsened intervening parts (IPs), with light blue crests (LBCs) seen in part of the marginal area (Fig. 10.19c). These findings do not differ greatly from those of typical chronic gastritis. Cyan-colored dilated veins can be seen beneath the mucosal epithelium.

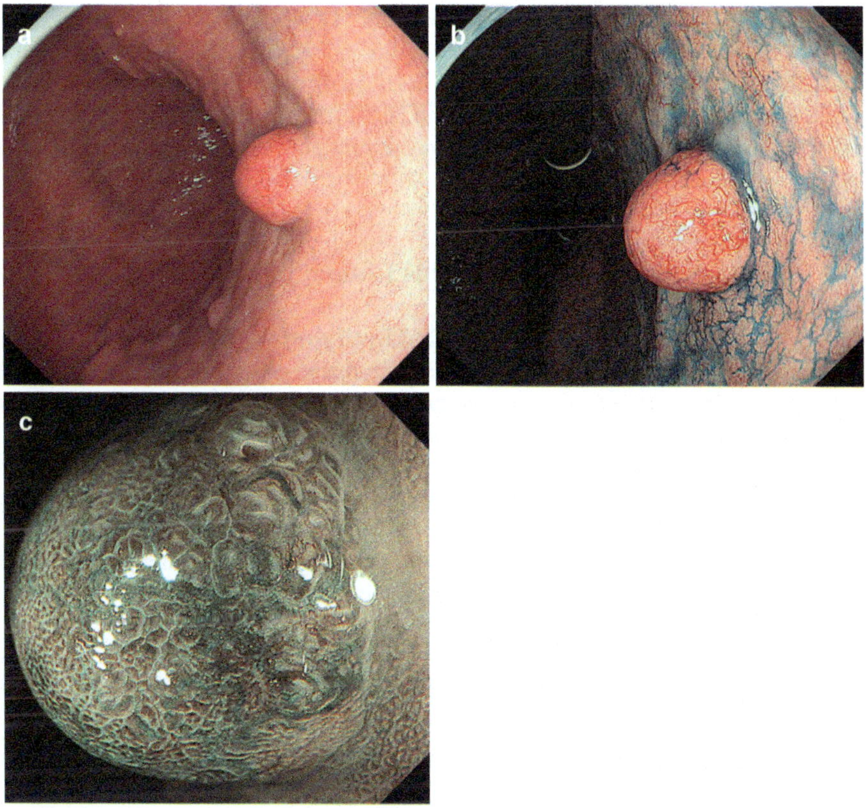

Fig. 10.19

10.18.1.3 Histological Findings

Figure 10.19d shows the ESD specimen. Tumor extends from the deep layers of the mucosa to the submucosa. Tumor cells have small round nuclei, with low grade atypia, and the tumor is composed of solid nests, ribbons, and glandlike structures. Although not shown in the figure, vascular infiltration was seen, so the ESD procedure was followed by a total gastrectomy with lymph node dissection.

10.18.2 Background Mucosa of This Tumor

10.18.2.1 M-NBI Findings (Maximal Magnifying Ratio)

In the fundic gland region (Fig. 10.19e), the marginal crypt epithelium (MCE) structure has disappeared, and we can see diffuse atrophic mucosa associated with irregular cyan-colored collecting venules (CVs). On the other hand, in the pyloric gland area (Fig. 10.19f), the normal microvascular pattern and microsurface pattern are completely preserved in the gastric antrum, with no pathological changes to be seen.

From the above magnifying endoscopic findings, we can diagnose atrophic gastritis predominately in the fundic gland region, i.e., type A gastritis.

10.18.3 Diagnostic Pointers for NBI

This tumor in itself has no specific features that would enable us to diagnose it as carcinoid. However, M-NBI examination allows us to accurately diagnose atrophic gastritis of the fundic gland region. The antral mucosa is normal, so we have atrophic gastritis predominately in the fundic gland region, or type A gastritis. It is a real benefit of NBI that carcinoid should be suspected in elevated lesions arising from a background of type A gastritis.

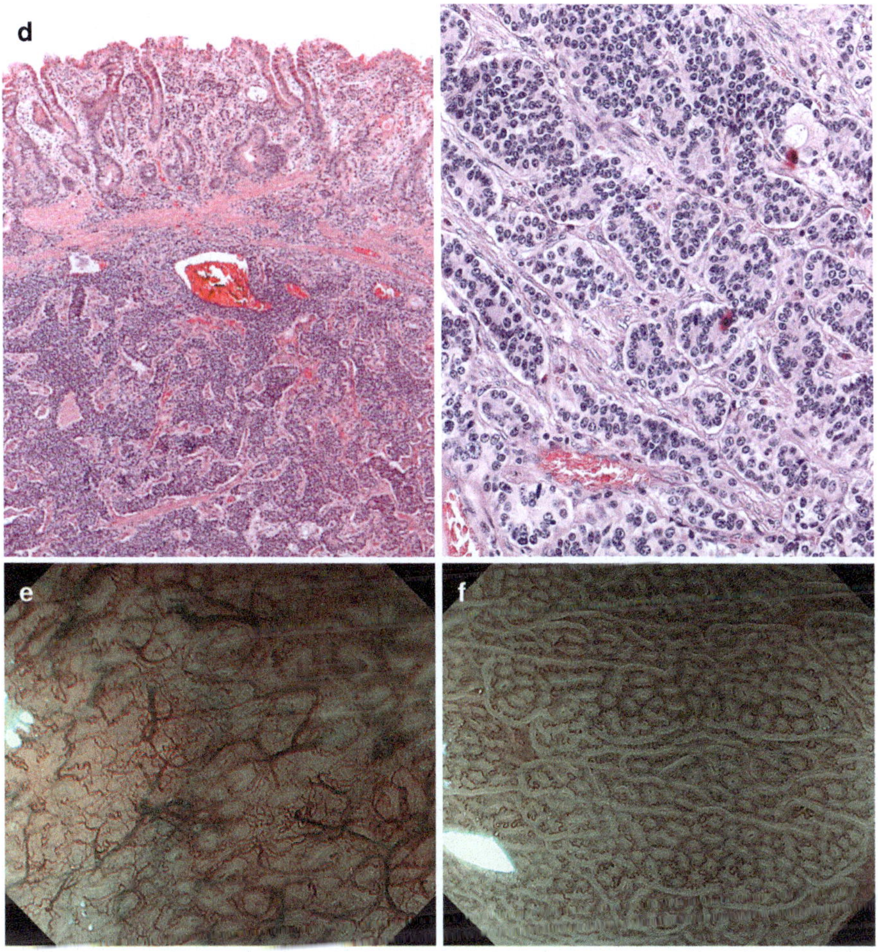

Fig. 10.19 (continued)

References

1. Yao K, et al. *Stomach and Intestine* 2010; **45:** 1159–1171
2. Kanemitsu T. Gastric Cancer 2014; 17: 469–477.
3. Maki S. Gastric Cancer 2013; 16: 140–146.
4. Yao K. Gastrointest Endosc 2008; 68: 574–580.
5. Nakamura M. Structure of gastric cancer (3rd edition), Igaku Shoin, 2005
6. Yao K (editor). Zoom gastroscopy, Springer 2013.
7. Ono S, et al. Gastrointest Endosc 2008; 68: 632–634

Atlas of Nonneoplastic Lesions in the Duodenum

11

Kenshi Yao

K. Yao
Department of Endoscopy, Fukuoka University Chikushi Hospital,
1-1-1 Zokumyoin, Chikushino 818-8502, Japan
e-mail: yao@fukuoka u.ac.jp

M. Muto et al. (eds.), *Atlas of Endoscopy with Narrow Band Imaging*,
DOI 10.1007/978-4-431-54243-8_11

11.1 Gastric Metaplasia

11.1.1 M-NBI Findings

1. Marginal area (demarcation line: present)
2. Lesion region (VS classification: regular MV pattern plus regular MS pattern, LBC+)

11.1.2 Explanation

Histologically, gastric metaplasia consists of only foveolar epithelium, whereas heterotopic gastric mucosa displays the fundic gland structure in addition to foveolar epithelium. When M-NBI of the surface reveals a tubular epithelial VS different from the duodenal villi, we can conclude that it is either gastric metaplasia or heterotopic gastric mucosa, although differentiation between the two is difficult.

11.1.2.1 Non-magnifying WLI Appearance

We can see a small inflamed reddish elevated lesion in the duodenal bulb (Fig. 11.1a).

11.1.2.2 M-NBI Appearance

The white bands of marginal villous epithelium (MVE) in the background mucosa (Figs. 11.1b, c) of the duodenal bulb are mainly curved, but do not show a typical villous structure, although light blue crests (LBCs) can be seen on the margins. However, LBCs are absent from the marginal area of the protrusion (demarcation line (DL), arrows). When we focus on the elevated area (Figs. 11.1c, d), the subepithelial microvascular pattern presents a coil-shaped morphology with a regular arrangement. The marginal crypt epithelium (MCE) has a curved to rounded morphology, without LBCs on the margins. From these findings, we can see that this lesion contains tubular crypts, unlike the normal duodenal mucosa.

11.1.2.3 Histological Findings

In the biopsy specimen stained with hematoxylin and eosin, the surface epithelium comprises crypt epithelium with a tubular structure (Fig. 11.1e). No fundic glands are visualized, so this is gastric metaplasia. Staining with Alcian blue PAS makes these findings clearer (Fig. 11.1f). Specifically, the duodenal epithelium, with goblet cells dyed blue by Alcian blue, has disappeared, replaced by foveolar epithelium dyed reddish-purple by PAS.

11.1.3 Diagnostic Pointers for NBI

Disappearance of LBCs at the margins of the MVE are characteristic of gastric metaplasia. The V and S morphology also resemble gastric mucosa.

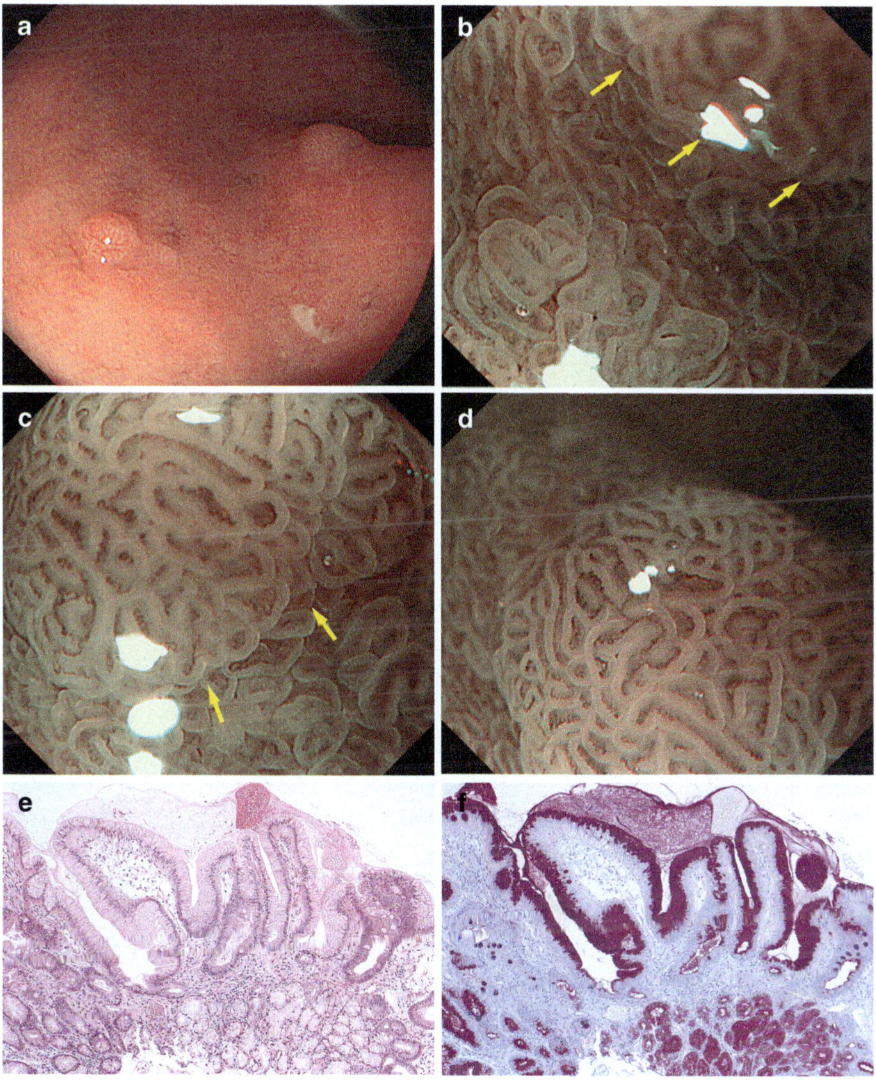

Fig. 11.1

Atlas of Neoplastic Lesions in the Duodenum

12

Hisashi Doyama and Kenshi Yao

H. Doyama
Department of Gastroenterology, Ishikawa Prefectural Central Hospital, Kanazawa, Japan

K. Yao (✉)
Department of Endoscopy, Fukuoka University Chikushi Hospital,
1-1-1 Zokumyoin, Chikushino 818-8502, Japan
e-mail: yao@fukuoka u.ac.jp

M. Muto et al. (eds.), *Atlas of Endoscopy with Narrow Band Imaging*,
DOI 10.1007/978-4-431-54243-8_12

12.1 Adenoma (Duodenal Papillary Region)

A variety of tumors occur in the duodenal papillary region. Of these, adenocarcinoma and adenoma are particularly common. However, differentiation between adenocarcinoma and adenoma is difficult using non-magnifying WLI. Furthermore, including the common problem of adenocarcinoma arising in adenoma, the false-negative biopsy rate is high.

12.1.1 M-NBI Findings

1. Marginal area (demarcation line: present)
2. Lesion region (VS classification: absent MV pattern plus regular MS pattern, WOS+)

12.1.2 Explanation

12.1.2.1 Non-magnifying WLI Appearance

In the duodenal papillary region, we can see a pale polypoid lesion 15 × 13 mm in size, adjacent to the duodenal papilla (Fig. 12.1 (a) side-viewing endoscopy, (b) forward-viewing endoscopy, (c) indigo carmine spraying). A distinct demarcation line (DL) can be seen in the non-magnified WLI images and the indigo carmine dye image.

12.1.2.2 M-NBI Appearance

M-NBI examination at low magnification (Fig. 12.1d) reveals the presence of WOS over the entire tumor. Accordingly, the microsurface pattern can be evaluated to some extent, but the microvascular pattern cannot be evaluated at all. Under M-NBI examination at the maximal magnifying ratio (Fig. 12.1e), the image of the vasculature is almost entirely obstructed by the presence of white opaque substance (WOS), rendering evaluation of the microvascular pattern impossible. Looking at the surface microstructure, WOS is widely present, so we are also unable to evaluate the marginal crypt epithelium (MCE). All of the WOS displays a ribbonlike morphology, with no irregularity or variability characteristic of cancer. Although mild nonuniformity in size is evident, the directionality, distribution, and arrangement are relatively regular. Accordingly, using WOS as a marker of the microsurface pattern, this is assessed as a regular MS pattern. VS discordance cannot be judged due to the presence of the WOS.

12.1.2.3 Histological Findings

Histological examination of the EMR specimen yields the diagnosis of tubulovillous adenoma (Fig. 12.1f).

12.1.3 Diagnostic Pointers for NBI

WOS is often identified in association with duodenal adenoma and adenocarcinoma. When WOS obscures the entire tumor, it is impossible to evaluate the microvascular pattern.

When WOS is used as the marker, adenoma can be diagnosed through evaluation of a regular MS pattern.

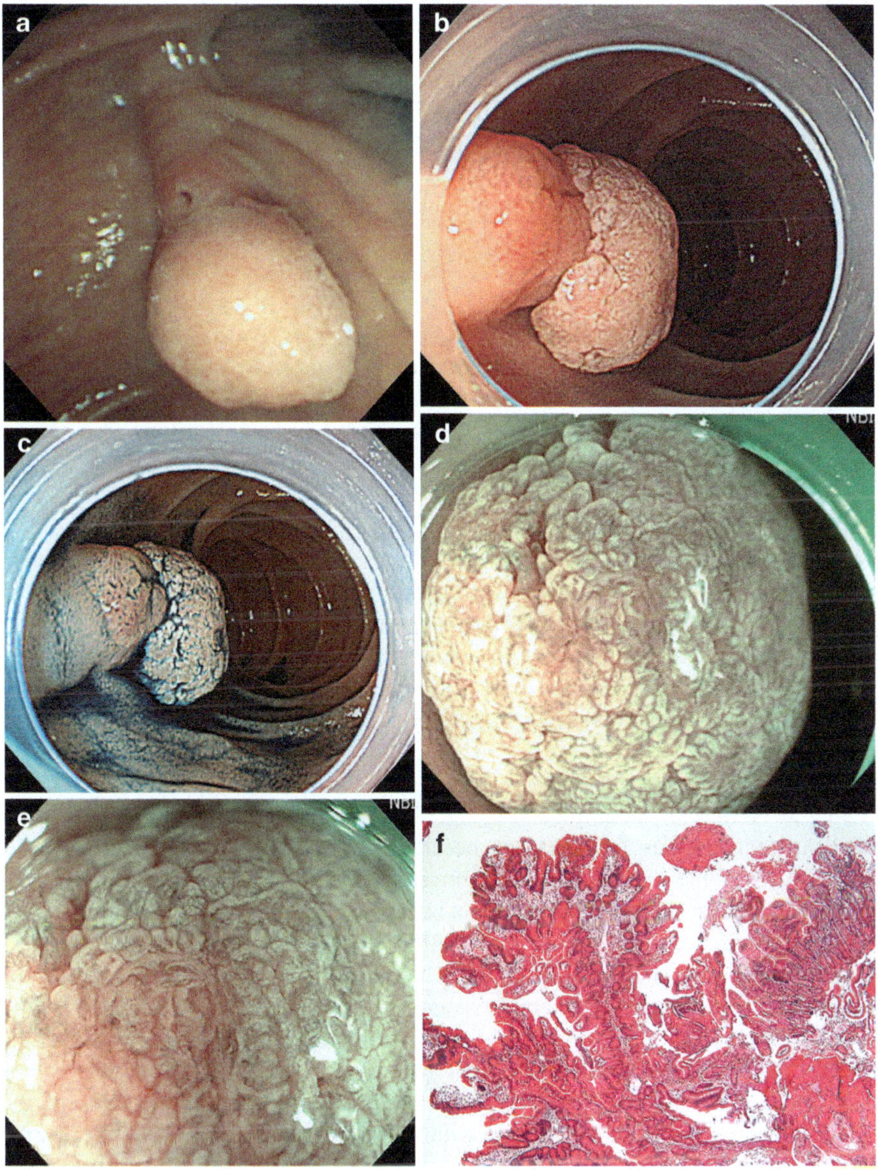

Fig. 12.1

12.2 Adenoma (Duodenal Non-papillary Region)

Detection of lesions in the duodenal non-papillary region has increased with advances in and diffusion of endoscopic examinations. As for the papillary region, however, differentiation between adenocarcinoma and adenoma is difficult using only non-magnifying WLI endoscopy.

12.2.1 M-NBI Findings

1. Marginal area (demarcation line: present)
2. Lesion: region with WOS (VS classification: absent MV pattern plus regular MS pattern, WOS+)
3. Lesion: region without WOS (VS classification: regular MV pattern plus regular MS pattern)

12.2.2 Explanation

12.2.2.1 Non-magnifying WLI Appearance

A pale flat 8 × 5 mm elevation is present on the anterior wall of the duodenal bulb. We can see a distinct demarcation line (DL) using both non-magnifying WLI (Fig. 12.2a) and indigo carmine spraying (Fig. 12.2b).

12.2.2.2 M-NBI Appearance

Using M-NBI at low magnification (Fig. 12.2c), the lesion surrounded by the normal duodenal villous structure can be clearly visualized. WOS covers approximately 2/3 of the entire lesion, and in areas free of WOS, the marginal crypt epithelium (MCE) and microvessels can be visualized. However, at this magnifying ratio, evaluation of the MV pattern and MS pattern is not possible.

Figure 12.2d, e shows the M-NBI findings (water immersion technique) at the maximal magnifying ratio. In areas covered by WOS, vessels and MCE cannot be visualized, and the WOS displays a regular reticular pattern. Using WOS as the marker, this was assessed as a regular MS pattern. VS concordance cannot be assessed because vessels cannot be visualized. In areas where WOS is absent, the MCE is round to oval, with a uniform width. The intervening part surrounded by the MCE is slightly nonuniform in size but with regular directionality, distribution, and arrangement. The morphology of the vessels in the intervening parts (IPs) is comparatively uniform. They show a symmetrical distribution and regular arrangement. No dissociation is seen between the MCE and microvessels, so there is no VS discordance. Detailed examination using M-NBI of areas with and without WOS allows us to diagnose the entire lesion as an adenoma.

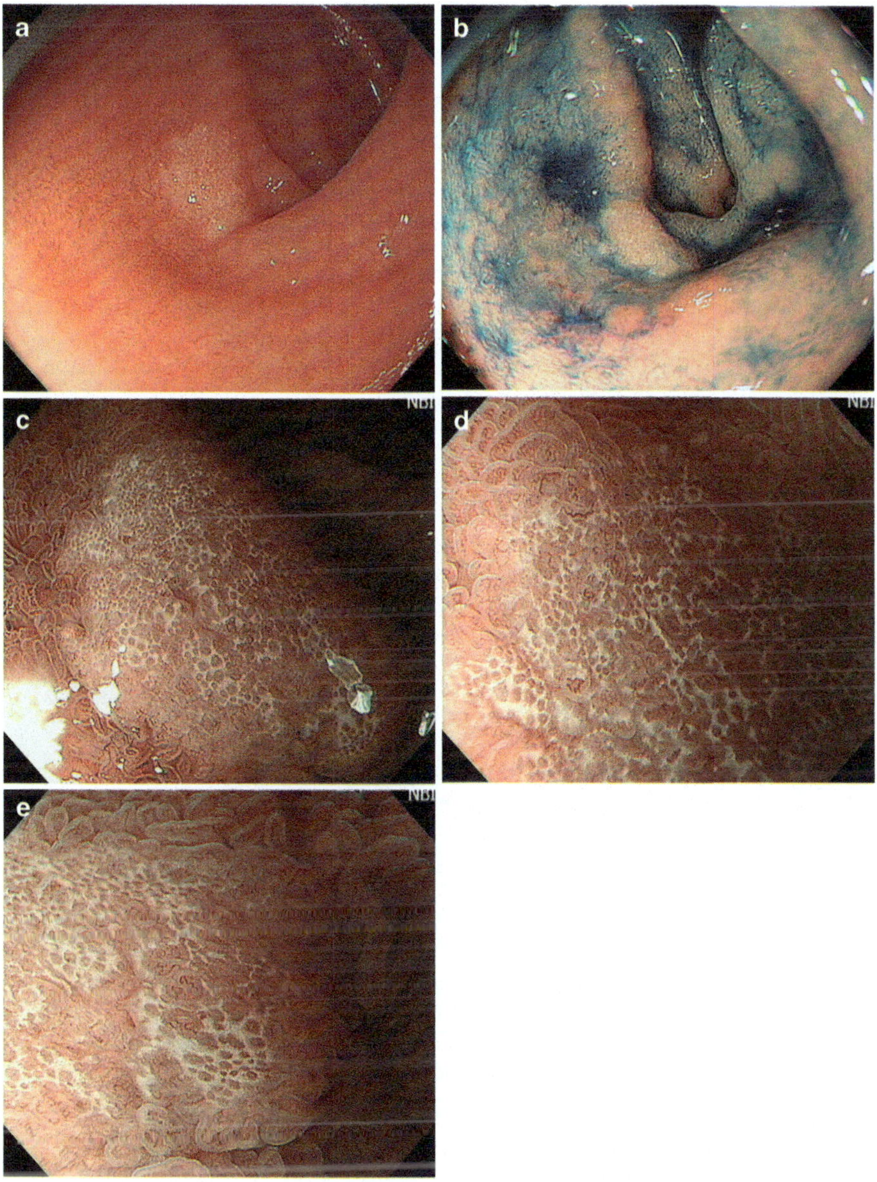

Fig. 12.2

12.2.2.3 Histological Findings

Histological examination of the EMR specimen reveals a tubular adenoma with moderate atypia (Fig. 12.2f).

12.2.3 Diagnostic Pointers for NBI

The MV pattern cannot be evaluated in areas with WOS, but using WOS as the marker, we can assess this as a regular MS pattern.

Areas without WOS have both a regular MV pattern and a regular MS pattern.

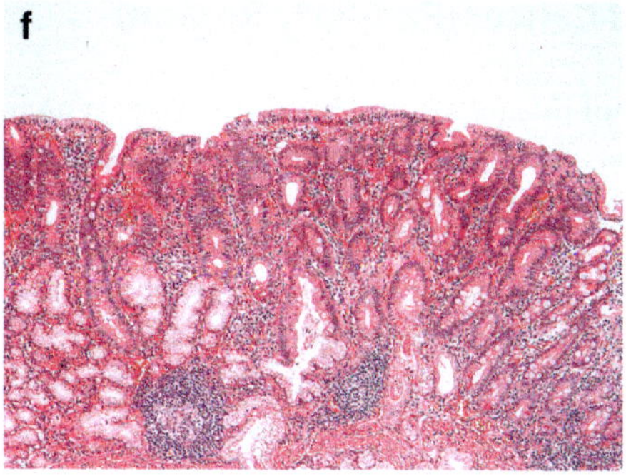

Fig. 12.2 (continued)

12.3 Duodenal Cancer (Papillary Region)

The rate of detection of duodenal tumors has increased with improvements in endoscopic equipment performance in recent years. The differential diagnosis between adenocarcinoma and adenoma is often difficult using non-magnifying WLI endoscopy and biopsy, and endoscopic treatment is often performed for the purpose of total biopsy. However, complications such as perforation (including delayed onset) and hemorrhage are common with endoscopic treatment of duodenal lesions, creating a need for the most rigorous preoperative diagnostic ability possible.

12.3.1 M-NBI Findings

1. Marginal area (demarcation line: present)
2. Lesion (VS classification: absent MV pattern plus irregular MS pattern, WOS+)

12.3.2 Explanation

12.3.2.1 Non-magnifying WLI Appearance

We can see a pale elevated 30 × 20 mm lesion in the region of the major duodenal papilla (Fig. 12.3a: side-viewing endoscopy image). The margins are distinctly visualized only using non-magnifying WLI. A depressed area is present within the lesion on the anal side, with a slightly bumpy irregular surface.

12.3.2.2 M-NBI Appearance

M-NBI examination at low magnification (Fig. 12.3b) reveals the presence of WOS over the entire tumor, and the difference in the MS patterns of the surface of the depression and its periphery can be evaluated to a certain extent, although evaluation of the MV pattern is not possible. Examination of the MS pattern of the depressed area using M-NBI at maximal magnifying ratio (Fig. 12.3c) reveals abundant WOS, and the MCE cannot be evaluated. Accordingly, using WOS as the marker, this is assessed as an irregular MS pattern. Due to the WOS, very few vessels can be visualized, so the MV pattern and VS discordance cannot be evaluated.

Examining the lesion outside the depression using M-NBI at maximal magnifying ratio (Fig. 12.3d), the WOS shows few characteristics typical of cancer such as irregularity or variability. Although there is slight nonuniformity of size, the directionality, distribution, and arrangement are relatively regular. A distinct difference can be seen between the depression and the rest of the lesion in the MS pattern.

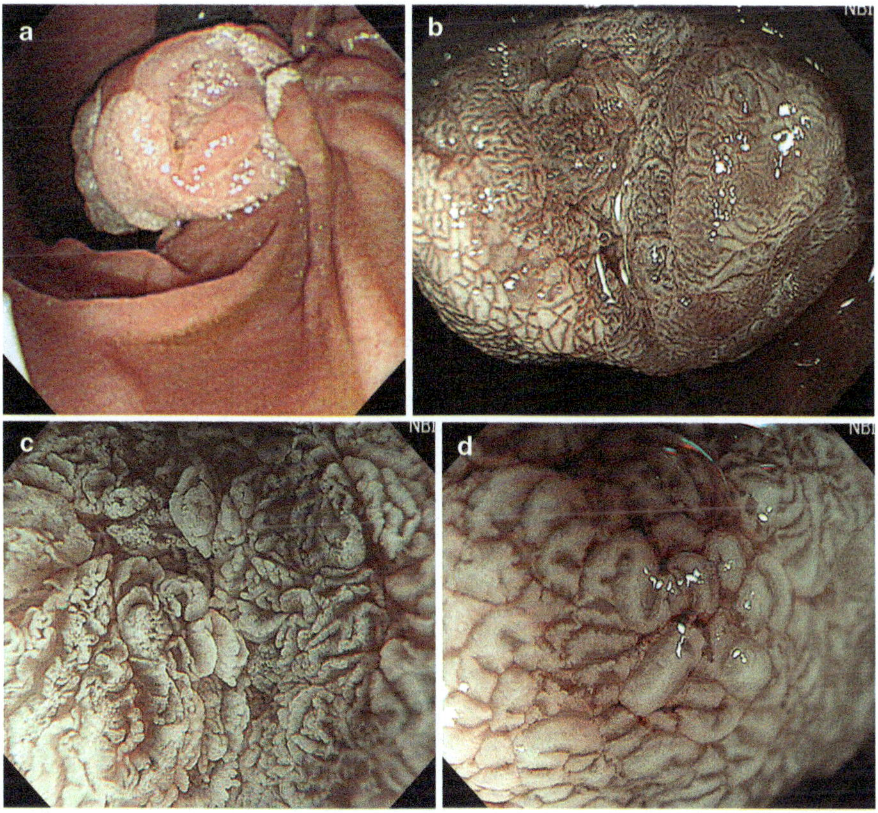

Fig. 12.3

12.3.2.3 Histological Findings

Histological examination of the biopsy specimen taken from the depressed area shown in Fig. 12.3c yields the diagnosis of papillary adenocarcinoma in the area shown in Fig. 12.3e. The biopsy specimen taken from the area shown in Fig. 12.3d has weaker atypia than the depressed area, and the histological findings are closer to adenoma (Fig. 12.3f).

12.3.3 Diagnostic Pointers for NBI

It is an easy matter to diagnose cancer in the depressed area from evaluation of the irregular MS pattern using WOS as the marker. Differences in histological differentiation between the depression surface and its periphery can be accurately determined from differences in the MS pattern.

The presence of WOS covering the entire tumor makes evaluation of the MV pattern impossible.

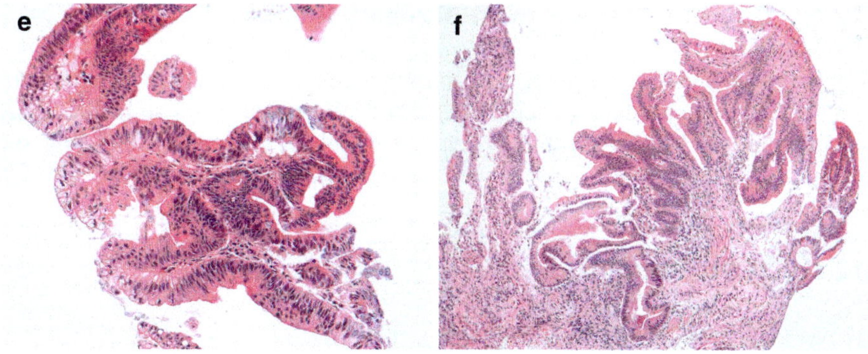

Fig. 12.3 (continued)

12.4 Duodenal Cancer (Non-papillary Region)

Cancer of the duodenum outside the papillary region is extremely rare. Although a diagnostic system for duodenal epithelioma has still not been firmly established, we have applied the VS classification system to the analysis of the M-NBI findings and here present the findings for an elevated early duodenal cancer.

12.4.1 M-NBI Findings

1. Marginal area (demarcation line: not examined)
2. Lesion (VS classification: absent/irregular MV pattern plus irregular MS pattern, WOS+)

12.4.2 Explanation

12.4.2.1 Non-magnifying WLI Appearance

We can see a pedunculated elevated lesion in the second part of the duodenum (Fig. 12.4a). The head of the polyp is predominantly white colored, with one reddish part. Indigo carmine dying (Fig. 12.4b) shows that the surface structure of the white area comprises a papillary to granular morphology, whereas the reddish part is close to nonstructured.

12.4.2.2 M-NBI Appearance (Water Immersion Technique)

Under low magnification (Fig. 12.4c), the findings are similar to those obtained using chromoendoscopy. When we examined the white area at the maximal magnifying ratio (Fig. 12.4d), compared to the width of the marginal villous epithelium (MVE), marginal crypt epithelium (MCE) in neoplasia is wider than the normal duodenal mucosa and forms rough papillary to tubular structures. This forms an irregular MS pattern with nonuniform sizes and irregular morphologies. The mucosal subepithelial vessels cannot be visualized due to the presence of WOS. On the other hand, examining the brown-colored area at the maximal magnifying ratio (Fig. 12.4e), we can visualize the subepithelial microvessels, proliferating in a rich and irregular variety, forming an irregular MV pattern.

12.4.2.3 Histological Findings

In the ESD specimen (Fig. 12.4f), we can see tumor glands with marked structural and cellular atypia, proliferating in tubular to papillary shapes.

12.4.3 Diagnostic Pointers for NBI

In the resected specimen, the tumor was localized within the mucosa. More detailed examination reveals a region with a high glandular density, corresponding to the reddish area (brown with NBI), and a region of rough tubular adenocarcinoma, corresponding to the white area (WOS+ with NBI). We should always imagine such histological architecture when we investigate endoscopic appearance.

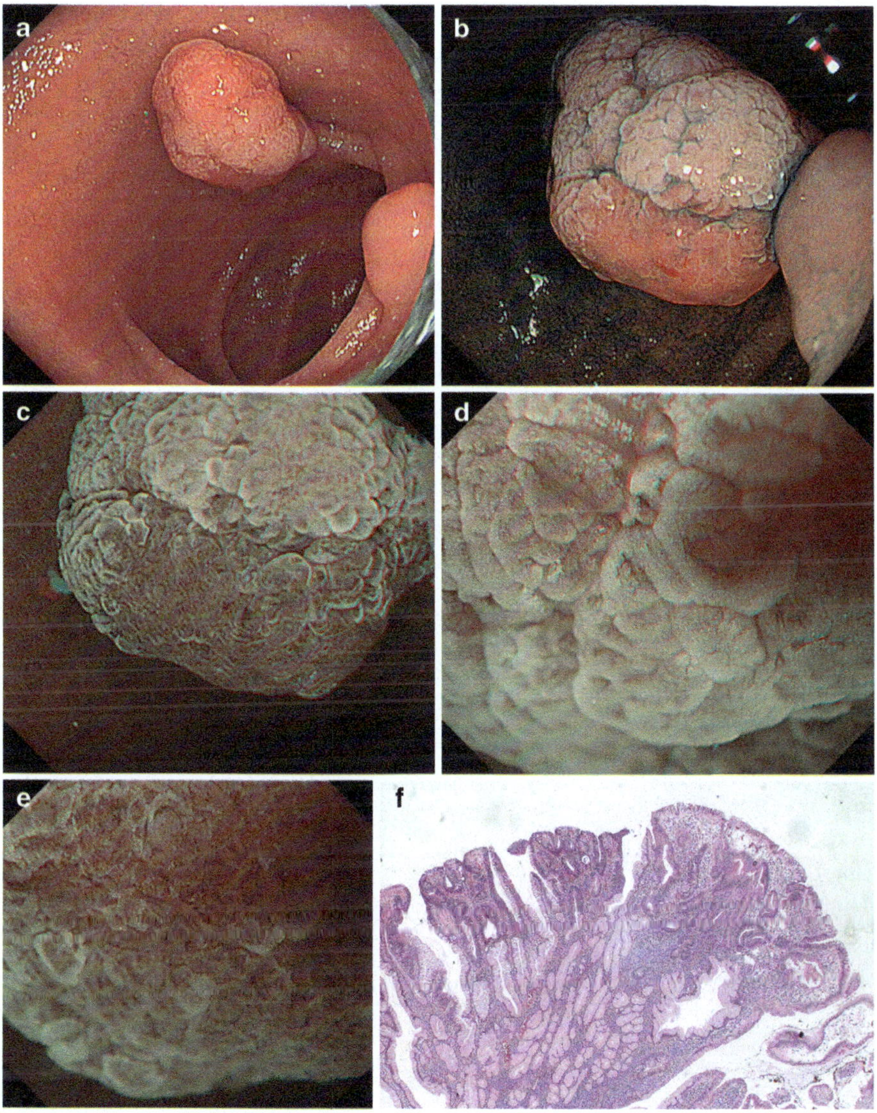

Fig. 12.4

Part IV

Atlas of NBI: Colon to Rectum

Overview

13

Yasushi Sano and Shinji Tanaka

13.1 Diagnostic System

13.1.1 Improved Polyp Detection Rates Using New-Generation NBI System (ELITE) in Screening Colonoscopy

A number of studies examining a possible add-on effect for NBI in colorectal tumor detection rates had not confirmed improved detection rates for colorectal polyps.

However, a recent prospective study in a multicenter trial in Japan showed that the new-generation NBI system (ELITE) with brighter light improved polyp detection rates significantly. Accordingly, in screening colonoscopy, it is preferable to detect a lesion using the new-generation NBI system [1].

13.1.2 Capillary Pattern Classification

The normal colorectal mucosa comprises intestinal crypts surrounded by a regular capillary network in a regular hexagonal or honeycomb-like pattern (Fig. 13.1a).

In general, on the surface of a neoplastic lesion, we see dilatation of these vessels, neovascular proliferation, or destruction of the vascular structure. In nonneoplastic lesions such as hyperplastic polyps, except inflammatory polyps, we do not see any definite vessel changes. Examination of microcapillary patterns associated with neoplastic lesions using NBI reveals brownish meshed vessels, dilated more than normal vessels. The authors refer to these as "meshed capillary (MC) vessels."

Y. Sano (✉)
Gastrointestinal Center, Sano Hospital, 2-5-1 Simizugaoka, Tarumi-ku, Kobe, Hyogo 655-0031, Japan
e-mail: ys_endoscopy@hotmail.com

S. Tanaka
Department of Endoscopy, Hiroshima University Hospital, Hiroshima, Japan

M. Muto et al. (eds.), *Atlas of Endoscopy with Narrow Band Imaging*,
DOI 10.1007/978-4-431-54243-8_13

Furthermore, for the purpose of qualitative assessment, we classify MC vessels into the following three types (capillary patterns (CPs); Fig. 13.2).

13.1.2.1 CP Type I

These are capillaries surrounding each crypt, with a regular hexagonal or honeycomb-like morphology. These vessels have a diameter of approximately 10 μm, making them difficult to discern with the resolution of presently available endoscopes. This pattern is seen in the normal mucosa or hyperplastic polyps.

13.1.2.2 CP Type II

With a diameter somewhat larger than that seen in the normal mucosa, these capillaries encircle the tubular or oval intestinal crypts. The honeycomb-like morphology may be preserved in places. These vessels are discernable with the resolution of presently available endoscopes. This pattern is seen in adenomatous polyps.

13.1.2.3 CP Type III

With a diameter somewhat larger than that seen in the normal mucosa, these capillaries irregularly encircle the intestinal crypts. Findings of capillaries with nonuniform diameters, interruptions, or increased density may be seen. The honeycomb-like morphology may be destructed. These vessels are discernable with the resolution of presently available endoscopes. This pattern is seen in cancer.

CP type III subgroups

III A: Lesions with vessels with marked irregularity (nonuniform diameters, tortuous, branching, or interrupted) over a circumscribed area

III B: Lesions with a circumscribed area with indistinct microvessels

13.1.3 Clinical Usefulness of the CP Classification

A therapeutic flowchart for NBI examinations is shown in Fig. 13.3.

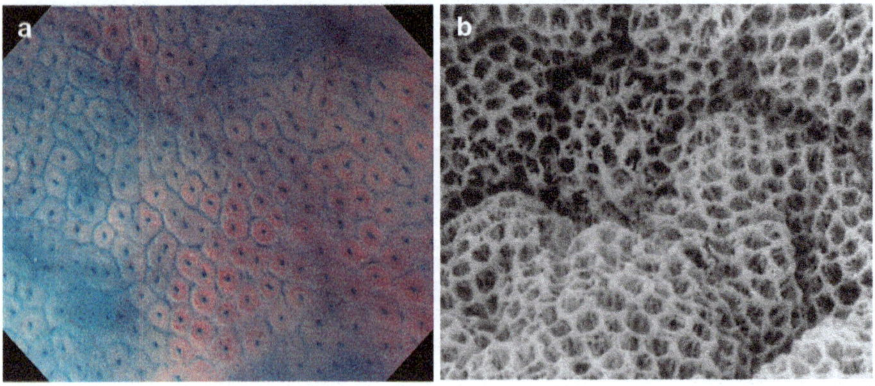

Fig. 13.1 (**a**) Capillary network in the normal colorectal mucosa. Indigo carmine dye sprayed appearance of the normal colorectal mucosa. We can see dot-shaped intestinal crypt openings (Kudo's type I pit pattern) and hexagonal grooves surrounding each crypt. (**b**) Capillary architecture of normal colorectal mucosa (scanning electron microscope (SEM) image). The vessels surround each crypt opening (honeycomb-like pattern)

Capillary pattern	I	II	IIIA	IIIB
Schema	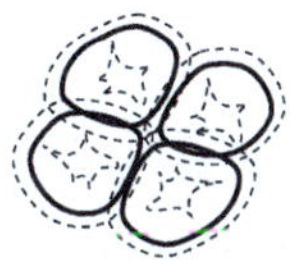	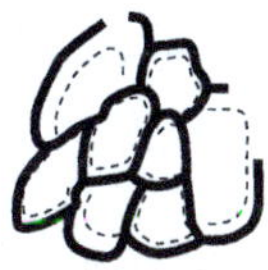	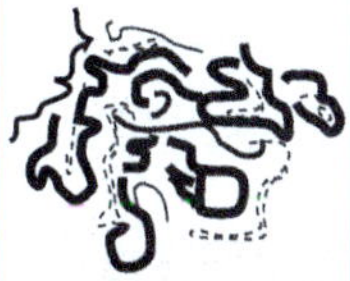	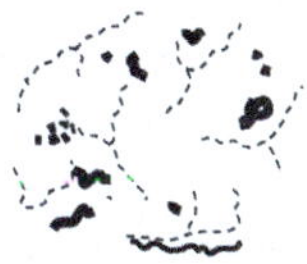
Endoscopic findings	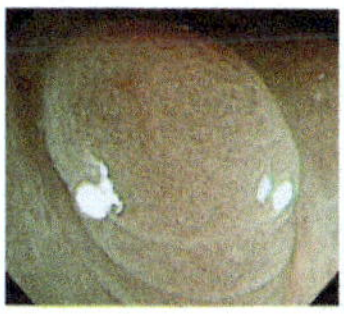	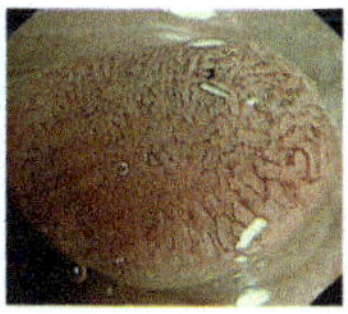	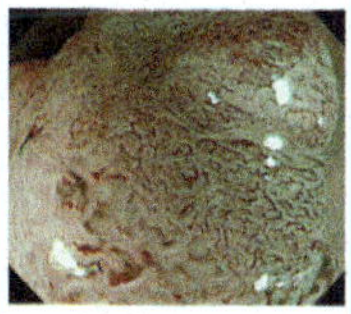	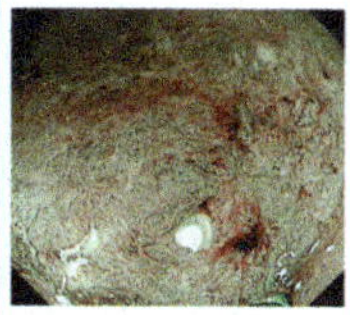
Capillary characteristics	Meshed capillary vessels (-)	• Meshed capillary vessels (+) • Capillary vessel surrounds mucosal glands	Meshed capillary vessels characterized by: blind ending, branching and curtailed irregularly • Lack of uniformity • High density of capillary vessels	• Nearly avascular or loose micro capillary vessels

Capillary pattern	Accuracy	Sensitivity	Specificity	PPV	NPV
Type I vs II [1, 2]	95.3 %	96.4 %	92.3 %	97.3 %	90.0 %
type II vs III [3]	95.5 %	90.3 %	97.1 %	90.3 %	97.1 %
type IIIA vs IIIB [4, 5]	87.7 %	84.8 %	88.7 %	71.8 %	94.5 %

Fig. 13.2 Capillary pattern classification (Sano's classification)

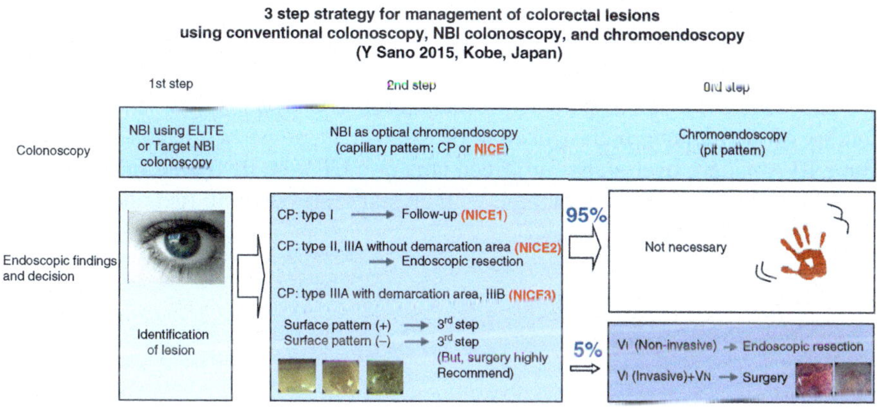

Fig. 13.3 Flowchart for diagnosis and treatment using NBI colonoscopy (3-step strategy) (Y Sano 2014, Kobe, Japan)

13.1.3.1 Differentiation Between Neoplastic and Nonneoplastic Lesions (Capillary Pattern Type I Versus Type II)

Determination of whether MC vessels are present or not is extremely useful in differentiating between neoplastic and nonneoplastic lesions. In a prospective trial, we found that the presence of MC vessels yielded an accuracy of 95.3 %, sensitivity of 96.4 %, and specificity of 92.3 % in diagnosing a neoplastic lesion [2]. A validation study conducted at another institution found that detection of MC vessels using NBI was also of benefit to less-experienced endoscopists [3]. Accordingly the use of NBI is thought to render chromoendoscopy, e.g., with indigo carmine, all but unnecessary for the decision whether to resect a lesion.

13.1.3.2 Differentiation Between Adenoma and Cancer (Capillary Pattern Type II Versus Type III)

Detection of a brown MC vessel structure is useful in differentiating between adenoma and cancer. The results of a prospective study of the correlation between CP type and tissue type showed that CP type II corresponds to adenomas with mild to moderate atypia and CP type III to adenomas with severe atypia or adenocarcinoma [4]. It is therefore possible to predict the tumor tissue type without performing chromoendoscopy.

13.1.3.3 Determination of the Depth of Invasion (Capillary Pattern Type III A Versus Type III B)

A detailed examination of a CP type III lesion, subclassified into type III A or III B, is useful in determining the depth of invasion of the lesion. The authors performed multiple regression analysis of the variability of atypical vessels identified using magnifying NBI, finding that vessel regularity and vessel density are independent predictors of SM cancer [5]. Furthermore, the prospective study by Ikematsu et al. found that these findings (CP types III A and III B) correlate with SM cancer [6].

However, the diagnostic ability of these patterns does not surpass the diagnostic ability of the pit pattern classification of Kudo et al., so when a lesion shows a CP type III A pattern over a circumscribed area or a CP type III B pattern, chromoendoscopy should be performed, e.g., with crystal violet staining (detailed examination of the type V pit pattern).

13.2 NBI International Colorectal Endoscopic (NICE) Classification (CTNIG Consensus)

13.2.1 Present State of Classification of NBI Colonoscopy Findings

At present, considerable debate occurs at scientific meetings concerning the magnifying NBI findings of colorectal tumors. Several classifications exist, with a variety of different definitions and interpretations, and a uniform classification of magnifying NBI colonoscopy findings has yet to be established.

On the other hand, even without using a magnifying endoscope, close examination using a modern high-resolution electronic endoscope allows us to discern the surface pattern of a colorectal tumor to some extent [7]. Similarly, we can discern the blood vessels to a certain extent using non-magnifying NBI. We can also see the surface pattern more clearly due to the NBI structure enhancement function [8]. Magnifying endoscopy is rarely used in the general clinical setting in Western countries, and even in Japan, it could not be said that magnifying endoscopy is widely used in the colorectal field.

13.2.2 NICE Classification

Against this background, we developed a simple classification of the NBI findings of colorectal tumors, suitable for use not only with magnifying endoscopy but also with close examination using a high-resolution electronic endoscopy system. We are presently conducting joint research with Western endoscopist colleagues [9].

As shown in Table 13.1, the classification is a simple one with three categories. It is based on three parameters: (1) color of the lesion (color), (2) microvascular pattern (vessels), and (3) microsurface pattern (surface pattern).

Type 1 is considered a marker of hyperplastic lesions, type 2 of adenomas, and type 3 of SM invasive cancer (Fig. 13.4).

NICE classification corresponds to CP classification (NICE type 1 ≒ CP type I, NICE type 2 ≒ CP type II or IIIA, NICE type 3 ≒ CP type IIIB). A validation study, conducted at six institutions in Japan and Western countries with the aim of objectively confirming the clinical usefulness of this classification, was recently completed, yielding favorable results [10, 11]. The six members of the Colon Tumor NBI Interest Group (CTNIG) are Drs. Shinji Tanaka and Yasushi Sano (Japan), Drs. Douglas K. Rex and Roy M. Soetikno (USA), Dr. Thierry Ponchon (France), and Dr. Brian P. Saunders (UK).

A great advantage of this NICE classification is that it can be used to perform NBI examinations of colorectal tumors, without employing magnifying endoscopy. Of course, magnifying NBI is needed to accurately differentiate between adenoma and cancer or to determine the depth of invasion by a cancer, but this would require wider use of magnifying endoscopes and the development of a uniform classification of magnifying NBI findings, as mentioned above. We believe this NICE classification has the potential to become the basis for a magnifying NBI classification.

We are confident that as more endoscopists adopt and gain an understanding of this classification, it will serve as an introduction to magnifying NBI for those not yet employing magnifying endoscopy.

Table 13.1 NBI International Colorectal Endoscopic (NICE) classification[a]

	Type 1	Type 2	Type 3
Color	Same or lighter than background	Browner relative to background (verify color arises from vessels)	Brown to dark brown relative to background; sometimes patchy whiter areas
Vessels	None, or isolated lacy vessels may be present coursing across the lesion	Brown vessels surrounding white structures[b]	Has area(s) of disrupted or missing vessels
Surface pattern	Dark or white spots of uniform size, or homogeneous absence of pattern	Oval, tubular or branched white structures[b] surrounded by brown vessels	Amorphous or absent surface pattern
Most likely pathology	*Hyperplastic and sessile serrated polyp (SSP)*[c]	*Adenoma*[d]	*Deep submucosal invasive cancer*

[a]Can be applied using colonoscopes with/without optical (zoom) magnification

[b]These structures (regular or irregular) may represent the pits and the epithelium of the crypt opening

[c]In the WHO classification, sessile serrated polyp and sessile serrated adenoma are synonymous

[d]Type 2 consists of Vienna classification types 3, 4 and superficial 5 (all adenomas with either low- or high-grade dysplasia, or with superficial submucosal carcinoma). The presence of high-grade dysplasia or superficial submucosal carcinoma may be suggested by an irregular vessel or surface pattern and is often associated with atypical morphology (e.g., depressed area)

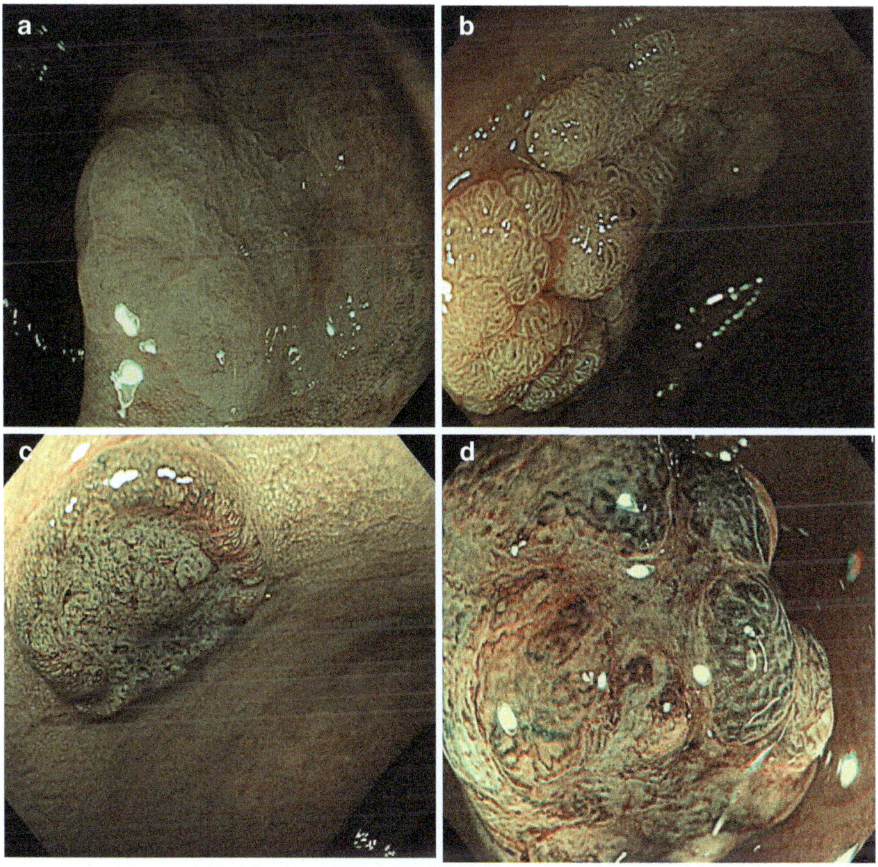

Fig. 13.4 Examples of types 1–3. (**a**) Same or lighter color than the background, microvessels cannot be discerned (type 1). (**b**) The surface pattern is indirectly distinct and regular, through brownish coloration around the crypts and structure enhancement (type 2). (**c**, **d**) Irregular microvessels with nonuniform diameters are seen as brown colored; no surface pattern can be discerned (type 3)

References

1. Horimatsu T, et al: Int J Colorectal **30**: 947–954, 2015
2. Sano Y, et al: Gastrointest Endosc **69**: 278–283, 2009
3. Higashi R, et al: Gastointest Endosc **72**: 127–135, 2010
4. Katagiri A, et al: Aliment Pharmacol Ther 27: 1269–1274, 2008
5. Fukuzawa M, et al: World J Gasroenterol **16**: 1727–1734, 2010
6. Ikematsu H, et al: BMC Gastroenterol **10**: 33, 2010
7. Tanaka S, et al. Stomach and Intestine 34: 1635–1644, 1999
8. Tanaka S, et al: Dig Endosc **18** (Suppl): S52–56, 2006
9. Oba S, et al: Digestion **83**: 167–172, 2011
10. Hewett DG et al. Gastroenterology. 2012;143:599–643.
11. Hayashi N, et al. Gastrointest Endosc 78, 625–38, 2013

14 Atlas of Normal Appearance

Hirohisha Machida and Yasushi Sano

H. Machida
Machida Gastroenterical Hospital, Osaka, Japan
e-mail: h-machida@med.osaka-cu.ac.jp

Y. Sano (✉)
Gastrointestinal Center, Sano Hospital, Kobe, Japan

M. Muto et al. (eds.), *Atlas of Endoscopy with Narrow Band Imaging*,
DOI 10.1007/978-4-431-54243-8_14

14.1 Peyer's Patches

Peyer's patches are an important part of the intestinal immune system and are involved in the uptake and presentation of antigens. Individual lymph nodes first appear in the jejunum, and in the ileum the lymphoid tissue increases, forming 20–30 Peyer's patches within the mucosa along or opposite the line of mesenteric attachment. Each Peyer's patch comprises approximately 20 lymph nodules.

Unlike regions without Peyer's patches, microfold cells (M cells) are scattered throughout the mucosal epithelium covering a Peyer's patch. M cells have a pocket-like structure on their basolateral side in which T cells and B cells are located. M cells take up antigenic substances from the intestinal lumen and present them to the T cells and B cells, thereby transmitting information to immunocytes within the Peyer's patch. This processing of antigens is the main role played by M cells, and it is characteristic of the epithelium covering the Peyer's patches that intestinal villi do not develop there and microvilli are not present.

14.1.1 Explanation

14.1.1.1 Non-magnifying Endoscopic Appearance

Non-magnifying endoscopic examination reveals Peyer's patches as pale islets in the ileum (Fig. 14.1a, seen in the lower ileum). As villi are absent over the patches, they appear on close examination as depressed areas paler or the same color as the surrounding mucosa (Fig. 14.1b). They also appear as depressed areas lacking villi using non-magnifying NBI (Fig. 14.1c).

14.1.1.2 Magnifying Endoscopic Appearance

Magnifying endoscopic examination reveals no clear surface pattern, giving an unstructured appearance, with no irregular vessels (Fig. 14.1d). Magnifying NBI examination reveals a white smooth surfaced area where a surface pattern cannot be visualized, with vessels showing no irregularity thought to be located in the submucosal layer (14.1e).

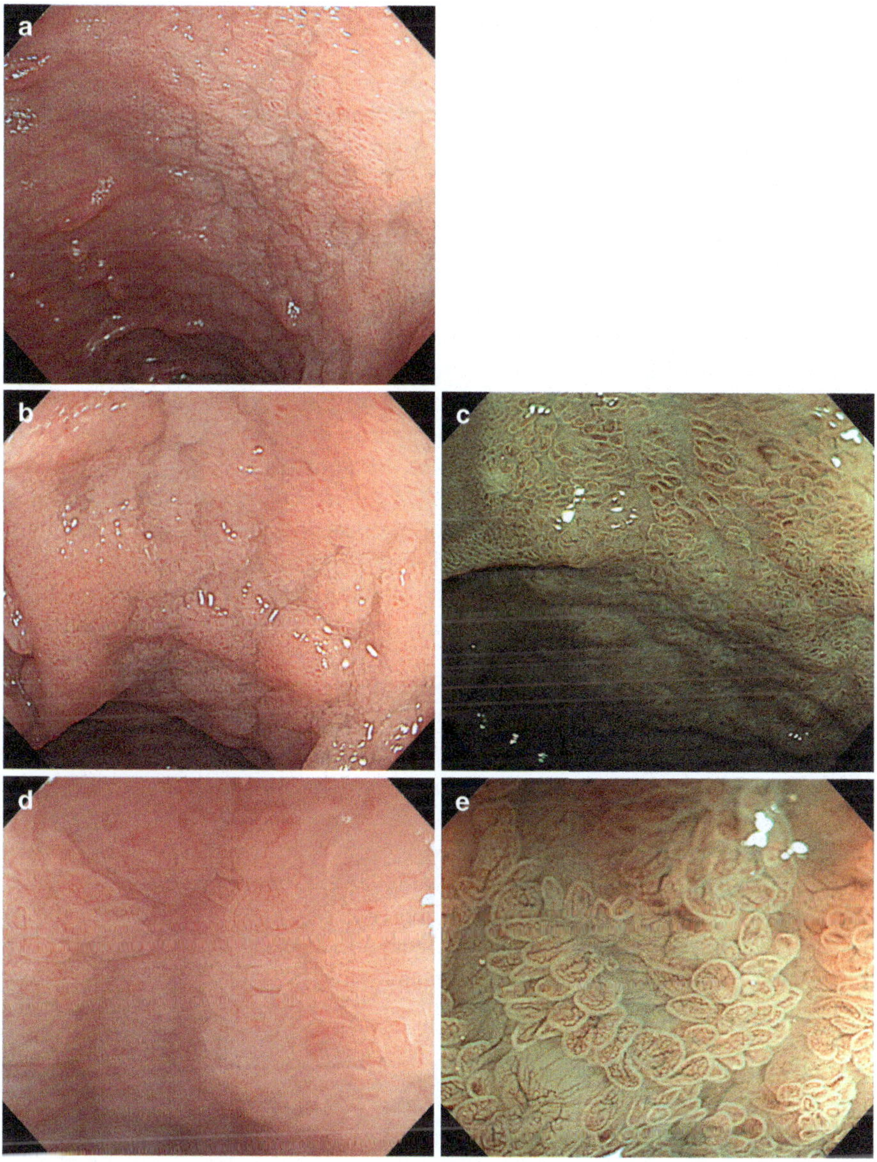

Fig. 14.1 Peyer paches

14.2 Normal Colonic Epithelium

More detailed examination of the capillaries and the surface microstructure has become possible with changing the spectral characteristics of the light source in gastrointestinal endoscopes over to a narrow band, or NBI.

14.2.1 Explanation

14.2.1.1 Endoscopic Examination

Examination of the normal colorectal mucosa using NBI allows us to see the capillary network of the normal mucosa more clearly than with WLI (Fig. 14.2a WLI, Fig. 14.2b NBI) [1]. If a lesion is present, it will be easier to detect using NBI because visibility of the capillaries will be improved.

Magnifying endoscopic examination of the normal colorectal mucosa shows normal intestinal crypts in a regular arrangement and honeycomb-like pattern with no nonuniformity of size. In the center of each section can be seen an oval crypt opening 0.07 ± 0.02 mm in diameter [2]. The crypt openings are visualized as white using NBI (Fig. 14.2c) and are also clearly delineated by chromoendoscopy using indigo carmine (Fig. 14.2d) or crystal violet (Fig. 14.2e).

14.2.1.2 Electron Microscopic and Histological Findings

In the normal colorectal mucosa, capillaries showing a regular hexagonal or honeycomb-like pattern (Fig. 14.2f, g) are located in the stroma directly beneath the epithelium (Fig. 14.2h, i), surrounding the crypt openings [3, 4]. The vascular network of the normal mucosa (Fig. 14.2f) is made up of arterioles running perpendicularly up from the submucosa and venules running parallel to the arterioles (Fig. 14.2g). Vascular endothelium staining for CD31 is located immediately beneath the normal mucosal epithelium (Fig. 14.2i arrow). However, these capillaries are 12.0 ± 0.1 μm in diameter, making them difficult to visualize with the resolution of presently available gastrointestinal endoscopes.

14.2.2 Diagnostic Pointers for NBI

When magnifying NBI examination is able to visualize few or no capillaries surrounding crypt openings, we can be confident that we are looking at normal mucosa, or a hyperplastic polyp.

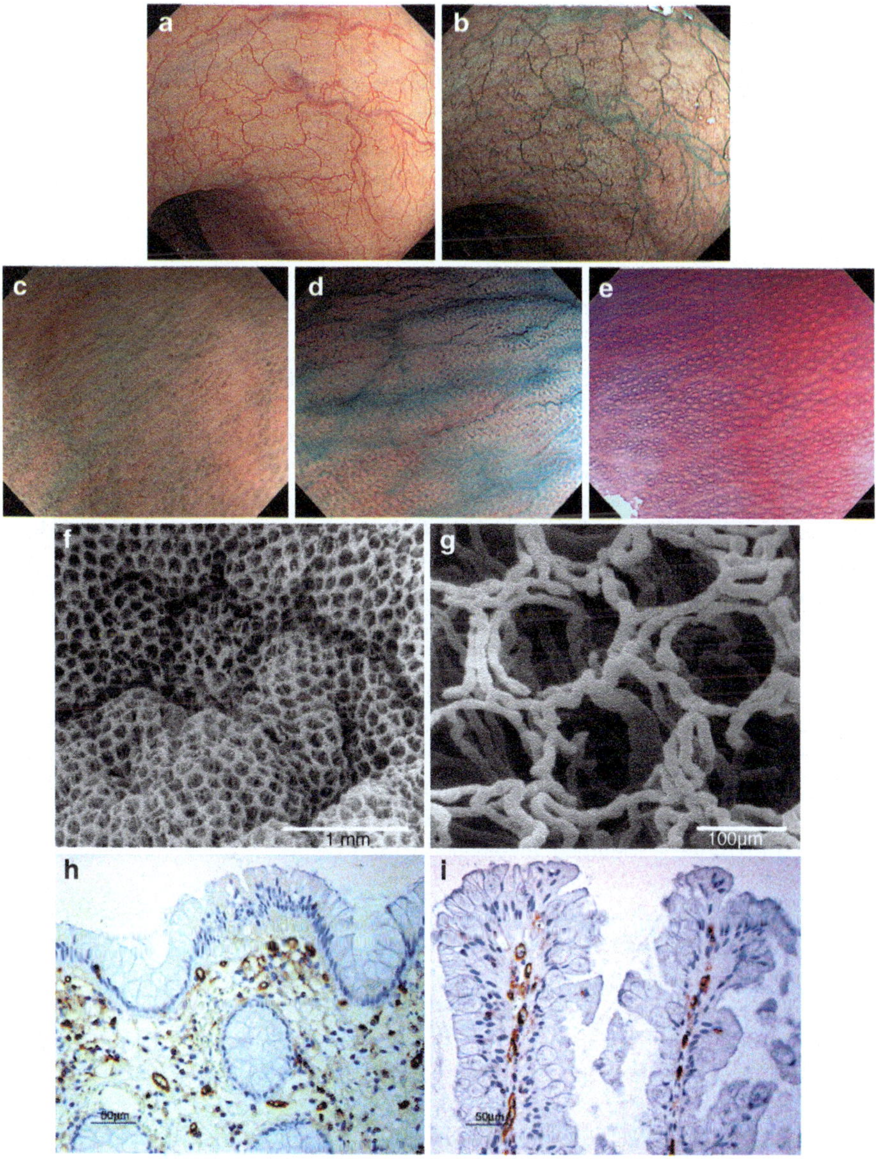

Fig. 14.2 Normal colorectal mucosa

14.3 Anal Canal Epithelium

The anal canal can be defined in two different ways, as the surgical anal canal or anatomical surgical canal (Fig. 14.3). Clinically, examination of the surgical anal canal is important in terms of considering possible surgical procedures. Accordingly, it is important to know the histological structures from the anorectal ring to the anal verge.

14.3.1 Histological Structures of the Surgical Anal Canal

The dentate line, the boundary between the ectodermal proctodeum (primitive anus) and endodermal hindgut (primitive rectum), is formed by raised areas, the anal papillae, and depressed areas, the anal crypts (Fig. 14.3). These extend as far as the anorectal ring (where they disappear is also called Herrmann's line). The anal crypts are 6–11 in number, on average 8, extending around the entire circumference of the anal canal. The anal crypts contain the openings of the anal glands and anal ducts (infection of the anal glands can lead to perianal abscesses or anal fistulae). The anatomical anal canal extends from the anal verge to the dentate line and has sensation through branches of the pudendal nerve; there is no sensation above the dentate line.

The anal canal is lined by a simple columnar epithelium above the dentate line and a stratified squamous epithelium below it. The gap between the inner and outer anal sphincters is referred to as the intersphincteric groove, and the area between the intersphincteric groove and the dentate line as the zona cutanea. The zona cutanea is lined by stratified squamous epithelium (anal epithelium). Distal to the intersphincteric groove is found cutaneous epithelium.

14.3.2 Advantages of NBI Examination

Using NBI, as with the gastroesophageal junction, the dentate line is easily identified as the distinct boundary between squamous epithelium and columnar epithelium. The vascular findings are similar to those in the esophageal and rectal mucosae.

Non-magnifying WLI examination of the lower rectum reveals a dentate line somewhat indistinct in its entire circumference (Fig. 14.4a), whereas the dentate line is clearly discernible using magnifying NBI (Fig. 14.4b arrows).

Magnifying NBI examination of the boundary between the lower rectum and the anal canal shows the transition zone between simple columnar epithelium and stratified squamous epithelium as distinct brown- and greenish-white-colored areas. Figure 14.4c shows the greenish-white zona cutanea, and Fig. 14.4d clearly shows the dentate line and the border of the columnar epithelial mucosa (arrows indicate the dentate line, columnar epithelial mucosa to the right).

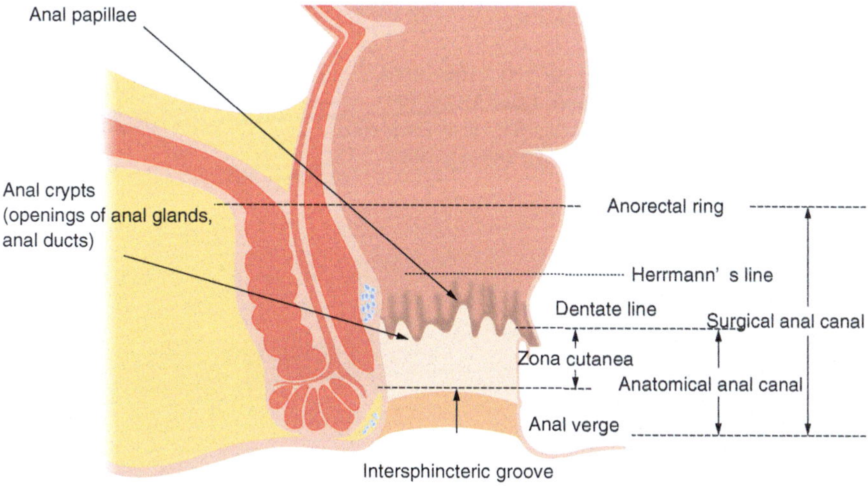

Fig. 14.3 Anatomical chart of anal canal

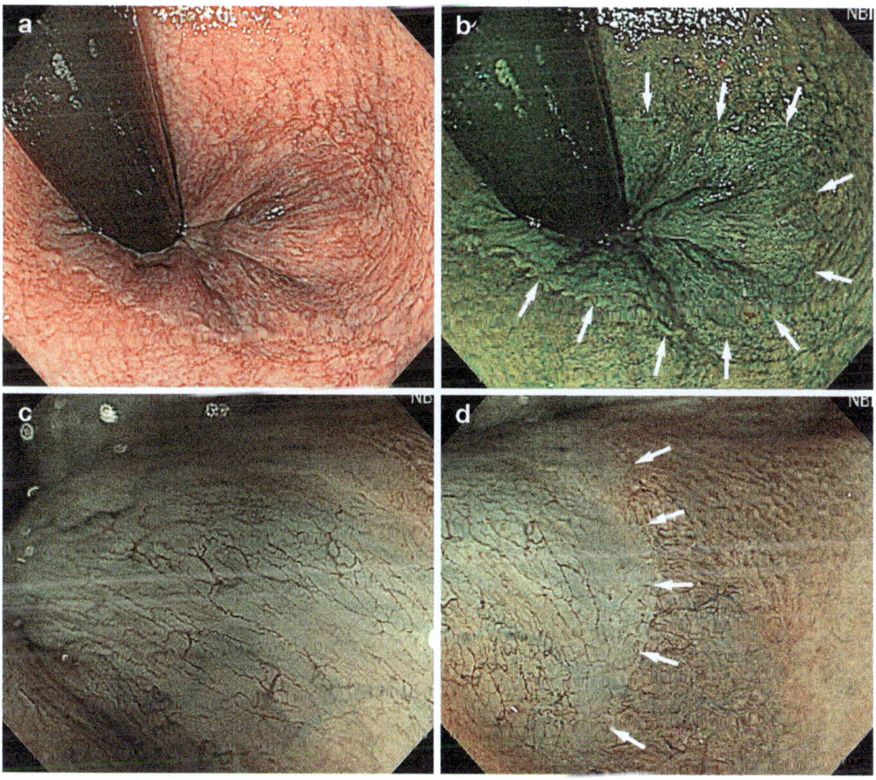

Fig. 14.4 Lower rectum

References

1. Machida H, et al: Endoscopy **36**: 1094–1098, 2004
2. Kudo S. Early colorectal cancer. Igaku Shoin, 1993
3. Konerding MA, et al: Br J Cancer **84**: 1354–1362, 2001
4. Sano Y, et al: Endosc **18** (Suppl 1): S44–51, 2006

Atlas of Nonneoplastic Lesions

15

Hirohisa Machida, Kougi Fu, Nobuo Aoyama,
Takashi Narabayashi, and Yasushi Sano

H. Machida (✉)
Machida Gastroenterical Hospital, Osaka, Japan
e-mail: h-machida@med.osaka-cu.ac.jp

K. Fu
Kamma Memorial Hospital, Nasushiobara, Japan

N. Aoyama
GI Endoscopy and IBD Center, Aoyama Clinic, Kobe, Japan

T. Narabayashi
Department of Gastroenterology, Narabayashi Hospital, Kobe, Japan

Y. Sano
Department of Gastrointestinal Center, Sano Hospital, Kobe, Japan

M. Muto et al. (eds.), *Atlas of Endoscopy with Narrow Band Imaging*,
DOI 10.1007/978-4-431-54243-8_15

15.1 Feces

The feces remaining within the gastrointestinal tract (residual feces) often give the appearance of red- to scarlet-colored superficial raised lesions (Fig. 15.1a, b), and bowel preparation fluid is seen as a reddish liquid (Fig. 15.1c, d) using NBI. Either may be confused with blood, but switching over from NBI to WLI makes it easy to differentiate between them.

The NBI system setup comprises an NBI filter that can be introduced or withdrawn from between the RGB rotating filter and xenon lamp within the light source unit. Though three primary colors red (R), green (G), and blue (B) used in WLI, NBI comprises light with two wavelengths, blue (415 nm) and green (540 nm). To produce a color image, a WLI video processor allocates red input to the R channel on the monitor, green to the G channel, and blue to the B channel. In an NBI system, out of consideration of human visual characteristics, the images taken with 415 nm incident light are allocated to the B and G channels and those taken with 540 nm incident light to the R channel [1].

Residual feces and bowel preparation fluid are seen as yellow using WLI, and on the endoscopy system monitor, yellow is displayed using red (R) and green (G). This suggests that no light that would be allocated to the blue (B) channel is emitted by residual feces or bowel preparation fluid. In other words, residual feces and bowel preparation fluid strongly absorb blue (B) wavelengths.

When a substance that absorbs blue (B) wavelengths is examined using NBI, of the two wavelength components of NBI, blue (central wavelength 415 nm) and green (central wavelength 540 nm), the blue wavelengths are absorbed, and only the green wavelengths return to the charge-coupled device (CCD) in the endoscope tip. In an NBI system, green (central wavelength 540 nm) incident light is allocated to the R channel, so in the end residual feces and bowel preparation fluid are seen as red on the monitor.

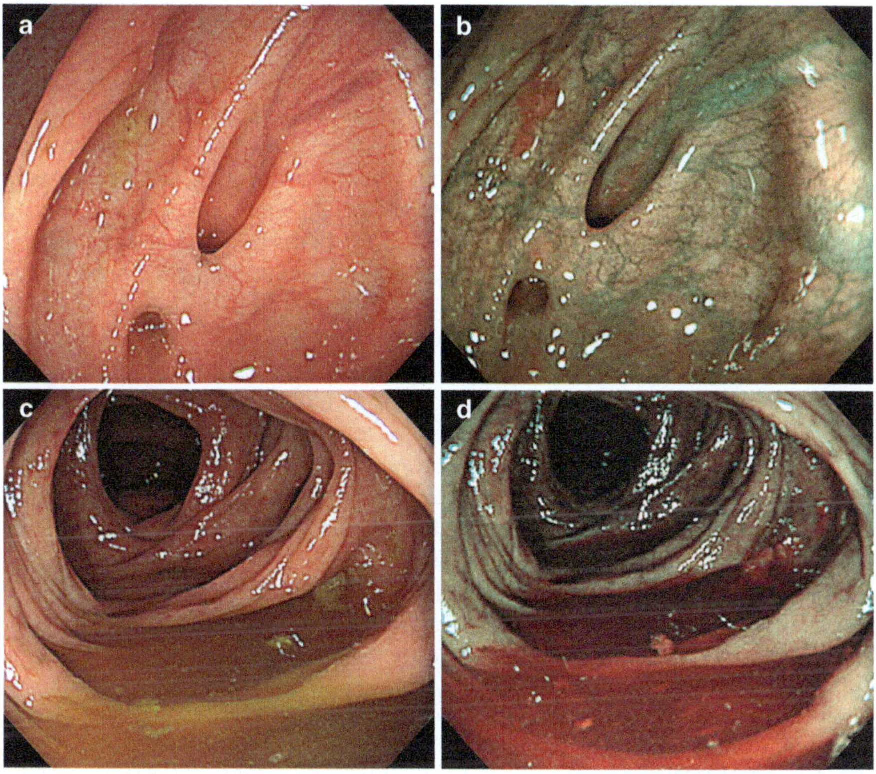

Fig. 15.1 Residual feces

15.2 Inflammatory Polyp [2]

Inflammatory polyps can arise throughout the colon. Polypoid lesions (mucosal protuberances) are formed secondary to colonic inflammation, such as inflammatory bowel disease or infectious enterocolitis. They are broadly classified into acute and chronic inflammatory polyps. Acute inflammatory polyps, or pseudopolyps, are areas of residual mucosa relatively elevated in comparison to multiple erosions or ulcers. Chronic inflammatory polyps arise as a regenerative reaction in the damaged mucosa, forming protuberances with no muscularis mucosae, showing fingerlike, stringlike, or other morphologies. Their coloration varies widely with the degree of inflammation, from pale to reddish. As they are the result of inflammation or ulceration, chronic inflammatory polyps range in size from microscopic to large enough to cause obstructive symptoms.

Typical inflammatory polyps are seen in the colonic mucosa in patients with ulcerative colitis, and multiple lesions are also referred to as inflammatory polyposis. Apart from ulcerative colitis, with a prevalence of 10–30 %, inflammatory polyps are also seen in patients with Crohn's disease, tuberculosis, ischemic colitis, and infectious colitis, e.g., amebic dysentery. Inflammatory polyps are also seen postoperatively at enteroenteric anastomosis sites.

The main pathohistological feature of inflammatory polyps is inflammation of the lamina propria; little or no nuclear atypia is seen, and they arise from near-normal glandular epithelium. They arise as single or multiple lesions, whether inflammation is active or has already receded [1].

15.2.1 Explanation

This 4 mm reddened small protuberance can be seen on the anal side of an area of ischemic colitis in the descending colon (Fig. 15.2a). Non-magnifying WLI examination reveals crypt openings appearing as white dots, with reddened surrounds (Fig. 15.2b).

Low-magnifying NBI examination visualizes the area seen as reddish with WLI as green in color (Fig. 15.2c). At higher magnification, surface vessels cannot be visualized, and this was assessed as CP type 1 (Fig. 15.2d). Indigo carmine spraying shows that the lesion pits are the same size as the pits in the surrounding mucosa, corresponding to type I pits in Kudo's classification. Accordingly, an inflammatory polyp associated with ischemic colitis was suspected (Fig. 15.2e).

The histological findings of hyperplastic colon mucosa were not inconsistent with an inflammatory polyp (Fig. 15.2f).

15.2.2 NBI Characteristics

NBI delineates vessels in the mucosal surface layers as brown and vessels in the deep mucosal layers as green. Inflammatory polyps are nonneoplastic lesions, so brown-meshed capillary vessels in the superficial layers, as found in neoplastic lesions, are not visualized (CP type I, NICE type 1).

One reason this lesion was visualized as green in color using NBI was thought to be vasodilatation, particularly in the deep mucosal layers. Histological examination of the resected specimen also showed dilatation and filling of deep mucosal vessels (Fig. 15.2f).

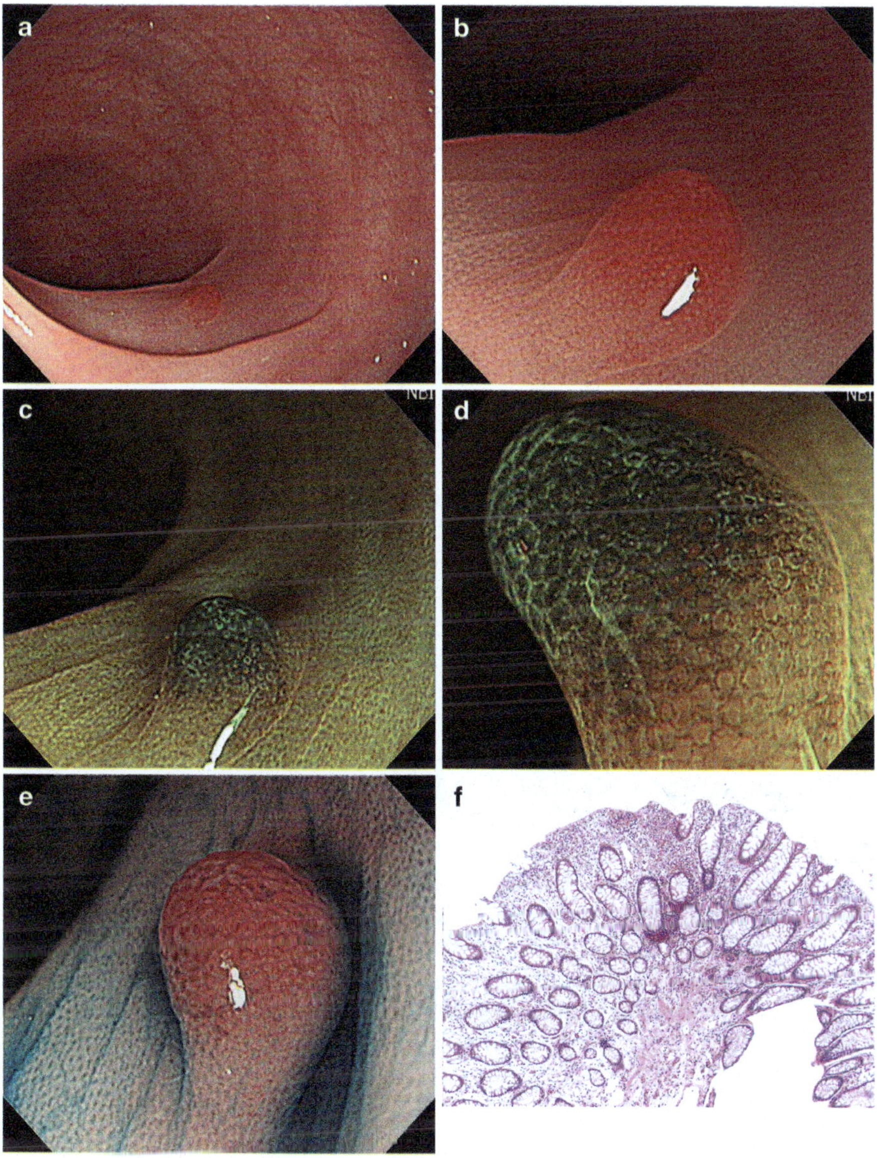

Fig. 15.2 Inflammatory polyp

15.3 Hyperplastic Polyp

Polyps are the most commonly seen lesions during colonoscopies. When a polyp is detected, in the first place a qualitative differential diagnosis, determining whether it is neoplastic or nonneoplastic, is essential in deciding treatment. This is because if the lesion is assessed as nonneoplastic (excluding some specific types, like large lesions), it is possible that no treatment will be an option (periodic monitoring), with no need for endoscopic treatment. Most of the nonneoplastic lesions are hyperplastic polyps 5 mm in size, and most of the neoplastic lesions are adenomas.

15.3.1 Explanation

For non-magnifying WLI examinations, this qualitative assessment is generally based on the lesion color and surface characteristics. Hyperplastic polyps are smooth surfaced, whitish in color, sometimes with mucus adherent to the surface (Fig. 15.3a). Magnifying endoscopy following dye spraying reveals a type II pit morphology (Fig. 15.3b), thought to correspond histologically to serrated glands. This qualitative assessment using magnifying chromoendoscopy has been reported to yield a greater than 95 % diagnostic accuracy.

On the other hand, because NBI uses short-wavelength incident light, it can clearly delineate the surface microvascular pattern and morphological changes. Neovascularization is seen in neoplastic lesions, increasing the vascular density, and the vessel diameters also increase, making them appear as brown blobs using NBI.

The authors refer to the dilated meshed vessels seen in neoplastic lesions as meshed capillary (MC) vessels. As little or no neovascularization is seen in hyperplastic polyps (CP type I, NICE type 1) (Fig. 15.3c–e), we can make the qualitative differential diagnosis between neoplastic and nonneoplastic lesion based on whether MC vessels are present or not. This is a useful and extremely simple method reported to have a diagnostic accuracy similar to that achieved with magnifying chromoendoscopy. Furthermore, the use of immunostaining in histological examinations (Fig. 15.3f) has demonstrated significantly higher vascular density in adenomas in comparison with hyperplastic polyps (particularly significant for vessels with diameters $\geq$10 μm).

15.3.2 Future Challenges

A future challenge is the endoscopic differential diagnosis between hyperplastic polyps and sessile serrated adenomas/polyps which have histologically similar serrated glands.

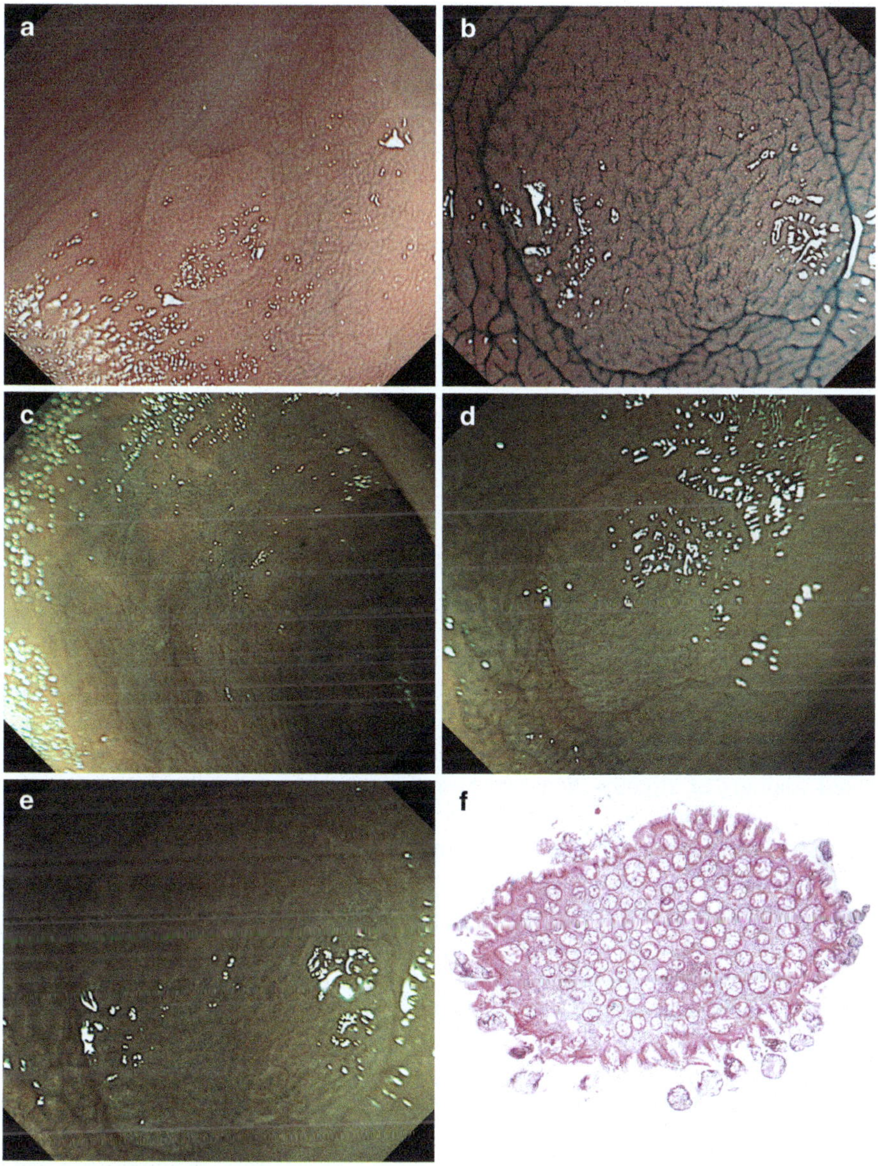

Fig. 15.3 Hyperplastic polyp

15.4 Ulcerative Colitis

Because there are no definite diagnosis regarding pathognomonic, endoscopic, or pathohistological findings for ulcerative colitis (UC), so in general the diagnosis is based on confirmation (= eliciting a history) of persistent (includes intermittent), diffuse, and continuous colitis and exclusion of other forms of inflammatory bowel disease.

NBI can be used to detect increases and decreases in superficial vessels and structural changes, so magnifying NBI may assist in differentiating between UC and the other inflammation, with limitations. At present, magnifying NBI can be used to detect mucosal healing, differentiate between unaffected areas and areas in remission, and detect neoplastic lesions, thereby contributing to qualitative assessments.

15.4.1 Explanation

Although determination of the margins of erosions and ulcers and evaluation of disease activity are readily performed using WLI, NBI is more useful in patients with milder disease. In non-magnifying examinations of a case of mild active UC, in comparison with WLI (Fig. 15.4a), in the marginal area of an active lesion, NBI delineates the affected mucosa as a distinct aggregation of brownish areas (Fig. 15.4b). Magnifying NBI examination of the affected mucosa shows the main pathology to be increased vascularity around the pits (Fig. 15.4c). At first, magnifying NBI examination of an apparently inactive area (Fig. 15.4d) also shows scattered findings of slightly increased vascularity and irregularity around the pits, indicating the importance of an accurate assessment of the degree of inflammation that can directly affect the choice of therapy.

Figure 15.4e, f shows the findings in a 30-year-old patient with a 10-year history of UC. Non-magnifying (color enhanced) WLI examination of the mucosa affected by UC reveals multiple coarse nodules, sufficient to diagnose not sporadic, but colitic cancer (Fig. 15.4e). Magnifying NBI clearly delineates neoplastic pits like gyrus on the surface of the coarse nodules.

15.4.2 Future Challenges

Colitic cancer is difficult to be diagnosed, rapidly progressive, and on the rise, with more patients living longer with UC due to advances in medical treatment. Because it is common in patients with persistent inflammation, unfortunately even with NBI it is often difficult to detect colitic cancer, and in atypical cases it may be difficult to differentiate from sporadic cancer. The decision whether to treat with a total colectomy or localized resection with endoscopic submucosal dissection (ESD) or endoscopic mucosal resection (EMR) should be an overall decision made with due consideration of the patient's history. There is an urgent need for accumulated evidence concerning endoscopy performed using image-enhanced endoscopy (see Sect. 16.13 and 16.14).

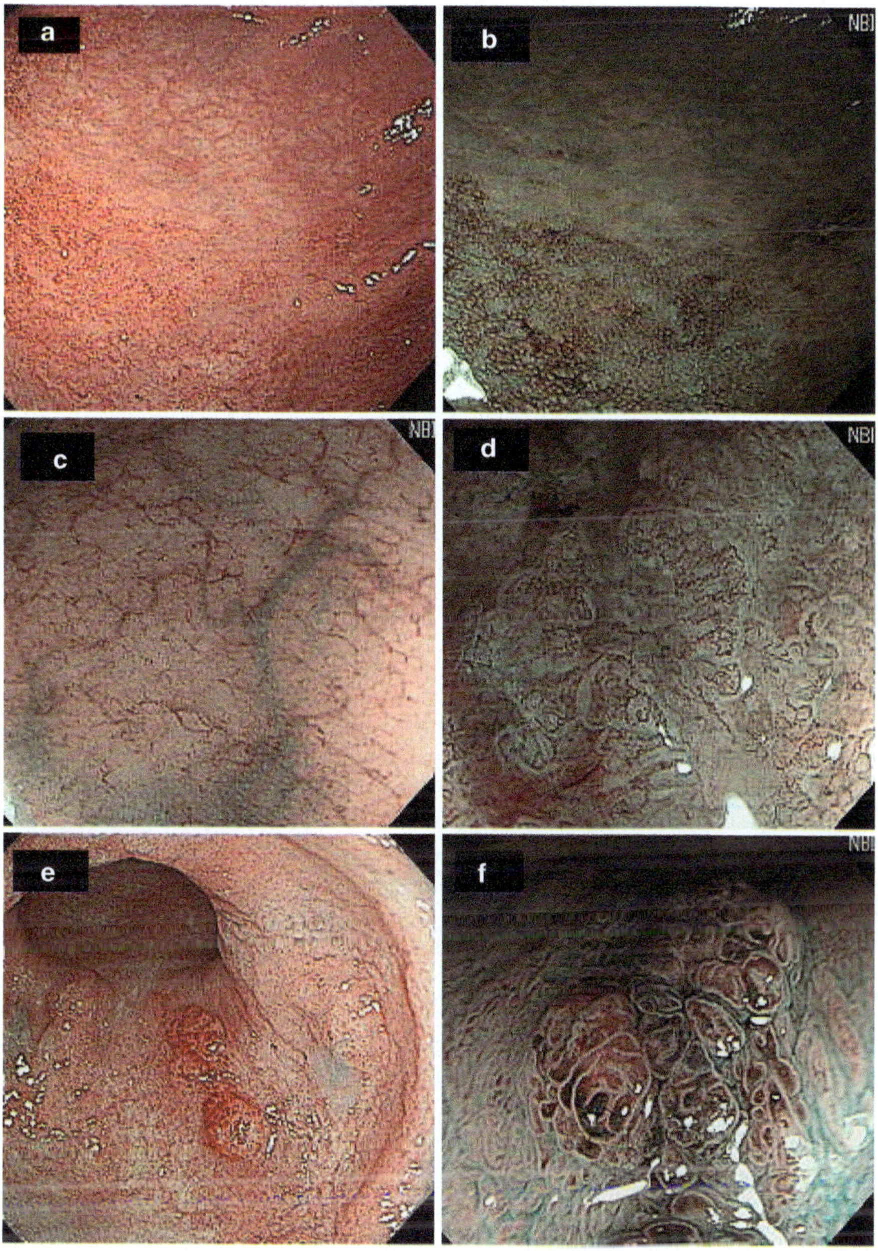

Fig. 15.4 Ulcerative colitis

15.5 Lymphoid Follicular Hyperplasia

Under normal physiological conditions, lymphoid tissue is located in the gastrointestinal tract beneath the mucosal epithelium, formed in response to outside antigenic stimulation before or after birth. They take the form of discrete lymph nodes or aggregations of lymphoid nodules (Peyer's patches). Only the former are found in the colorectal region and are common in the cecum, ascending colon, and rectum.

These lymph nodes are the site for proliferation of B-cell lymphocytes, and those with a germinal center are referred to as lymphoid follicles. In conditions such as infections or autoimmune disease associated with activation of the B-cell-mediated immune system, reactive germinal centers enlarge and increase in number, leading to hyperplasia of the lymphoid follicles [3, 4].

Reactive lymphoid follicular hyperplasia is visualized using non-magnifying WLI as multiple small whitish protrusions of similar sizes. The endoscopic findings are sometimes similar to those observed with lymphoproliferative disorders such as follicular lymphoma, mantle cell lymphoma, or mucosa-associated lymphoid tissue (MALT) lymphoma; however, lesions are uniform in size in cases of hyperplasia and often nonuniform in lymphoproliferative disorders.

15.5.1 Explanation

In the distant view using non-magnifying WLI (Fig. 15.5a), it is difficult to discern the scattered pale ring-shaped red haloes. Examining the same region using non-magnifying NBI (Fig. 15.5b), 2–3 mm small protrusions with a whitish center and brown ring-shaped margins are easily discerned. M-NBI examination (Fig. 15.5c) reveals vessels, slightly larger in diameter than those in the surrounds, extending from the lesion margins toward the center, although the center is almost no vascularity. Magnifying chromoendoscopy with indigo carmine dye (Fig. 15.5d) demonstrates type I pits in the protrusion, as in the margins. As the main part of the lesions was deeper than the mucosal epithelium and lesion sizes were uniform, lymphoid follicular hyperplasia should be diagnosed. Histopathological examination using HE staining (Fig. 15.5e) showed enlargement of the germinal centers of the subepithelial lymphoid follicles. Immune staining with anti-Bcl-2 protein antibodies (Fig. 15.5f) was negative in the germinal centers and positive in the mantle zone, confirming the diagnosis of lymphoid follicular hyperplasia.

15.5.2 NBI Characteristics

The distant view showed lesions with a whitish center and brown ring-shaped margins, with markedly improved visualization in comparison with WLI.

The close view shows slightly enlarged vessels extending from the margins of the protuberance toward the center. As these findings are also seen in hyperplastic polyps, we can assess this as a nonneoplastic lesion.

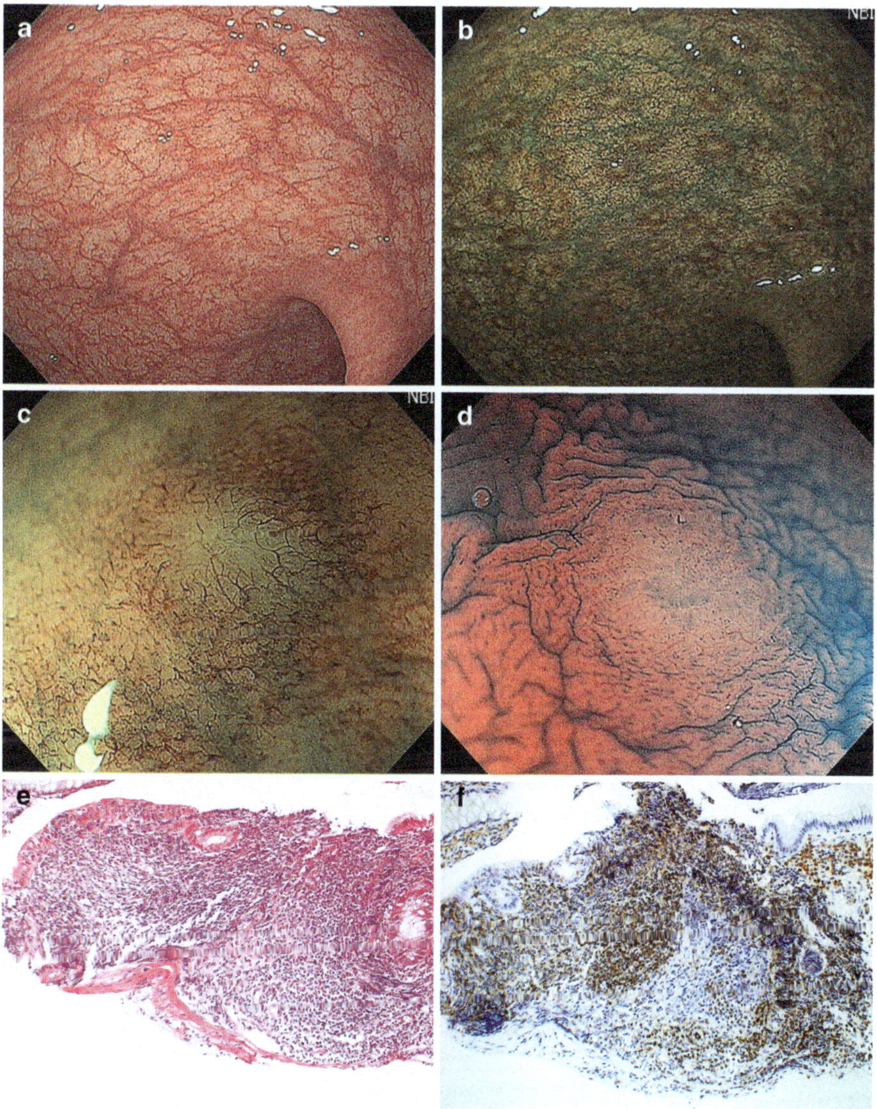

Fig. 15.5 Lymphoid follicular hyperplasia

References

1. Tajiri H (ed.): Atlas of new endoscopic imaging technologies. Japan Medical Center, 2006
2. Nakamura S (ed.): Interpretation of pathology specimens from the gastrointestinal tract. Japan Medical Center, 1999
3. Iwashita A: Early colorectal cancer. 8: 349–351, 2004
4. Nimura S, et al.: Early colorectal cancer. 8: 379–390, 2004

Atlas of Neoplastic Lesions

16

Reiji Higashi, Toshio Uraoka, Taku Sakamoto, Takahisa Matsuda, Takahiro Fujii, Takahiro Horimatsu, Yutaka Saito, Takaya Aoki, Yoshiki Wada, Shinei Kudo, Wataru Sano, Masahito Kotaka, Mineo Iwatate, Atsushi Katagiri, Hiroaki Ikematsu, Yasuhiro Ono, Kenji Watanabe, Masakazu Nishishita, Hirokazu Yamagami, Santa Hattori, Takahiro Fujimori, Hirohisa Machida, Yoshinobu Yamamoto, Hogara Nishisaki, and Yasushi Sano

R. Higashi (✉)
Department of Internal Medicine, Hiroshima City Hospital,
7-33 Motomachi, Naka-ku, Hiroshima 730-8518, Japan

T. Uraoka
Department of Gastrointestinal Medicine, Tokyo Medical Center, Tokyo, Japan

T. Sakamoto • T. Matsuda • Y. Saito
Endoscopy Division, National Cancer Center Central Hospital, Tokyo, Japan

T. Fujii
Department of Gastroenterology, Takahiro Fujii Clinic, Tokyo, Japan

T. Horimatsu
Department of Gastroenterology and Hepatology, Kyoto University Graduate School of Medicine, Kyoto, Japan

T. Aoki
Department of Gastrointestinal Medicine, Makino Memorial Hospital, Kanagawa, Japan

Y. Wada
Department of Gastroenterology and Hepatology, The Tokyo Medical and Dental University School of Medicine, Tokyo, Japan

S. Kudo
Digestive Disease Center, Showa University Northern Yokohama Hospital, Yokohama, Japan

W. Sano • M. Kotaka • M. Iwatate • S. Hattori
Gastrointestinal Center, Sano Hospital, Kobe, Japan

A. Katagiri
Department of Gastroenterology, Showa University School of Medicine, Tokyo, Japan

H. Ikematsu • Y. Ono
Division of Digestive Endoscopy and Gastrointestinal Oncology, National Cancer Center Hospital East, Kashiwa, Japan

M. Muto et al. (eds.), *Atlas of Endoscopy with Narrow Band Imaging*,
DOI 10.1007/978-4-431-54243-8_16

K. Watanabe • H. Yamagami
Department of Gastroenterology, Osaka City University Graduate School of Medicine, Osaka, Japan

H. Machida
Machida Gastroenterical Hospital, Osaka, Japan

M. Nishishita
Department of Gastroenterology, Nishishita Gastrointestinal Hospital, Osaka, Japan

T. Fujimori
Department of Pathology, Shinko Hospital, Kobe, Japan

Y. Yamamoto
Department of Gastrointestinal and Hepato Biliary Oncology, Hyogo Cancer Center, Akashi, Japan

H. Nishisaki
Department of Gastroenterology, Hyogo Prefectural Kaibara Hospital, Hyogo, Japan

Y. Sano
Department of Gastrointestinal Center, Sano Hospital, Kobe, Japan

16.1 Protruded-Type Adenoma

The majority of colorectal cancers arise from adenomas, following the "adenoma-carcinoma sequence." Accordingly, resection of all neoplastic polyps ("clean colon") can be expected to reduce the cumulative incidence of colorectal cancer by 76–90 %. However, attempts to achieve a "clean colon" may result in an increase in unnecessary polypectomies, making differentiation between neoplastic and non-neoplastic polyps extremely important.

Sano et al. refer to dilated meshed vessels on the surface of neoplastic lesions, as visualized using M-NBI, as "meshed capillary vessels" (MC vessels). With the aim of application in qualitative assessments, they further classify MC vessels into three types of capillary pattern (CP: four types including two subtypes). Classifications by Hirata and Tanaka et al., as well as classifications by Wada and Kudo et al. along with their diagnostic ability, have also been published. We await the results of efforts to standardize these classifications.

16.1.1 Explanation

In this case, non-magnifying WLI examination reveals a sessile lesion with a smooth surface and markedly reddened in a partial part (Fig. 16.1a). Non-magnifying NBI examination visualizes this lesion as a brownish area (Fig. 16.1b). M-NBI shows MC vessels, with no signs of irregularity such as nonuniform diameters, tortuosity, or interruption, enclosing the pits in a honeycomb pattern (CP type II, NICE type 2) (Fig. 16.1c, d). In a partial area of the lesion, we can see intensely brown-colored areas corresponding to the stroma, the dense pattern proposed by Wada and Kudo et al. as characteristic of adenoma (Fig. 16.1c). Magnifying chromoendoscopy with indigo carmine dye reveals a type III_L pit pattern (Fig. 16.1e, f).

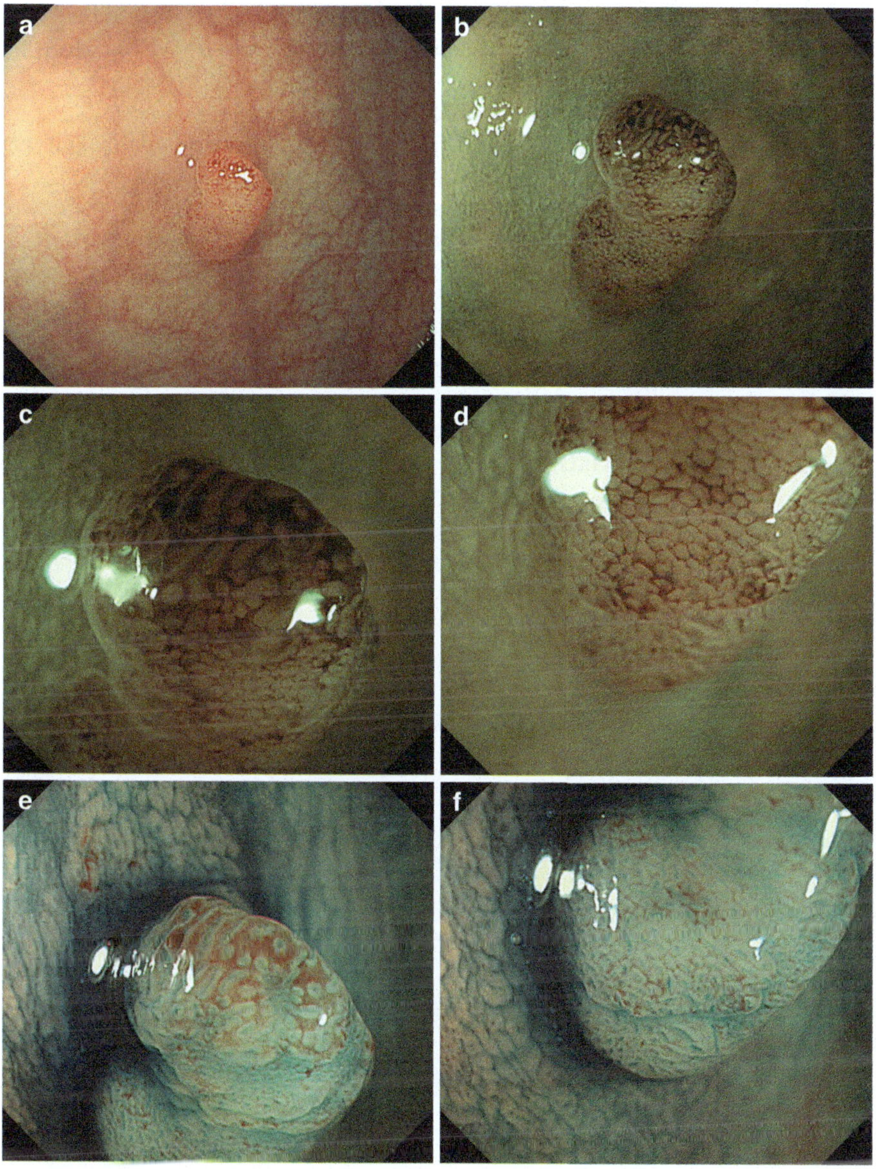

Fig. 16.1 Protruded-type adenoma

Adenoma was diagnosed from the above findings, and EMR was performed. The histopathohistological diagnosis was a tubular adenoma with mild atypia (Fig. 16.1g, h).

16.1.1.1 Points for Interpretation of Findings

- Adenomatous lesions are visualized as brownish areas using non-magnifying NBI.
- M-NBI examination, with the emphasis on whether MC vessels are present or not, differentiates more accurately between neoplastic and nonneoplastic lesions.
- NBI findings of MC vessels irregularly encircling pits, or with nonuniform diameters, tortuosity, interruptions, or increased vascular density, or loss of the honeycomb pattern, are indicative of invasive cancer, so we add a chromoendoscopic examination to determine the pit pattern.

16.1.2 NBI Characteristics

M-NBI examination reveals tubular or oval-shaped enlarged pits, surrounded by dark brown capillaries with no signs of irregularity. A dense pattern, corresponding to the stroma, is visualized as an intense dark brown.

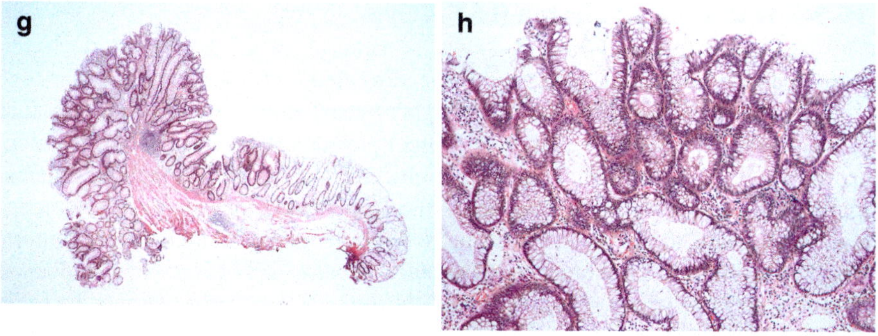

Fig. 16.1 (continued)

16.2 Flat-Type Adenoma (LST-NG)

In comparison to granular-type lateral spreading tumor (LST-G), nongranular-type lateral spreading tumor (LST-NG) has a higher rate of submucosal invasion. Another characteristic of LST-G is that it is difficult to identify the site of invasion in approximately 30 % of lesions, due to multicentric growth. Although the clinical importance of superficial tumors such as LST-G is becoming more widely recognized worldwide, they are considered more difficult to detect than polypoid tumors. Non-magnifying WLI examination usually reveals LST-G as low reddened protruding lesions with a smooth surface, but some lesions will be almost the same height and color as the nonneoplastic mucosa. In other words, they may be overlooked unless during the examination we pay close attention to findings such as "gathering of the surrounding mucosal folds, catch light (uneven mucosal surface), and vessel visibility." Clinical studies are under way aimed at improving detection rates, concentrating on refinement of optical digital methods.

16.2.1 Explanation

This lesion is located in the transverse colon. Non-magnifying WLI examination (distant view) reveals a lesion sitting across a fold, making it difficult to detect. Drawing near to the lesion, it is visualized as an area of "reddish color, mild surface unevenness (catch light), and loss of vessel visibility" (Fig. 16.2a). Non-magnifying NBI examination reveals little color contrast with the surrounding mucosa, indicating NBI does little to increase the discernibility of this lesion (Fig. 16.2b).

In an M-NBI examination from a medium magnification, we can see dense vessels with roughly equal diameters (Fig. 16.2c). Raising the magnification as we examine the vessels, the findings are roughly the same as at medium magnification, with the exception of a partial area where the vessel paths are slightly irregular compared to their surrounds, and the vessel diameters are nonuniform in diameter (larger vessels) (Fig. 16.2d). However, looking at the lesion as a whole, this area is extremely small in extent, and the histopathological finding as determined by the vessel pattern is adenoma (>intramucosal cancer) (CP type II, NICE type 2). Endoscopic resection was considered appropriate for this lesion. At present, we perform magnifying endoscopy not only with NBI but also with chromoendoscopy, and in this case the predominant pit pattern was type III_L, with some type III_S in a partial area (Fig. 16.2e).

The diagnoses based on the pit pattern and the NBI findings were similar, and en block resection using the ESD method was performed (Fig. 16.2f, g). The final histopathological diagnosis was a "tubular adenoma, low and high grade."

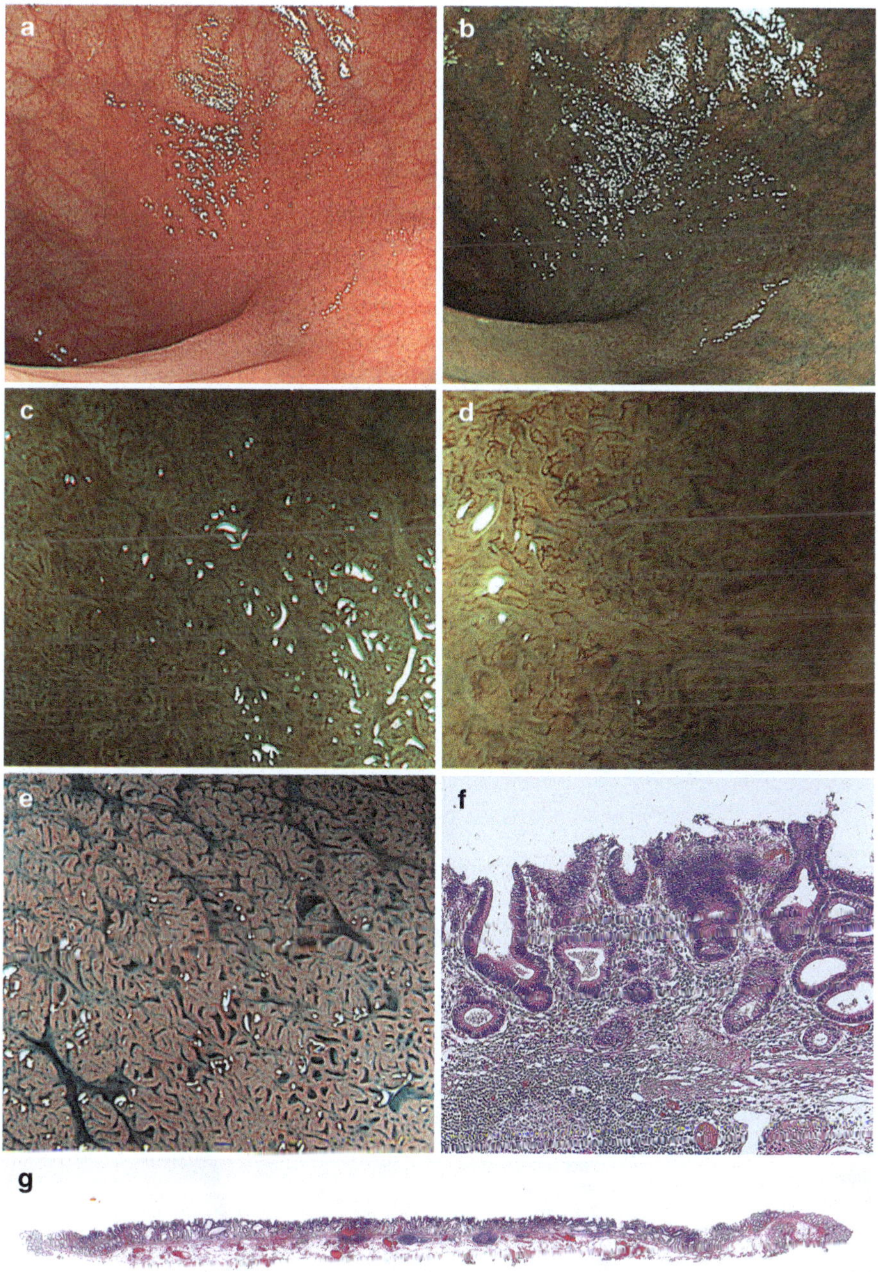

Fig. 16.2 Flat-type adenoma (LST-NG)

16.2.2 NBI Characteristics

In an M-NBI examination, we should first gain an overall grasp of the vascular pattern of the entire lesion at medium magnification, then examine any areas of interest at high magnification, paying attention to features such as any irregularities of vessel paths or alterations in vascular density.

A variety of studies have examined the usefulness of NBI in the colorectal field. Consistent evidence concerning differentiation between neoplastic and nonneoplastic lesions has been produced, and a consensus has been reached. However, there remains considerable room for debate concerning improvement in detection rates and determination of the depth of invasion. In particular concerning the latter, we should be aware that the diagnostic ability of NBI in determining the depth of invasion is not superior to that of chromoendoscopy.

In general, if non-magnifying WLI or M-NBI examination indicates a lesion is an adenoma or intramucosal cancer, there should be no problem with proceeding to endoscopic resection. If submucosal invasive cancer is suspected on the basis of the non-magnifying WLI or M-NBI findings, however, more detailed information is required, so there should be no hesitation in determining the pit pattern using crystal violet staining.

16.3 Depressed-Type Adenoma

Endoscopic detection of depressed colorectal tumors (type IIc) has hitherto involved picking up slight mucosal changes during a non-magnifying WLI examination, such as loss of capillary visibility, slight reddening, or surface unevenness. This has been dependent on the skill and "craftsmanship" of the endoscopist, with not all able to detect these lesions. The authors have been considering this challenge of how to make it easier to identify these difficult to detect depressed tumors. Nothing has emerged so far in the way of a revolutionary method of detecting type IIc lesions, however. In recent years, expectations have risen that the use of image enhancement methods such as NBI, flexible spectral imaging color enhancement (FICE), and autofluorescence imaging (AFI) will prove applicable in detection as well as qualitative and quantitative assessments. Of these possibilities, we have concentrated on detection and diagnosis of superficial tumors using NBI.

16.3.1 Explanation

This case is a 40-year-old male who underwent colonoscopy for the purpose of screening for colorectal cancer (at the author's hospital, when we use a high vision format colonoscope, unless the bowel preparation was inadequate or melanosis coli is present, in all cases we insert the scope as far as the cecum using WLI, then change over to NBI for the withdrawal from the cecum).

In this case, using NBI we detected a superficial depressed tumor (type IIc) 6 mm in size in the sigmoid colon. As shown in Fig. 16.3a, we can see a ring-shaped brownish area, an important finding for the detection of type IIc lesions using NBI, that we call the O-ring sign. The center of the ring is visualized as the same color as the surrounding mucosa or slightly whitish. Non-magnifying WLI (Fig. 16.3b) and indigo carmine-sprayed (Fig. 16.3c) examination reveal the macroscopic features of a type IIc lesion, with type I pits and raised margins corresponding to the O-ring sign seen using NBI. The pattern is consistent with type I pits, with sparse vessels forming an immature network within the depression (CP type II, NICE type 2) (Fig. 16.3d). Magnified chromoendoscopy using crystal violet staining reveals type III_S pits densely packed on the surface of the depression and slightly widened and stretched type I pits on the raised marginal area (Fig. 16.3e).

Figure 16.3g shows the loupe findings, with a type II_C lesion. Tubular glands are densely packed on the surface of the depression, showing cellular atypia in all layers (Fig. 16.3g), yielding the diagnosis of an adenoma with mild atypia.

16.3.2 NBI Characteristics

This case supports the usefulness of NBI endoscopy for screening of type II_C lesions. Identification of a ring-shaped brownish area (O-ring sign) is important for the detection of colorectal type II_C lesions using NBI.

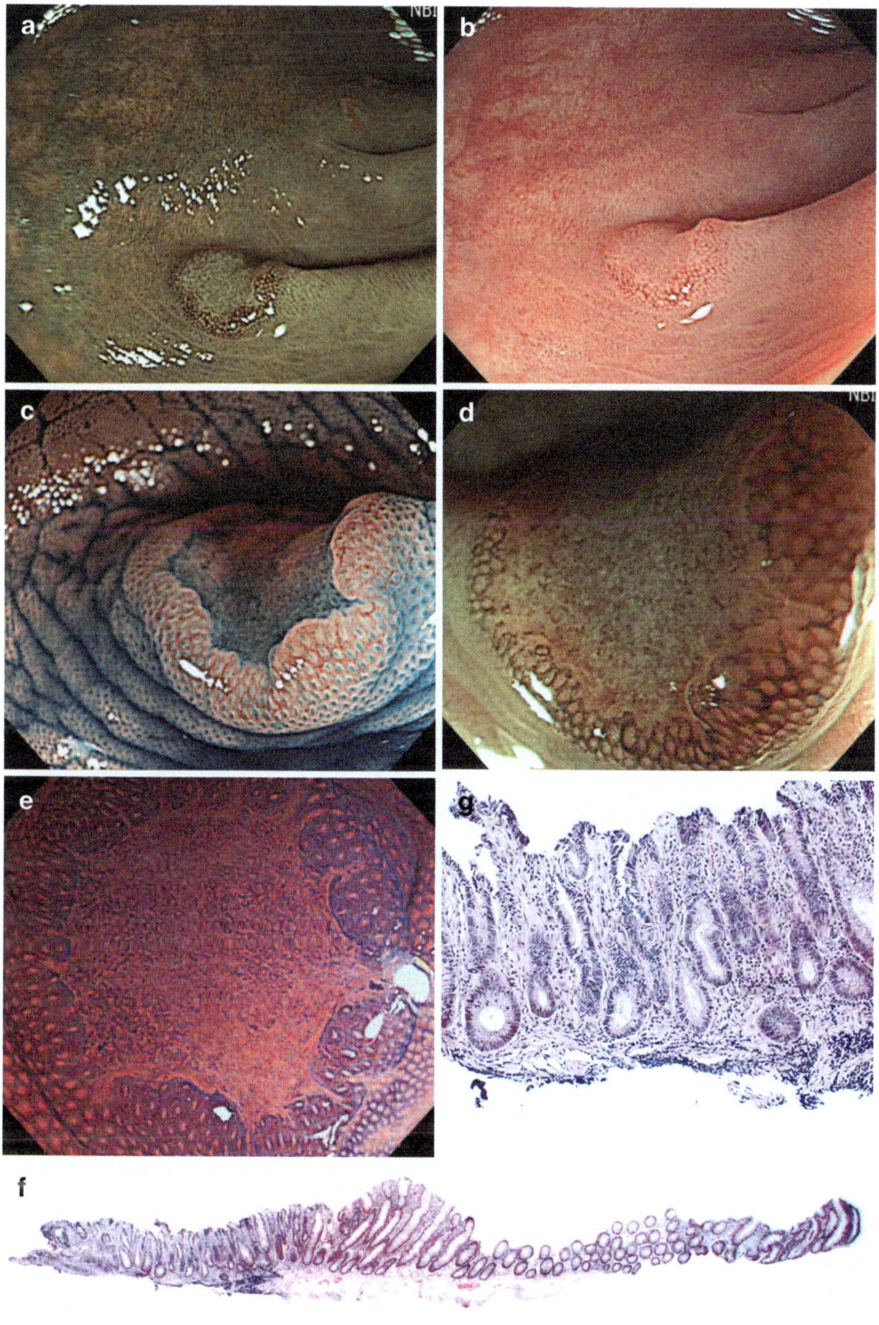

Fig. 16.3 Depressed-type adenoma

16.4 Early Colorectal Cancer: Type 0-I (1)

16.4.1 Explanation

Non-magnifying WLI examination reveals a slightly reddened protruded type 0-I_S lesion 10 mm in size, associated with white plaques on the surrounding mucosa, with a slight depression in the center (Fig. 16.4a). Following indigo carmine spraying, we can see a slightly depressed area in the center of the lesion, with some surface irregularity (Fig. 16.4b).

Non-magnifying NBI examination reveals irregular atypical vessels in the lesion marginal area, delineated as dark brown, but capillaries are clearly visible in the central area (Fig. 16.4c). Even with M-NBI, only a few dot vessels can be discerned in the lesion center, forming a rough vascular network, so this was assessed as a CP type III_B (NICE type 3) pattern (Fig. 16.4d).

Crystal violet staining showed pits with narrow lumens, irregular margins, and indistinct outlines, comprising a type V_I (severe irregularity) pit pattern (Fig. 16.4e).

From the above findings, this lesion was diagnosed as a highly invasive SM cancer, and it was resected surgically. Histopathological examination of the resected specimen revealed a moderately differentiated tubular adenocarcinoma with vascular invasion and deep submucosal invasion. The final histopathological diagnosis was type 0-Is, 10×10 mm, tub2, pSM (>6,000 μm), ly1, v2, pN0, pPM0, pDM0, and pRM0 (Fig. 16.4f).

16.4.2 NBI Characteristics

Sano et al. propose a three-step strategy for the treatment of colorectal lesions [1, 2]. When a lesion is detected using non-magnifying WLI, the capillary pattern (CP) should be determined using NBI, then lesions with a CP type I (NICE type 1) can be observed without treatment, and endoscopic resection is indicated for lesions with a CP type II or III_A (NICE type 2). Chromoendoscopy should be performed if a CP type III_B (NICE type 3) is seen, and endoscopic resection is indicated for lesions with a type V_I (mild irregularity) pit pattern. If a circumscribed type V_I (severe irregularity) or type V_N pit pattern is seen, SM deep invasive cancer is likely, and surgical resection is indicated.

In this case, M-NBI revealed a CP type III_B (NICE type 3) (surface pattern (+)) and crystal violet chromoendoscopy a type V_I (severe irregularity) pit pattern. With a preoperative diagnosis of SM deep invasive cancer, this lesion was resected surgically. The histological finding was SM deep invasive cancer, agreeing with the endoscopic findings. Furthermore, NBI showed a whitish grooved surface pattern, whereas the depth of invasion was pSM massive. Further studies of the usefulness of the surface pattern in determining the depth of invasion are needed.

The CP type III_B (NICE type 3) (surface pattern (−)) signifies destruction of the mucosal layer and exposure of SM cancer on the surface of an unstructured area, so it should be considered an SM deep invasive cancer, and surgical resection is strongly recommended.

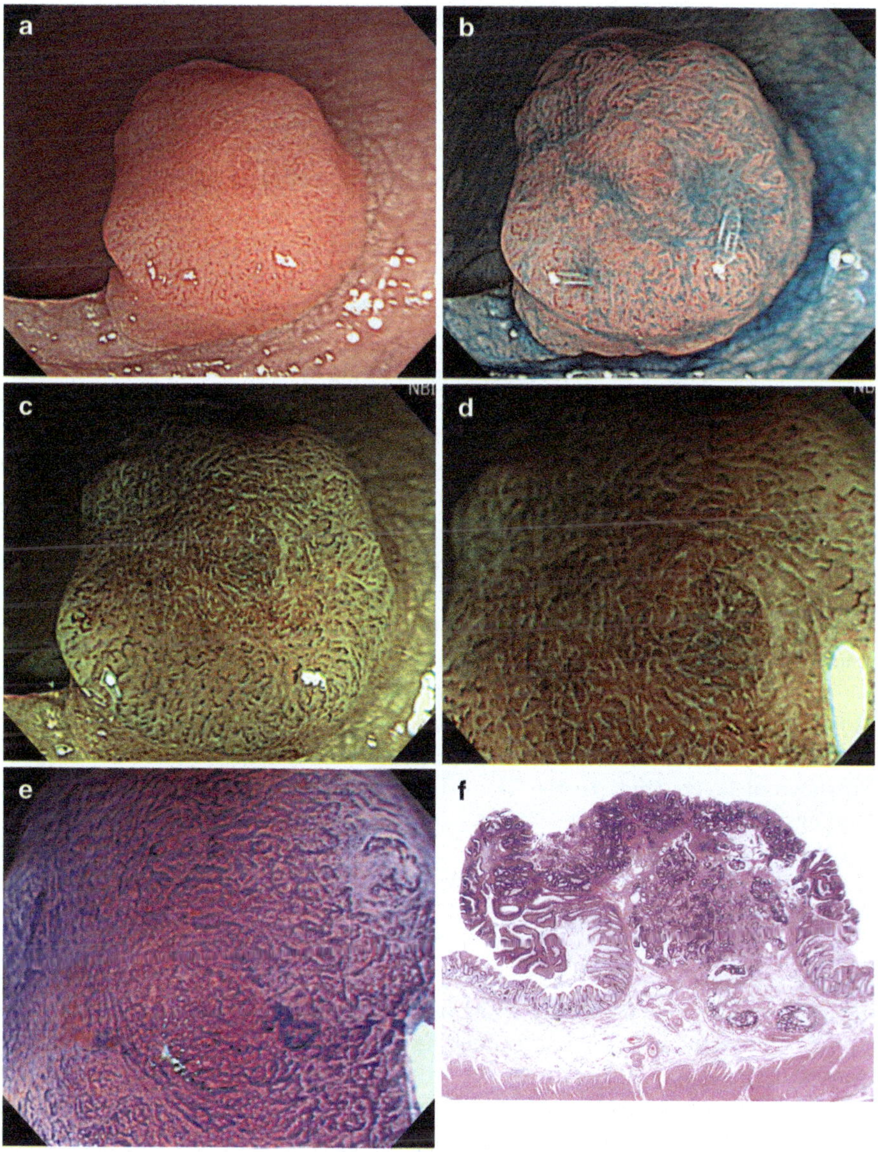

Fig. 16.4 Early colorectal cancer: Type 0-I

16.5 Early Colorectal Cancer: Type 0-I (2)

16.5.1 Explanation

Non-magnifying WLI examination reveals a reddened protruded lesion, 20 mm in size, in the lower rectum (Rb). White plaques are seen on the surrounding mucosa, and the protruded lesion has an irregular surface with a central depression (Fig. 16.5a). Following indigo carmine spraying, the central area is difficult to visualize as a depression, although it is at a different level to the surrounds, and we cannot rule out the possibility of invasion of the deep submucosal layer in that area (Fig. 16.5b).

Non-magnifying NBI examination reveals vessels with nonuniform diameters irregularly surrounding the pits in the depressed area (Fig. 16.5c). M-NBI of the same area shows vessels with nonuniform diameters, branching, and interruptions, but maintaining a normal vascular density. This corresponds to a CP type III_A in the Sano classification (NICE type 2), and these findings were consistent with an intramucosal or shallow submucosal invasive cancer (Fig. 16.5d).

Non-magnifying examination of the depressed area following indigo carmine spraying reveals a type V_I (mild irregularity) pit pattern, and the addition of magnification yields the diagnosis of an intramucosal or shallow submucosal invasive cancer (Fig. 16.5e).

This lesion was resected endoscopically. The histopathohistological diagnosis was a moderately differentiated tubular adenocarcinoma, reaching the muscularis mucosae in the depressed area, but remaining intramucosal without invading the submucosal layers (Fig. 16.5f). These findings agreed with the NBI endoscopic findings.

16.5.2 NBI Characteristics

M-NBI examination of the vascular architecture of the lesion surface has been reported to have the potential to assist in determining the depth of tumor invasion [2–4]. Although various classifications have been proposed, findings of densely packed irregular and abnormal vessels, with features including nonuniform diameters, branching, and interruptions, are indicative of intramucosal or shallow submucosal invasive cancer in all classifications. These findings can be considered typical regardless of the classification used.

When a submucosal deep invasive cancer cannot be excluded from the non-magnifying WLI findings, however, with NBI we can do no more than observe vascular changes associated with atypia, and confirmation of the lesion pit pattern, directly reflecting structural atypia, is still considered necessary.

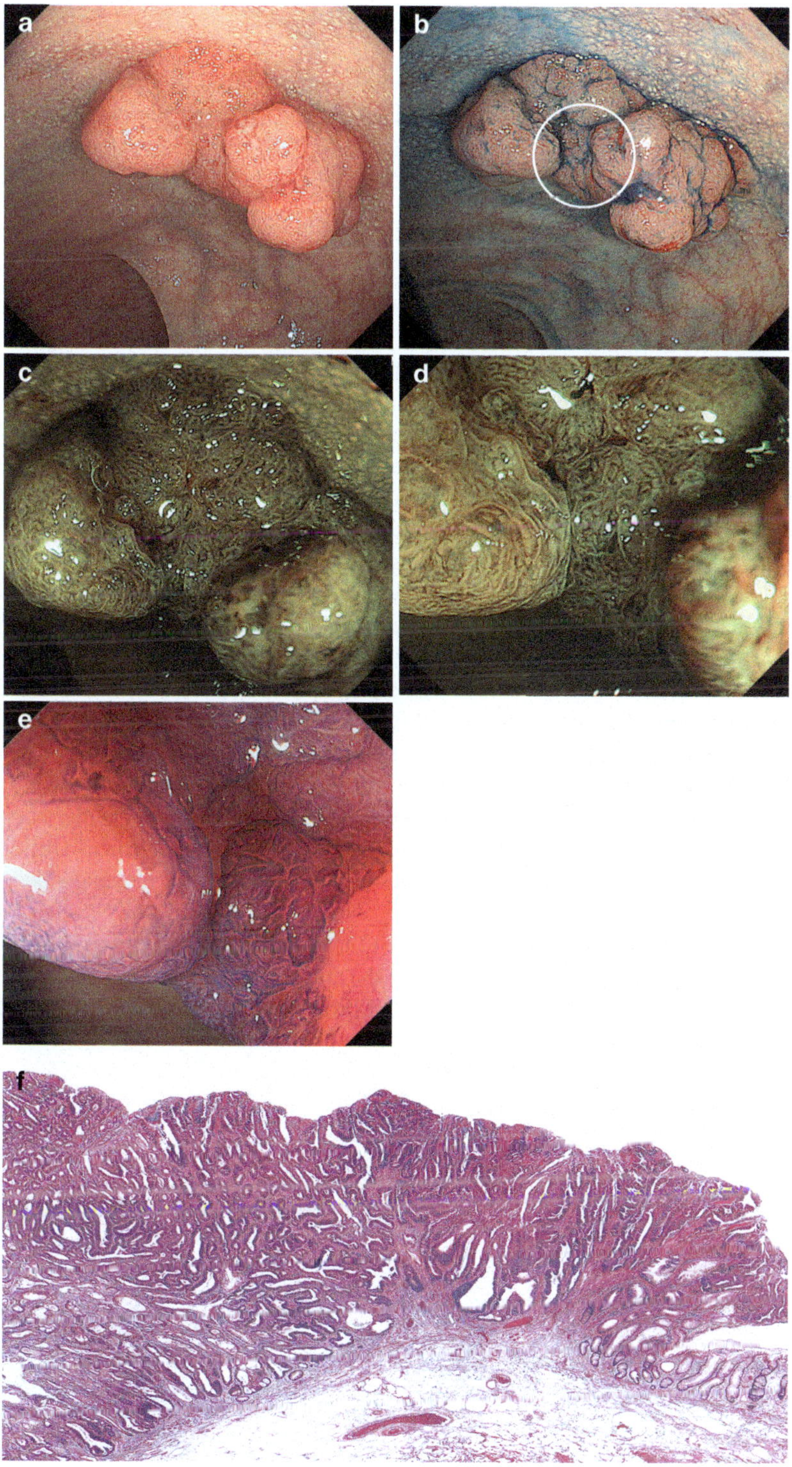

Fig. 16.5 Early colorectal cancer: Type 0-I

16.6 Early Colorectal Cancer: Type 0-IIa (1)

This is a case of type 0-IIa early colorectal cancer (depth of invasion pM, well-differentiated adenocarcinoma), previously presented at the 14th Tokyo Metropolitan Area Gastrointestinal Endoscopy Meeting.

16.6.1 Explanation

This case is a 74-year-old male. We can see a superficial elevated lesion 40 mm in size in the ascending colon. Non-magnifying WLI examination reveals this lesion as slightly reddish in color compared to the surrounding mucosa (retroflexed view, Fig. 16.6a). Mild bunching of the surrounding folds is seen (Fig. 16.6b, indigo carmine spraying), but this becomes less noticeable with stretching. A slightly raised area can be seen on the anal side of the lesion (retroflexed view, Fig. 16.6a).

Non-magnifying NBI examination shows the lesion as a brownish area in comparison to the surrounding mucosa and delineates the lesion margins more distinctly (Fig. 16.6c). M-NBI of the anal side raised area reveals meshed capillary vessels, slightly dilated in comparison with normal vessels, corresponding to CP type II or III_A in the Sano classification (NICE type 2) (Fig. 16.6d).

Magnifying examination following indigo carmine spraying revealed type III_L pits in the raised area (Fig. 16.6e) and type III_L to III_S pits even in the flat area. Similarly, magnifying examination following crystal violet staining showed type III_L pits in the raised area. This was assessed as a type V_I (noninvasive) pit pattern due to the nonuniform sizes and disturbed arrangement.

On the basis of the above findings, endoscopic treatment was considered appropriate, and en block resection using the ESD method was performed. During the procedure, moderate fibrosis was detected in the submucosa of the anal side raised area.

The hisotpathohistological diagnosis was a well-differentiated adenocarcinoma (Fig. 16.6f, g). This tumor was confined to the mucosa and was negative for vascular invasion. The reason for the submucosal fibrosis remains unclear, but may have been related to a biopsy taken by the referring physician.

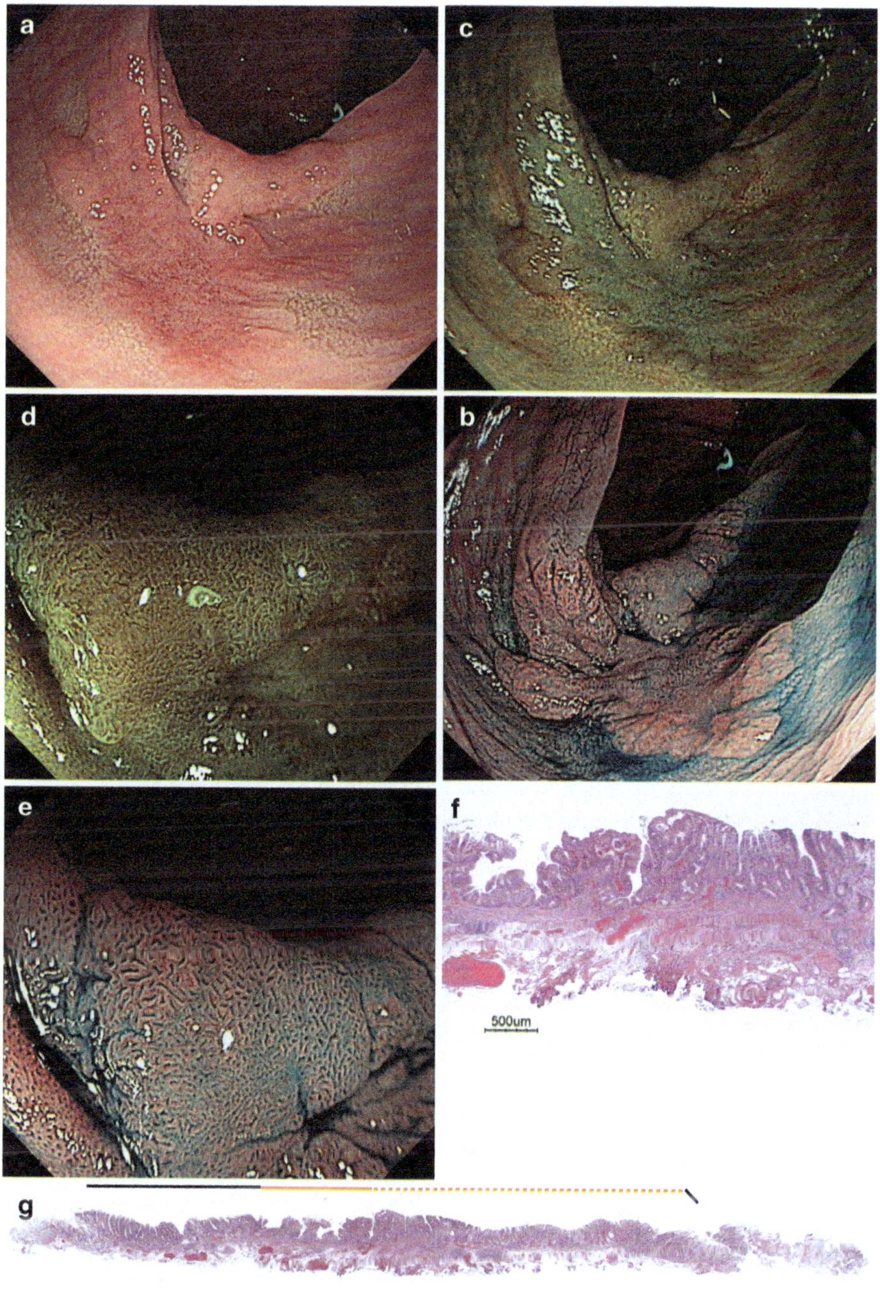

Fig. 16.6 Early colorectal cancer: type 0-IIa

16.7 Early Colorectal Cancer: Type 0-IIa (2)

This is a case of type 0-IIa early colorectal cancer (depth of invasion pM, well-differentiated adenocarcinoma).

16.7.1 Explanation

We can see a superficial elevated lesion, 20 mm in size, located in the sigmoid colon. Non-magnifying WLI examination reveals this lesion as slightly reddish in color compared to the surrounding mucosa (Fig. 16.7a, b indigo carmine spraying). This is associated with mild gathering of the surrounding mucosa, so SM invasion was considered possible on the basis of the WLI findings.

Non-magnifying NBI examination shows the lesion as a brownish area in comparison to the surrounding mucosa (Fig. 16.7c). M-NBI of the lesion surface reveals meshed capillary vessels, slightly dilated in comparison with normal vessels, surrounding the pits (Fig. 16.7d). These vessels show lack of uniformity, branching, and interruptions. These findings correspond to CP type III_A in the Sano classification (NICE type 2).

Magnifying examination following crystal violet staining revealed an irregular pit pattern over the entire lesion, which was assessed as a type V_I pit pattern (Fig. 16.7e). No patchiness was detected in the V_I pit pattern area, so it was assessed as a noninvasive pattern.

On the basis of the above findings, endoscopic treatment was considered appropriate, and en block resection using the ESD method was performed.

The histopathohistological diagnosis was a well-differentiated adenocarcinoma (Fig. 16.7f). This tumor was confined to the mucosa and was negative for vascular invasion.

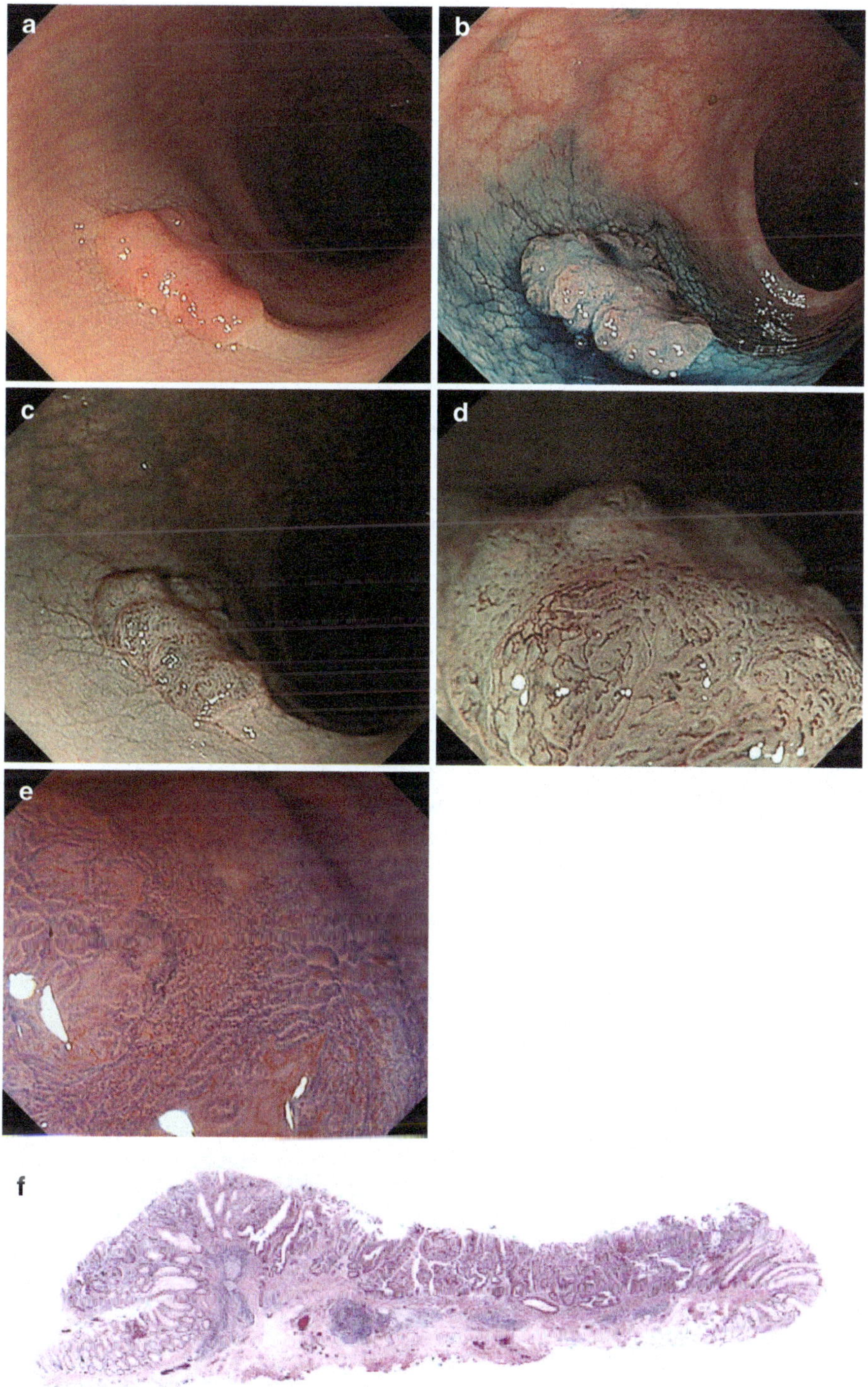

Fig. 16.7 Early colorectal cancer: type 0-IIa

16.8 Early Colorectal Cancer: Type 0-IIc (1)

The depressed lesion contains type IIc, IIc + IIa, IIa + IIc, and Is + IIc elements.

With an NBI system, it is possible to instantaneously change modes and obtain more information useful in the evaluation of the surface microvascular pattern. Recognition of characteristic vascular findings, not only in protruded and flat lesions but also in depressed lesions, makes a more accurate diagnosis possible.

In this section, I will present and explain the typical vascular pattern observed in depressed early colorectal cancers, in particular SM deep invasive cancers.

16.8.1 Explanation

This lesion, 9 mm in size, is located in the rectosigmoid colon (RS). At first glance, non-magnifying WLI delineates this as an elevated lesion with a slightly reddened area on its apex with an uneven surface (Fig. 16.8a). Indigo carmine spraying enhances the area thought to be a depressed section, so this was assessed as a type IIa + IIc morphology (Fig. 16.8b). The surface structure of the sides of the protruding lesion shows a type I pit pattern, so the entire lesion was thought to have arisen from a depressed lesion.

Non-magnifying NBI examination shows the vascular density to be low in the area assessed as a depressed section using indigo carmine spraying, in comparison with the areas thought to be the sides of the protruding lesion. The scattered vessels in the low vascular density area lack regularity, showing an irregular "sparse pattern" (CP type III_B, NICE type 3) (Fig. 16.8c, d). Crystal violet staining reveals a type V_I (severe irregularity) pit pattern, with narrow lumens and irregular margins, in the "sparse pattern" area (Fig. 16.8e), yielding the diagnosis of SM deep invasive cancer.

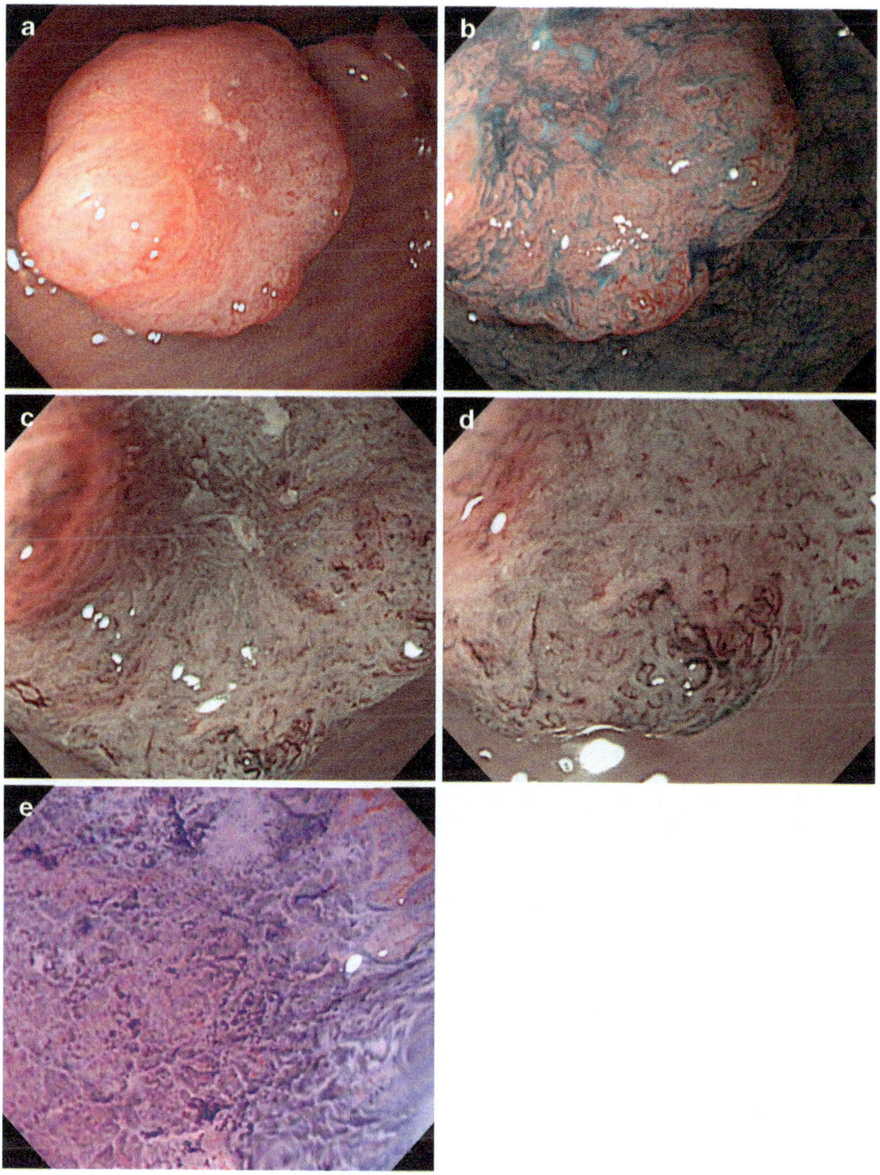

Fig. 16.8 Early colorectal cancer: type 0 IIc

This lesion was resected surgically with laparoscopic assistance. The histopathohistological diagnosis was an adenocarcinoma (tub 2>1), pSM 3,250 μm, ly1, v2, pN1, H1, pPM0, and pDM0 (Fig. 16.8f). The depressed section showing the sparse pattern and type V_I (severe irregularity) pit pattern was an exposed desmoplastic reaction, associated with disappearance of the muscularis mucosae in the invasive region.

16.8.2 NBI Characteristics

When an early colorectal cancer shows an area of surface unevenness, raising suspicion of deep submucosal invasion, vessels are often seen as sparse in that area. With high magnification, vessels with nonuniform diameters and abnormal paths will be visible in that sparse area.

This decrease in vascular density, where vessels become "sparse," is seen not only in depressed lesions but also when part of an elevated or flat lesion becomes cancerous and becomes depressed.

f

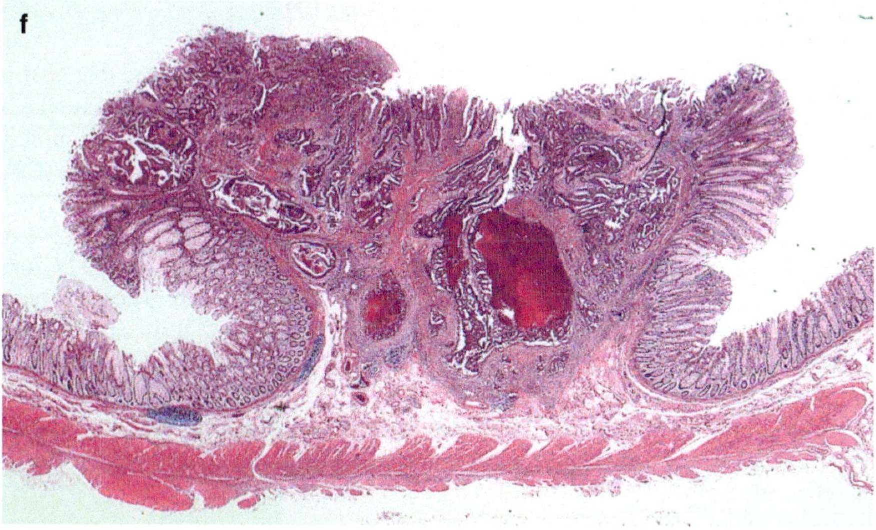

Fig. 16.8 (continued)

16.9 Early Colorectal Cancer: Type 0-IIc (2)

Machida et al. [5], Sano et al. [6], and Katagiri et al. [7] have reported that NBI is useful in the qualitative assessment. Ikematsu et al. [2] further reported that NBI is also useful in quantitative assessments, through differentiation between capillary patterns (CP) type III_A (NICE type 2) and III_B (NICE type 3) capillary patterns (CP). Ikematsu et al. conducted a study of 130 lesions diagnosed with type III CP. They found that 86 of the 91 lesions (94.5 %) assessed as CP type III_A (NICE type 2) were adenoma, M cancer, SM shallow invasive cancer, whereas 28 of the 39 lesions (71.8 %) assessed as CP type III_B (NICE type 3) were SM deep invasive cancer. They concluded that differentiation between the CPs type III_A and III_B enabled prediction of SM deep invasive cancer with a diagnostic accuracy of 87.7 %, sensitivity of 84.8 %, and specificity of 88.7 %.

A CP type III_B (NICE type 3) was also detected in this lesion, yielding a preoperative diagnosis of SM deep invasive cancer.

16.9.1 Explanation

Non-magnifying WLI examination revealed a slightly reddened elevated lesion, 8 mm in size, with a depressed area and white plaques on the surrounding mucosa, in the rectum (Fig. 16.9a).

NBI examination at low magnification revealed brown capillaries in the depressed area, indicating this is a neoplastic lesion (Fig. 16.9b) [5, 6]. High magnification of the depressed area shows slightly enlarged irregular capillaries with nonuniform diameters on the right side (CP type III_A, NICE type 2) and sparse, difficult to visualize, capillaries on the left (CP type III_B, NICE type 3) (Fig. 16.9c).

Strong magnification of the depressed area following crystal violet staining shows a type V_I (severe irregularity) pit pattern, with marked pit destruction, irregular pit margins, narrow lumens, and indistinct outlines (Fig. 16.9d).

On the basis of the above findings, SM deep invasive cancer was diagnosed, and this lesion was resected surgically.

Even at low magnification, histopathological examination confirms loss of the mucosal layer and exposure of SM cancer on the surface (Fig. 16.9e). High magnification (Fig. 16.9f) shows an SM deep invasive cancer, with rupture of the muscularis mucosae, and depth of invasion 2,000 μm from the surface. The final diagnosis was type 0-IIa+IIc, 8 mm, tub1, pSM (2,000 μm), ly0, v0, pN0.

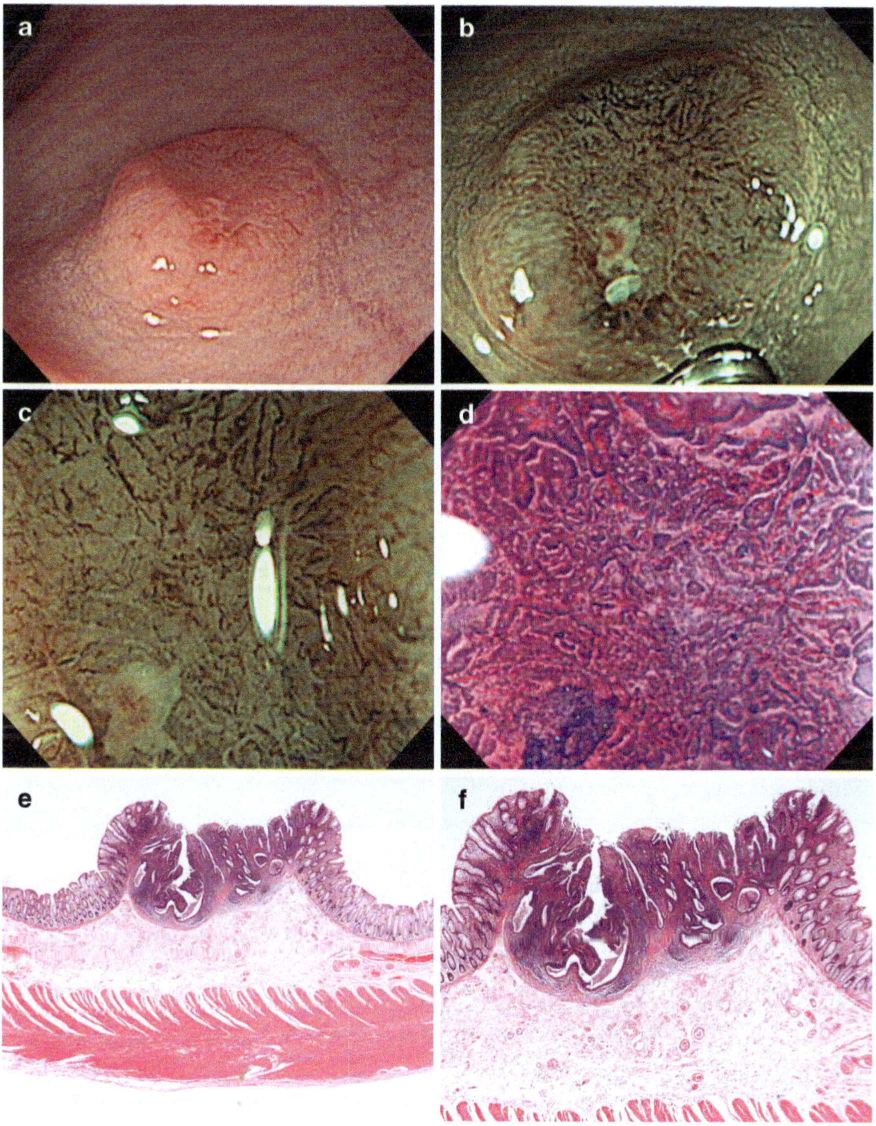

Fig. 16.9 Early colorectal cancer: type 0-IIc

16.10 Early Colorectal Cancer: Type 0-IIc (3)

Superficial depressed (type IIc) tumors are usually defined as lesions with a distinct depressed section lower than or at the same level as the surrounding mucosa. The incidence of type IIc lesions was 4.9 % in a multicenter retrospective study [8]. They should never be overlooked, as they tend to invade the submucosa while still small, markedly more often than other macroscopic types, 44 % of lesions 6–10 mm in size and 70.4 % 11–15 mm [9].

It is important to detect these lesions using non-magnifying WLI, and "mild reddening" is a particularly important finding. Caution is required because depressed areas are often associated with raised margins and are often initially thought to be a type IIa superficial elevated lesion [10, 11].

16.10.1 Explanation

Non-magnifying WLI examination revealed a depressed lesion, 4 mm in size, with a distinct boundary and raised margins. The depressed area is a light reddish color, with central adherent white substance (Fig. 16.10a).

Non-magnifying NBI examination revealed no visible vessels in the raised marginal area, as in the surrounding mucosa, indicating nonneoplastic mucosa (type I CP in the Sano classification) (Fig. 16.10b). M-NBI of the depressed area shows densely packed relatively small irregular meshed vessels on the left side (type III_A CP, NICE type 2) and an area of slight vessel sparsity (type III_B CP, NICE type 3), with severe atypia, on the right (Fig. 16.10c).

Crystal violet staining of the right side of the depressed area shows a type V_I (severe irregularity) pit pattern (Fig. 16.10d).

Histopathological examination of the crystal violet-stained right side of the depressed area in the resected specimen shows an intramucosal cancer with severe atypia (Fig. 16.10e, HE loupe image; Fig. 16.10f, high magnification of blue rectangle in Fig. 16.10e).

16.10.2 NBI Characteristics

The margins of this depressed lesion are nonneoplastic mucosa, with almost no vessels visible using NBI (type I CP, NICE type 1).

NBI examination of the depressed area reveals mainly densely packed meshed vessels that are relatively small, reflecting the short straight pits (type III_A CP, NICE type 2). However, in the SM invasive area, conversely, the vascular density becomes low, due to the desmoplastic reaction (type III_B CP, NICE type 3).

The reported diagnostic accuracy for lesions showing a type III_B CP (NICE type 3) predicting SM deep invasive cancer is rather low at 86.3 % for NBI alone, but combination with chromoendoscopy raises it to 91.5 % [12]. It is essential to pay close attention to the vascular density within the depressed area, and if a type III_B CP (NICE type 3) is detected, also perform crystal violet staining to determine the pit pattern, and base the treatment choice on all the available findings.

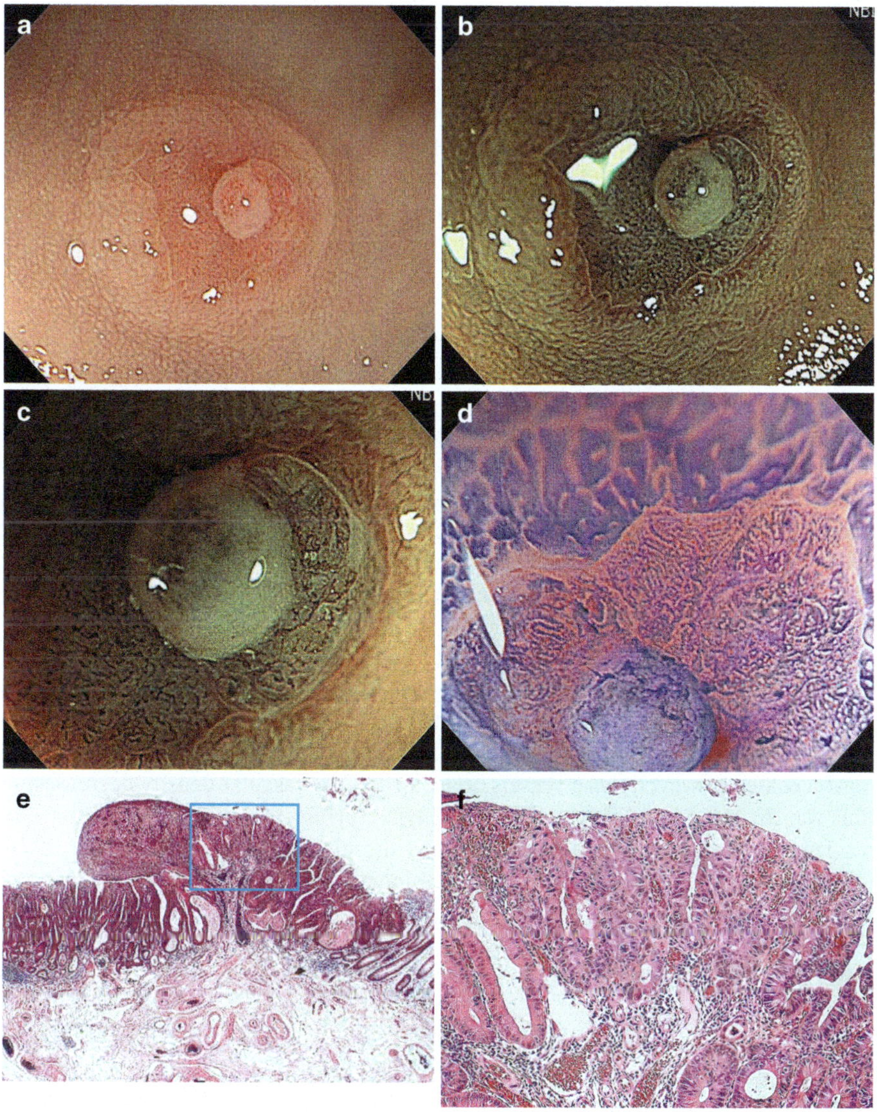

Fig. 16.10 Early colorectal cancer: type 0-IIc

16.11 Advanced Colorectal Cancer

Colorectal cancer is the third most common cause of all cancer-related death in Japan; it ranks third in men and first in women.

Although fecal occult blood testing is widely used as a cancer screening test, the final diagnosis must be made via colonoscopy and pathohistological examination of endoscopic biopsy specimens. Differentiated adenocarcinoma is the most common histological type and circumscribed ulcerated lesions the most common macroscopic type.

16.11.1 Explanation

In this retroflexed non-magnifying WLI view of the lower rectum (Rb), we can see a raised lesion, 15 mm in size, with steep sides and a deep central depression (Fig. 16.11a). Indigo carmine dye spraying delineates the margins of the depression more distinctly (Fig. 16.11b). The depressed area has an uneven surface, and the edge of the depressed area forms a circumferential raised margin, particularly on the right side. Based on these findings, a type IIa+IIc SM deep invasive cancer or type 2 advanced cancer (MP) is suspected.

With non-magnifying NBI, we can discern the vascular pattern of the lesion, particularly on the oral side of the depressed area (Fig. 16.11c). M-NBI examination of this area reveals a positive surface pattern (linear white zone) and markedly dilated abnormal vessels at the lesion margins (Fig. 16.11d). As we approach the lesion center, however, these vessels break up and the vascular density decreases, so this was assessed as a CP type III_B (NICE type 3) (Fig. 16.11e).

This lesion was resected surgically, and the histological findings were of Rb, type 2, moderately differentiated adenocarcinoma, pMP, n (+) (Fig. 16.11f).

16.11.2 NBI Characteristics

This is a typical case of CP type III_B (NICE type 3). Caution is required because sometimes, as in this case, a surface pattern can be discerned even in an advanced cancer.

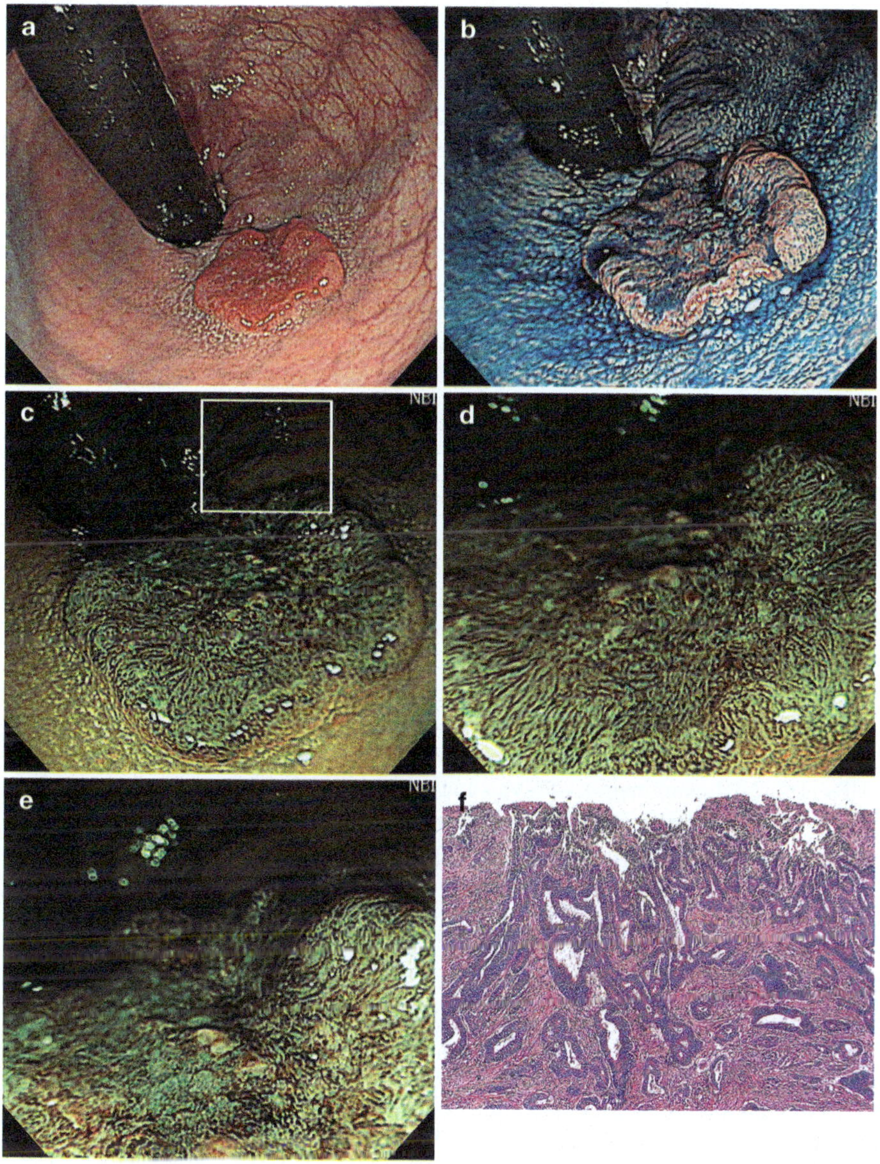

Fig. 16.11 Advanced colorectal cancer

16.12 Sessile Serrated Polyp

Although hyperplastic polyps (HPs) have been considered benign lesions with no malignant potential, in 1990 Longacre and Fenoglio-Preiser identified neoplastic lesions resembling an HP that they named serrated adenomas (SAs) [13]. Since that time, there has been discussion of a possible progression from HP to SA to colorectal cancer, the so-called serrated pathway. In 2003, Torlakovic et al. proposed a division of SAs into two subsets, sessile serrated adenoma/polyp (SSA/P) and traditional serrated adenoma (TSA) [14].

HPs and SSA/Ps were previously classified together under the broader definition of HPs, but the high risk of malignant change in SSA/Ps makes it necessary to differentiate them from the narrowly defined HPs. At present, however, the situation is unclear, with consistent pathological diagnostic criteria also lacking.

16.12.1 Explanation

16.12.1.1 Concerning Diagnosis

As outlined above, at present it is difficult to diagnose SSA/Ps endoscopically. It is possible, however, to distinguish between HPs and SAs to some extent, using magnifying chromoendoscopy.

Using NBI, we can diagnose HPs from the absence of discernible vessels. Fujii et al. proposed dividing SAs into a serrated villous (SV) subtype, with a pinecone-like morphology, and a serrated hyper (SH) subtype, with a similar morphology to HPs [15]. NBI examination of SVs shows vessels with no nonuniformity of diameter within the stroma. However, in almost all SHs, as with HPs, no vessels are seen. It is possible that SVs correspond to TSAs, and SHs to SSA/Ps, but further studies should elucidate this point.

16.12.1.2 Case Study

This case was a large hyperplastic polyp, 13 mm in size. The non-magnifying WLI and chromoendoscopic findings were indicative of HP, with a smooth whitish surface and adherent mucin. Magnifying chromoendoscopic findings showed a type II pit pattern, confirming the diagnosis of HP (Fig. 16.12a–c).

NBI examination was unable to discern any vessels, except a few vessels crossing the lesion (CP type I, NICE type 1) (Fig. 16.12d, e).

This lesion was resected using the EMR method, and histological examination revealed dilated and multibranching crypts, flattening of the crypt bases, and prominent nucleoli, yielding the diagnosis of SSA/P (Fig. 16.12f).

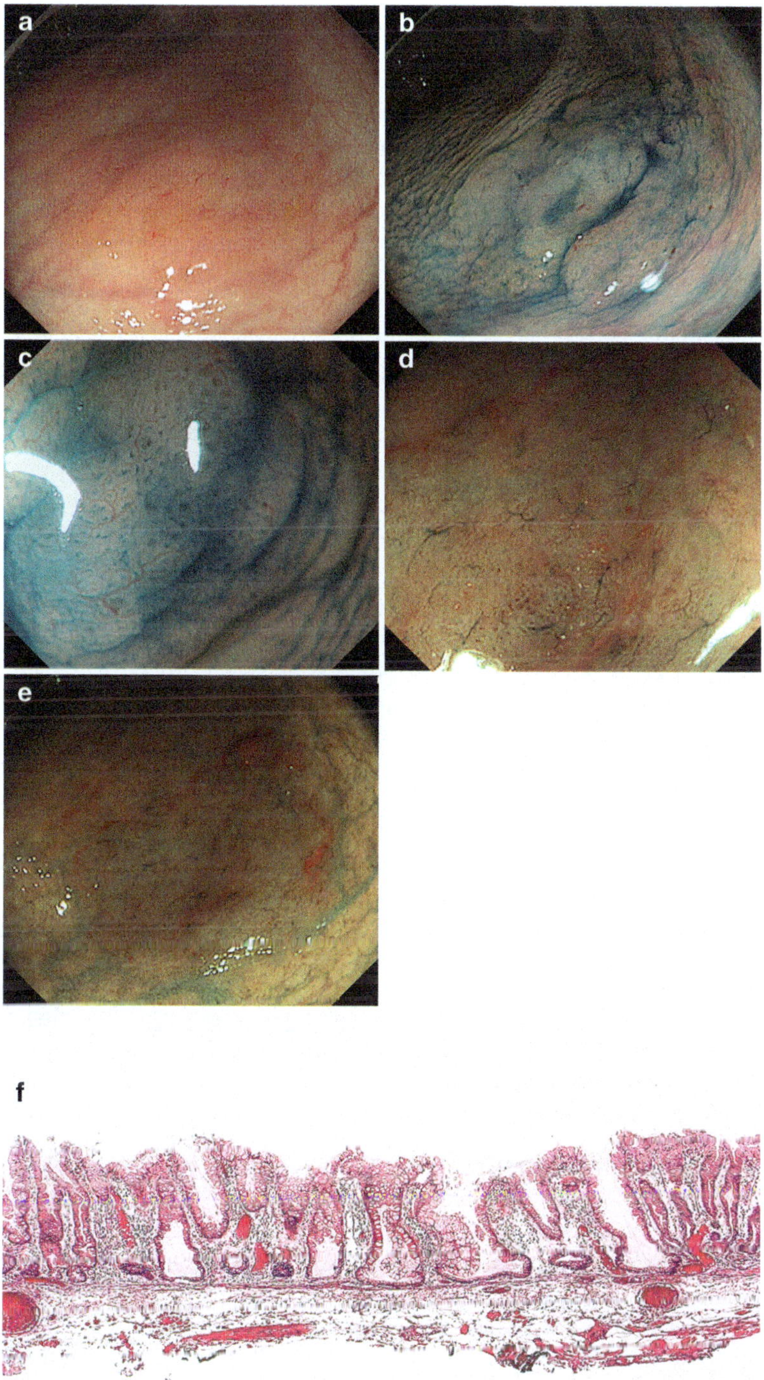

Fig. 16.12 Sessile serrated adenoma/polyp

16.13 Colitic Cancer (Ulcerative Colitis-Related High-Grade Dysplasia) [16, 17]

Seen in patients with long-term ulcerative colitis (UC), UC-related dysplasia/cancer (CC/D) is important as a potentially lethal complication of a benign condition. In Japan, the increasing number of patients with UC, and with long-term disease, has led us to reconsider how surveillance colonoscopies (SCs) should be conducted.

Based on the assumption that CC/D is difficult to visualize endoscopically, SC in Western countries with a large UC patient number has predominantly taken the form of random biopsies, of the order of 4 every 10 cm of bowel. However, doubts over the lack of efficacy of this method, and increased use of chromoendoscopy in recent years, have led to recognition of the usefulness of targeted biopsies using chromoendoscopy and magnified chromoendoscopy. There have been few reports of the benefits of SC using NBI, but it merits further study, and discussion regarding indications and techniques.

16.13.1 Explanation

This case was a 60-year-old female with a 16-year history of pancolitis (UC). During SC in the form of NBI total colonoscopy, a lesion was detected in the sigmoid colon (Fig. 16.13a). Switching over to M-NBI, a neoplastic lesion was suspected from the surface pattern (CP type III_A, NICE type 2) (Fig. 16.13b), and a detailed examination using chromoendoscopy was considered necessary. The protrusions on the oral side of the lesion show a nonneoplastic surface pattern (Fig. 16.13c). Non-magnifying WLI examination reveals nodular protrusions arising from the rough UC-affected background mucosa (Fig. 16.13d).

Autofluorescence imaging (AFI) delineates the oral side protrusions shown in Fig. 16.13c as green in color, confirming their nonneoplastic appearance. Raised lesions suspicious for CC/D are seen as magenta (Fig. 16.13e). Magnifying chromoendoscopic examination of the lesion reveals tubular pits, with a reduced pit density, yielding the diagnosis of CC/D (Fig. 16.13f).

Histological examination of a biopsy specimen revealed UC-related high-grade dysplasia (Fig. 16.13g), and the patient underwent total colectomy. Histological examination of the surgically resected specimen confirmed the diagnosis of UC-related high-grade dysplasia.

16.13.2 NBI Characteristics

Where possible, SC should be performed during endoscopic remission of UC. CC/D often arises in UC background mucosa that is scarred, atrophic, and degenerate. We may see a number of features in background mucosa with these characteristics suggesting the possibility of CC/D. When findings that suggest CC/D are identified using non-magnifying NBI, we should immediately switch over to M-NBI and examine the surface pattern with the aim of determining whether it is a lesion with a high likelihood of CC/D.

In this case, on the oral side of the highly dysplastic lesion was an area of nonneoplastic regenerative hyperplastic changes. Using NBI, we were able to delineate the demarcation line between the two.

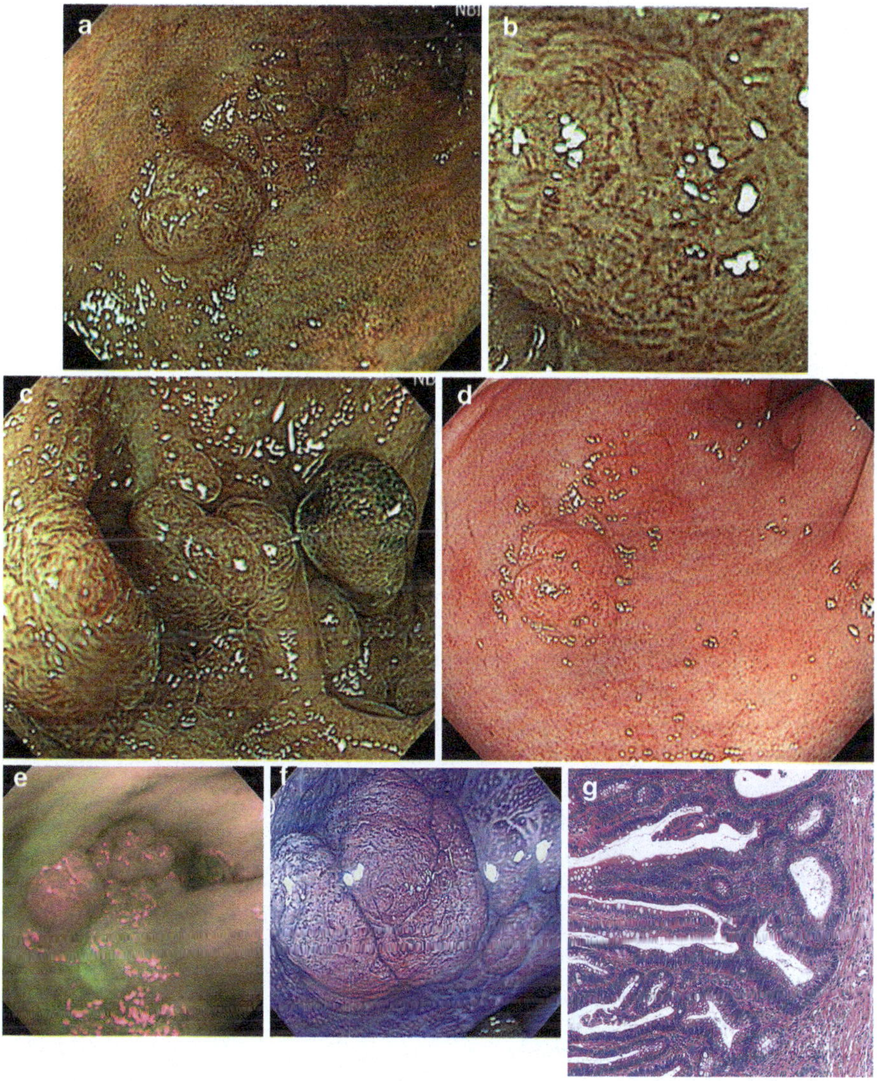

Fig. 16.13 Ulcerative colitis-related high-grade dysplasia

16.14 Colitic Cancer (Ulcerative Colitis-Related Low-Grade Dysplasia) [18, 19]

It is important that, where possible, surveillance colonoscopy (SC) in patients with ulcerative colitis (UC) should be performed during endoscopic remission. This is not only because the risk of post-endoscopic relapse is reduced but also because it allows a more detailed NBI or chromoendoscopic examination, as described below. Furthermore, the likelihood of successful histological differentiation between inflammatory atypia and neoplastic atypia increases, resulting in a more accurate SC procedure overall.

16.14.1 Explanation

This case was a 30-year-old male with an 8-year history of pancolitis (UC). During SC in the form of NBI total colonoscopy, a lesion was detected in the transverse colon (Fig. 16.14a). Switching over to M-NBI, a neoplastic lesion was suspected from the tubular surface pattern (CP type II, NICE type 2) (Fig. 16.14b), and a detailed examination using chromoendoscopy was considered necessary. Non-magnifying WLI examination reveals a superficial elevated lesion arising from within the UC-affected background mucosa with some scarring (Fig. 16.14c). Comparison with Fig. 16.14a shows that more detail is visible with NBI than with WLI. Magnifying chromoendoscopy using indigo carmine dye spraying reveals type III_L pits (Fig. 16.14d). Magnifying chromoendoscopy using crystal violet staining reveals type IV_H-like pits, with a fern leaf morphology and reduced pit density, in one part of the lesion, indicating a high likelihood of CC/D (Fig. 16.14e).

Histological examination of a biopsy specimen revealed UC-related low-grade dysplasia (Fig. 16.14f). Multiple CC/D lesions were detected in other sites, so the patient underwent total colectomy. Histological examination of the surgically resected specimen confirmed the diagnosis of UC-related low-grade dysplasia.

16.14.2 NBI Characteristics

With the application of NBI to SC, we anticipate improved ability to visualize findings associated with a high likelihood of CC/D (lesion detection) and the ability to make a qualitative assessment of any detected lesions. In this case, we can see from a comparison of Fig. 16.14a, c that more detail is visible using NBI. Debate is still controversial concerning detection of discolored CC/D lesions, but most CC/D lesions show red coloration, so visibility is improved as shown in this case.

When, as in this case, type IV_H-like neoplastic pits with a decreased pit density are observed within a UC-affected area, this should be considered a lesion with a high likelihood of CC/D and multiple biopsies taken from the lesion and the surrounding mucosa. Using M-NBI, we cannot perform a qualitative analysis of CC/D lesions with the same degree of confidence as with a sporadic neoplastic lesion, but as with lesion, it can be a useful first step.

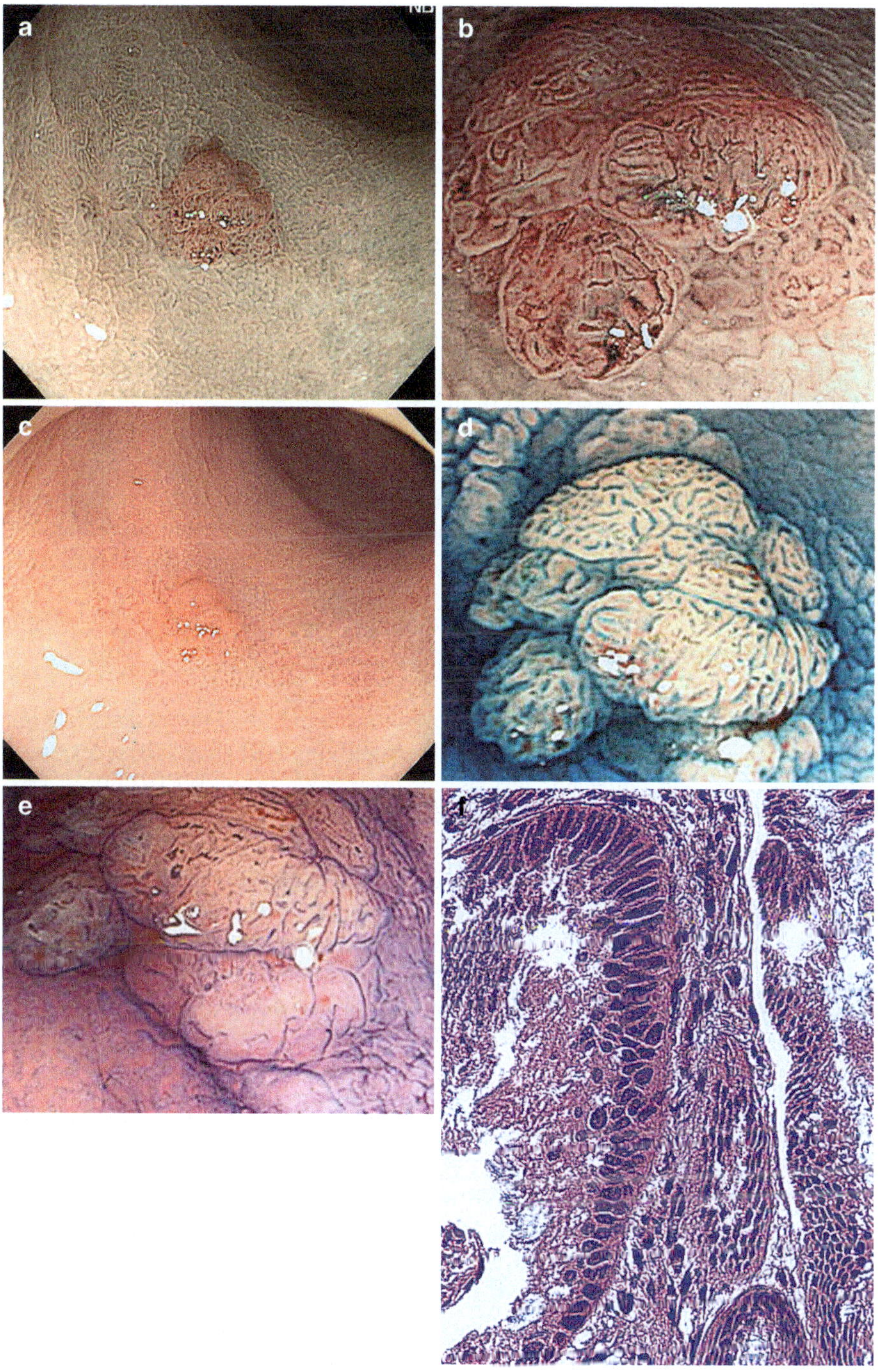

Fig. 16.14 Ulcerative colitis-related low-grade dysplasia

16.15 Familial Adenomatous Polyposis

Familial adenomatous polyposis (FAP) is an autosomal dominant inherited neoplastic condition characterized by numerous adenomas in the gastrointestinal tract, in particular the colon. Endoscopically, it is classified by the number of colorectal polyps, as severe or high density (>1,000), mild or low density (100–1,000), or attenuated (<100).

The main causative gene is the *APC* gene, with abnormalities seen in the *APC* gene in approximately 2/3 of individuals with definite clinical FAP. Of the remaining 1/3, some have been reported to have abnormalities in the autosomal recessive *MYH* gene [20], creating interest in MYH-associated polyposis (MAP).

The incidence of FAP is roughly 1 in 17,000 births. Colorectal cancer is rare before the age of 15, but the onset of malignancy rises steeply after the age of 20, reaching 50 % by the age of 40, and almost all individuals with FAP develop colorectal cancer during their lifetime. Iwama et al. analyzed the age at time of surgery and colorectal cancer in 1,162 patients who underwent surgery, finding that the median age of patients with (1) no colorectal cancer, (2) only early cancer, and (3) advanced cancer was (1) 28 years, (2) 31 years, and (3) 39 years, respectively [21].

16.15.1 Explanation

From a distance, non-magnifying WLI reveals scattered small protrusions 2–3 mm in size (Fig. 16.15a). From a distance, non-magnifying NBI shows these lesions as brownish areas and delineates lesions not discernible using WLI (Fig. 16.15b). M-NBI clearly reveals regular meshed capillary vessels (CP type II, NICE type 2) (Fig. 16.15c) and magnifying chromoendoscopy with indigo carmine dye spraying type IIIL pits (Fig. 16.15d), yielding the diagnosis of adenomas.

The pathohistological findings were of a dense glandular proliferation, with spindle-shaped nuclei, showing no nonuniformity in size, aligned with the basement membrane, so this was diagnosed as low-grade adenoma (Fig. 16.15e: HE stain, low magnification; Fig. 16.15f: high magnification of the area within the blue box in Fig. 16.15e).

16.15.2 NBI Characteristics

In comparison with WLI, more detail is visible with NBI. In particular, small flat lesions are difficult to discern using WLI, but are clearly delineated using NBI. Uraoka et al. reported NBI is particularly useful in detecting flat lesions <5 mm in size [22].

M-NBI revealed regular meshed capillary vessels, the so-called typical type II CP pattern in this lesion.

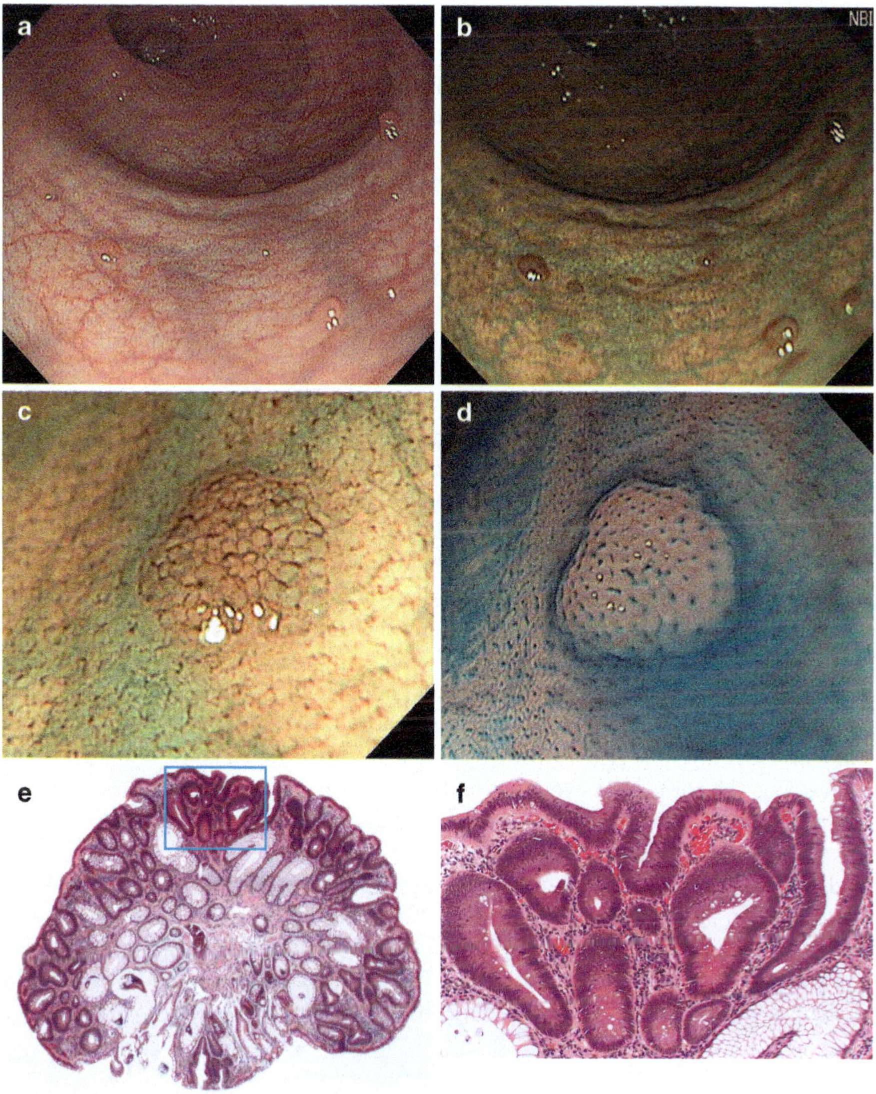

Fig. 16.15 Familial adenomatous polyposis

16.16 Malignant Lymphoma

Colorectal malignant lymphoma is relatively uncommon, accounting for approximately 23.8 % of malignant lymphoma of the gastrointestinal tract and 0.4 % of all malignancies of the lower gastrointestinal tract [23]. It most commonly affects the cecum and rectum. It can present a variety of morphologies: ulcerated, protruded, or diffuse. There are also a variety of histological types, including diffuse large B-cell lymphoma (DLBCL), mucosa-associated lymphoid tissue (MALT) lymphoma, mantle cell lymphoma, and follicular lymphoma.

16.16.1 Explanation

During a colonoscopy, once the cecum has been reached, the scope should be introduced into the terminal ileum. Lymphoid follicles are common in the small intestine, but if there are any that are coarser than their neighbors, or forming aggregations, malignant lymphoma should be suspected and biopsies taken. Lymphoid follicular hyperplasia of the cecum or rectum can also present with multiple small protuberances resembling submucosal tumors. Malignant lymphoma should be suspected in cases with isolated lesions, severe deformation, or central ulceration and biopsies taken.

In this case, we can see a coarse polypoid nodule with a markedly distorted morphology (Fig. 16.16a). Following indigo carmine dye spraying, the surface is smooth with no visible pits. Erosions can be seen on the top of some of the protuberances (Fig. 16.16b). NBI examination does not reveal any vessels on the coarse nodules, but we can see tortuous vessels with relatively uniform diameters on the small protuberances (Fig. 16.16c, d).

Biopsies failed to yield a tissue diagnosis, so polypectomy was performed, in part to obtain a diagnosis. Histological examination revealed a tumor follicle containing a large number of atypical lymphocytes with uniform sizes. Immune staining was CD20 (++), CD5 (−), bcl-1 (−), bcl-2 (++), CD3 (−), and CD10 (+). The diagnosis was follicular lymphoma (Fig. 16.16e, f).

16.16.2 NBI Characteristics

It is difficult to identify any characteristic NBI findings of colorectal malignant lymphoma because of the low number of patients and similar vascular patterns seen in nonneoplastic lymphoid follicles. At present, WLI examination is considered the most effective modality, although we hope to accumulate greater patient numbers.

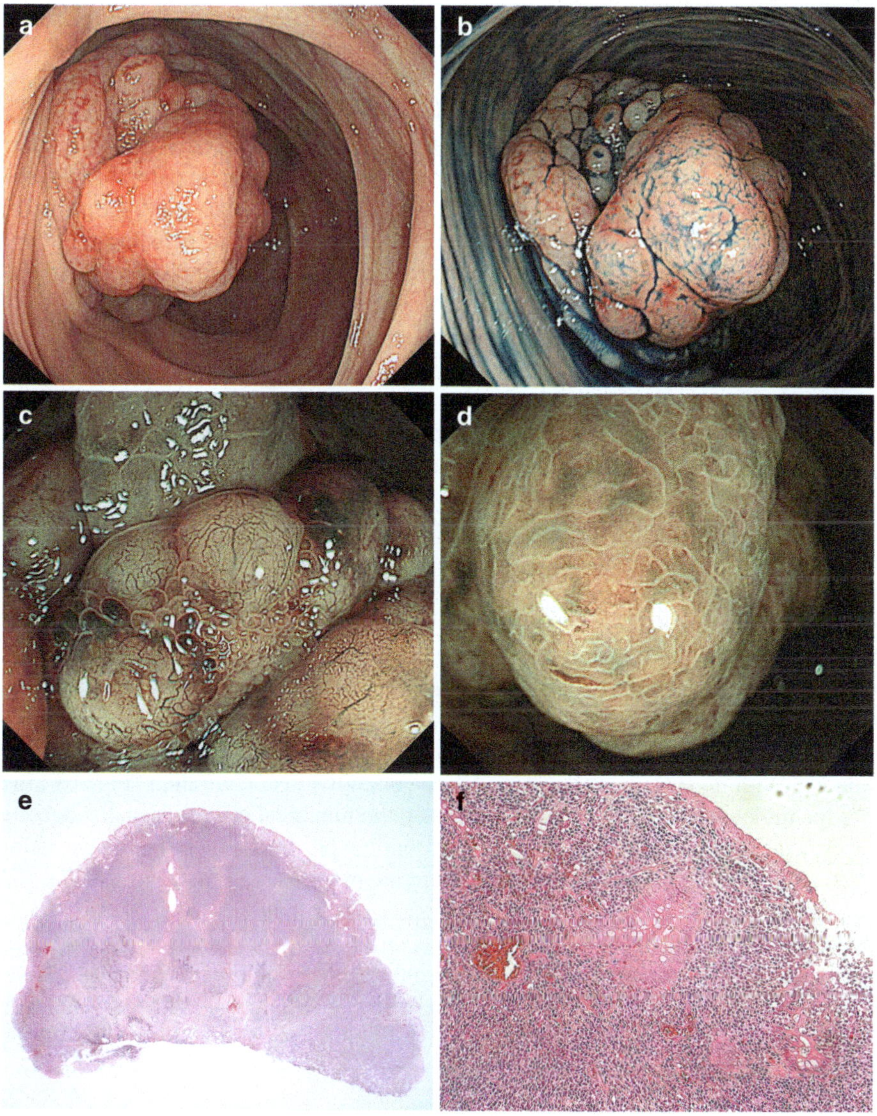

Fig. 16.16 Malignant lymphoma

16.17 Carcinoid Neoplasia

Carcinoid is an overall term for tumors arising from cells that differentiate into neuroendocrine cells. Carcinoid neoplasias do indeed sometimes display a carcinoma-like histological pattern and biological behavior. They are most often benign, or only locally invasive, but some show borderline malignancy, or metastasize, and are treated as malignant tumors. Carcinoid neoplasias usually arise in the gastrointestinal or bronchial mucosa, sites with neuroendocrine cells located in the mucosa. 90 % have their origin in the gastrointestinal tract, in particular the appendix, ileum, and rectum.

Gastrointestinal carcinoids arise from endocrine cells located in the intestinal gland bases and unlike cancers are considered slow-growing tumors with a low degree of atypia and therefore low malignant potential.

Pathohistological examination of biopsy or resected specimens is essential for the diagnosis of carcinoid. When carcinoid is suspected from the HE-stained findings, the diagnosis should be confirmed by additional special staining, including Grimelius staining and immune staining with anti-chromogranin A antibodies.

16.17.1 Explanation

Carcinoid neoplasias are covered in normal mucosa and grow from the deep mucosal layers, extending into the submucosa invasively and expansively [23]. They generally have the macroscopic appearance of non-pedunculated polypoid submucosal tumors, with no surface irregularity, and a yellow-whitish coloration (Fig. 16.17a). As the tumor surface is covered in normal epithelium, oval pits are visualized, but it is difficult to identify capillary vessels surrounding pits on the mucosal surface using NBI (Fig. 16.17b). Indigo carmine dye spraying reveals type I pits (Fig. 16.17c).

Although there are no characteristic vascular morphologies directly attributable to carcinoid on NBI examination, as the tumor grows expansively in the deep mucosa, large vessels in the submucosa compressed by the tumor become visible. These are vessels that were always present in the submucosa and are visualized through the epithelium thinned from compression by the tumor. Accordingly, they are not tumor vessels (neovascularization) and exhibit none of the irregularity seen with tumor vessels, such as nonuniform diameters.

M-WLI clearly delineates thick vessels in the submucosa compressed by the tumor, itself growing expansively in the deep mucosa (Fig. 16.17d). M-NBI delineates the vascular network more clearly, but does not reveal any vessels surrounding the crypts or any irregular vessels (Fig. 16.17e).

Histological examination of this lesion shows compression and thinning of the mucosa by a tumor located in the submucosa (Fig. 16.17f). Narrow cords of fibrous tissue can be seen within the stroma forming a dense follicular structure. In one part it forms pseudoglandular structures, with palisades and ribbonlike structures (Fig. 16.17g).

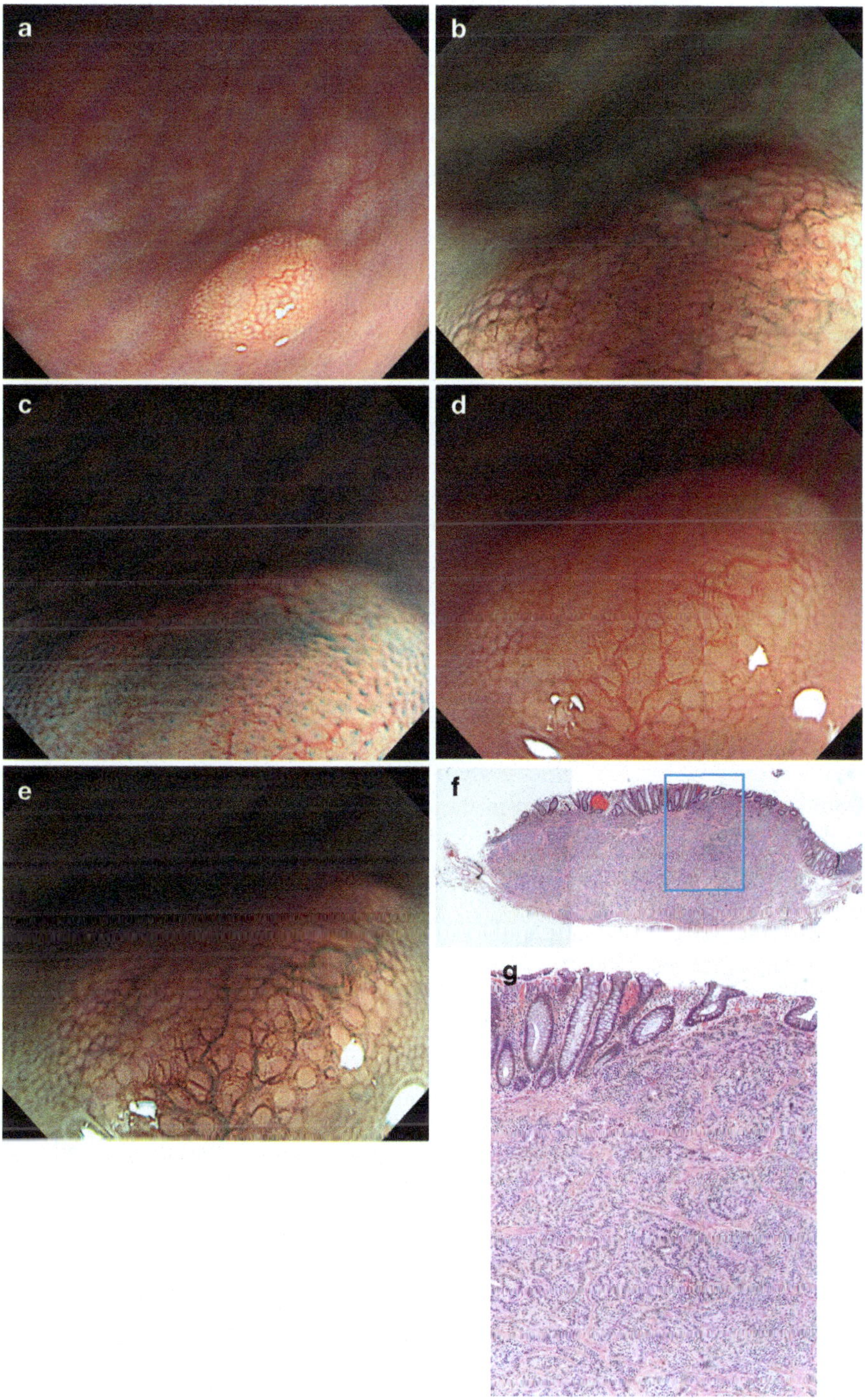

Fig. 16.17 Carcinoid neoplasia

16.18 Anal Condyloma Acuminata

Anal condyloma acuminata are caused by a localized infection with the human papillomavirus (HPV). They are more common in males, with a male to female ratio of 2:1. Onset is usually in young people aged between 20 and 30 years, with an average age in the late 30s. Sexual transmission is common; in particular, anal intercourse is considered to increase the risk of this condition. HIV antibodies are positive in 30 % of patients with anal condyloma acuminata.

The most common symptoms are a palpable lump, itchiness, bleeding, pain, and discharge. Lesions are usually multiple, favoring the skin from the genitals to the perianal area, although single anal lesions are sometimes seen. HPV types 6 and 11, considered low risk for cancer, are the most common cause of anal condyloma acuminata, but infections with high-risk types are also seen, with concomitant risk of malignancy. Malignant change has been reported in 30 % of cases of anal giant condyloma acuminata.

Apart from surgical excision, treatment modalities include cryotherapy, electrocoagulation therapy, CO_2 laser therapy, interferon therapy, interferon therapy, and topical 5FU, bleomycin, or imiquimod. Although surgical excision is said to provide the best cure rates, there have been reports of squamous cell carcinomas of the anal canal 5–10 years following surgical excision, so posttreatment follow-up is needed.

16.18.1 Explanation

Multiple warts are usually seen in the anal canal, upper anus, or perianal area, although single lesions sometimes occur. As they grow larger, some warts flatten out like velvet, others aggregate into a papillary morphology, and others form cauliflower-like protrusions. The most common coloration is a whitish hue. Non-magnifying WLI reveals a papillary or velvety surface structure, with dilated loop-shaped vessels. The cases presented in Fig. 16.18a, b show whitish superficial elevated lesions approximately 20 mm in size extending from the anal canal into the lower rectum (Rb). Their surfaces show papillary and nodular protuberances.

Dye spraying reveals a velvety surface with dilated pits. The lesion is stained by iodine, forming a distinct margin with the surrounding columnar epithelium (Fig. 16.18c). The presence of non-iodine staining areas suggests the possibility of squamous cell carcinoma or severe dysplasia.

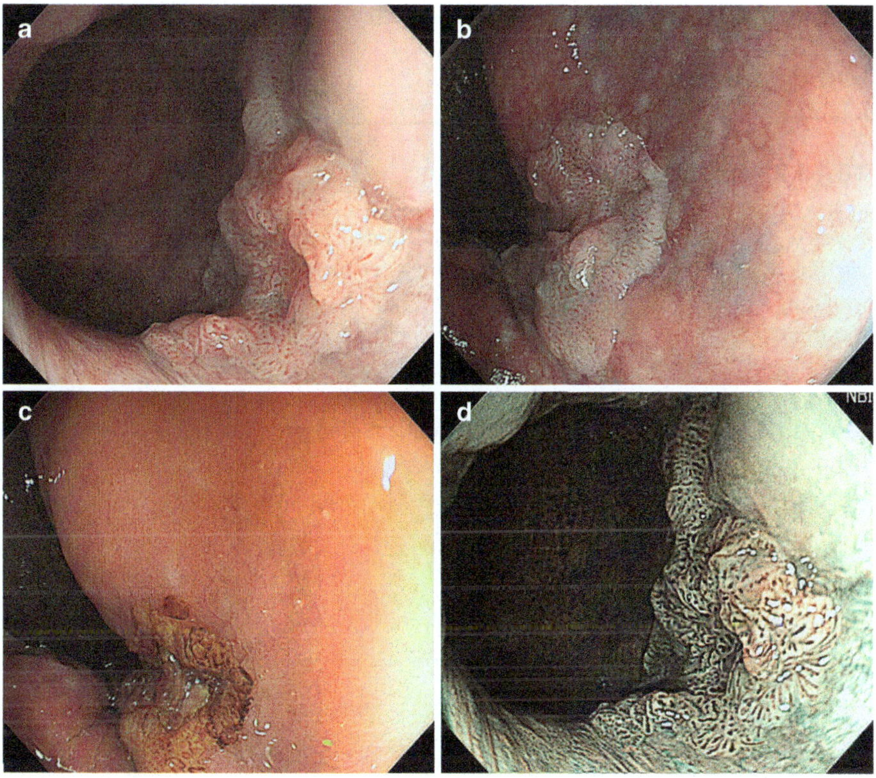

Fig. 16.18 Anal condyloma acuminata

Histological examination of an HE-stained specimen reveals proliferation of stratified squamous epithelium with a papillary morphology, associated with characteristic koilocytosis (Fig. 16.18f).

16.18.2 NBI Characteristics

Even without magnification, NBI reveals dilated brownish vessels on the lesion surface, with the entire lesion somewhat darker brown in coloration than the surrounding mucosa (Fig. 16.18d). M-NBI reveals characteristic vessels that resemble the dilated, elongated, branching intraepithelial papillary capillary loops (IPCLs) seen in esophageal squamous cell carcinomas. Unlike squamous cell carcinomas, however, these vessels have relatively uniform diameters and morphologies. The M-NBI image in Fig. 16.18e shows dilated and elongated loop-shaped vessels and the papillary, velvety surface morphology.

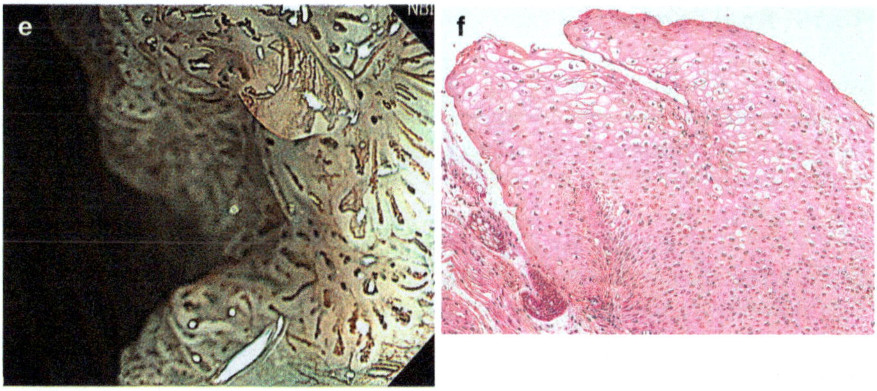

Fig. 16.18 (continued)

16.19 Anal Cancer

Anal cancer is relatively uncommon, only accounting for approximately 1.5 % of gastrointestinal cancers and 4 % of cancers of the lower gastrointestinal tract [25]. However, the incidence of anal cancer has without doubt risen in recent years. Approximately 80 % of anal cancers are squamous cell carcinomas, with many reported to be attributable to human papillomavirus (HPV, in particular HPV-16 and HPV-18) [26]. Almost all patients with anal cancer undergo invasive treatments such as chemotherapy and/or surgical excision, with a 5-year survival rate of 58.0 % [27]. Accordingly, there have been few reports of the NBI findings of anal intraepithelial cancer.

16.19.1 Explanation

Examination of the anal canal is relatively difficult, requiring measures such as retroflexing the scope in the lower rectum and attachment of a transparent hood to the scope tip [28]. Retroflexion of the scope in the lower rectum requires insufflation with sufficient air to fully expand the rectum. On the other hand, attachment of a transparent hood allows us to examine the rectum with relative ease.

In this case, we are unable to identify any definite abnormalities with retroflexed non-magnifying WLI examination (Fig. 16.19a). Non-magnifying NBI reveals a brownish area (Fig. 16.19b). M-NBI reveals dilated tortuous vessels that resemble the intraepithelial papillary capillary loops (IPCLs) seen in the esophagus [29] (Fig. 16.19c, d). Iodine staining of the same area delineates the lesion as a nonstaining area, with distinct margins (Fig. 16.19e). A local (perianal) resection was performed.

Histological examination revealed an intraepithelial tumor with severe atypia, with one area of squamous cell carcinoma, also confined to the epithelium (Fig. 16.19f).

16.19.2 NBI Characteristics

As with the esophagus, detection of a brownish area is important in NBI examination of the anal canal. When a brownish area is identified, we should immediately change over to M-NBI to determine whether any vascular irregularities are present. As with IPCLs in the esophagus, we examine the vessels for dilatation, tortuosity, nonuniformity of diameter, and nonuniform morphology. If any of these findings are present, anal cancer should be suspected and biopsies taken.

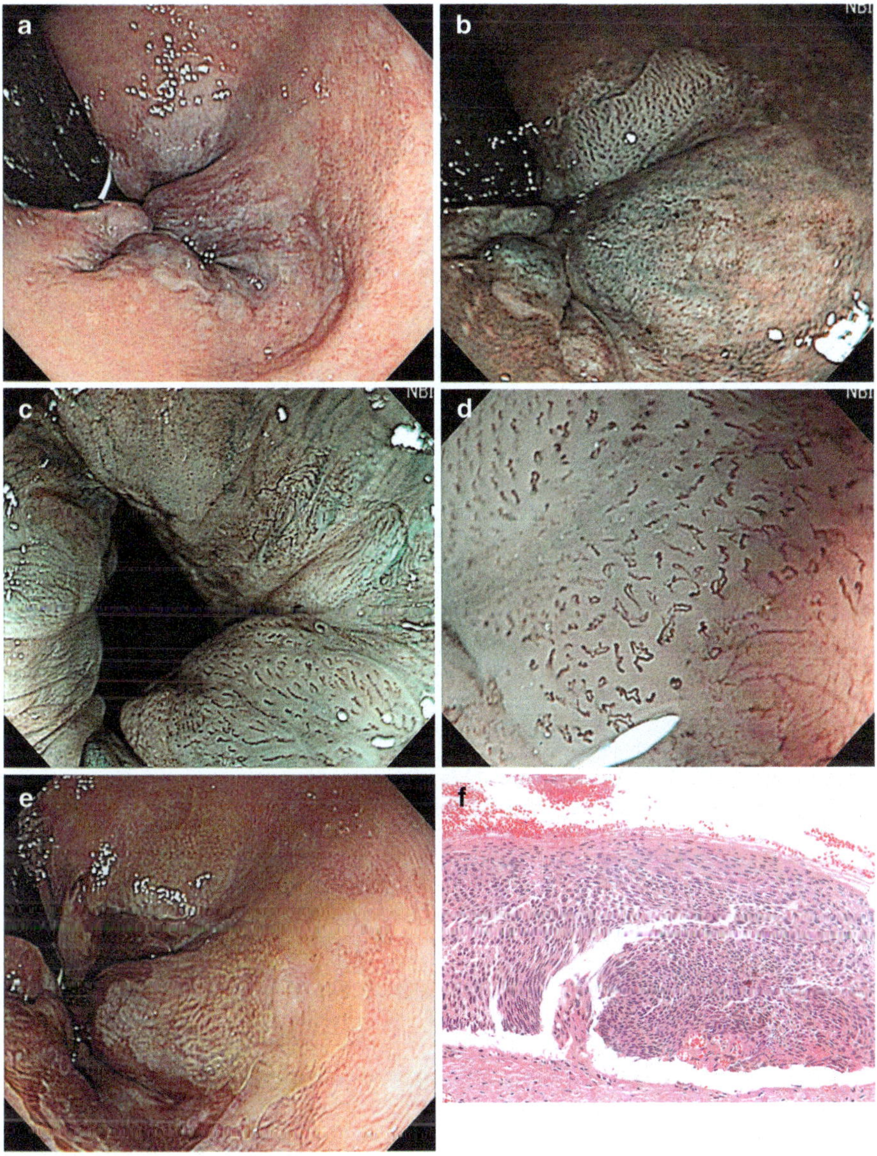

Fig. 16.19 Anal squamous cell carcinoma

Acknowledgments We thank Dr. Hidenobu Watanabe, Professor Emeritus at Niigata University, Special Consultant at the PCL Pathology and Cytology Laboratories, who kindly provided the pathohistological images.

References

1. Sano Y, et al: Dig Endosc 18 (Suppl): S44–S51, 2006
2. Ikematsu H, et al: BMC Gastoenterol **10**: 33, 2010
3. Horimatsu T, et al: Gastrointestinal Endoscopy **65**: AB270, 2007
4. Fukuzawa M, et al: World J Gasroenterol **16**: 1727–1734, 2010
5. Machida H, et al: Endoscopy **36**: 1094–1098, 2004
6. Sano Y, et al: Gastrointest Endosc **67**: 278–283, 2009
7. Katagiri A, et al: Aliment Pharmacol Ther **27**: 1269–1274, 2008
8. Okuno T et al.: Early Colorectal Cancer 8: 21–27, 2004
9. Kudo S: Colorectal pit pattern diagnosis. Igaku Shoin, 1993
10. Kudo S et al.: Stomach and Intestine 29: 45–54, 1994
11. Ito M: Early Colorectal Cancer 2: 15–23, 1998
12. Ikematsu H et al.: Early Colorectal Cancer 12: 389–394, 2008
13. Longacre TA, et al: Am J Surg Pathol **14**: 524–537, 1990
14. Torlakovic E, et al: Am J Surg Pathol **27**: 65–81, 2003
15. Fujii et al.: Stomach and Intestine **34**: 1653–1664, 1999
16. Niwa H (sup. ed.): Image-Enhanced Endoscopy Atlas. Japan Medical Center, 2010
17. Tanaka N (ed.): Upskilling in Colonoscopy (Diagnosis), Chugai Igakusha, 2010
18. Watanabe K et al.: GI Research 17: 236–240, 2009
19. Watanabe K et al.: Stomach and Intestine 43: 1320–1324, 2008
20. Sieber OM, et al: N Engl J Med **348**: 791–799, 2003
21. Iwama T, et al: Int J Clin Oncol **9**: 308–316, 2004
22. Uraoka T, et al: J Gastroenterol Hepatol **23**: 1810–1815, 2008
23. Iwashita A: Stomach and Intestine 30: 869, 1995
24. Nakamura S (ed.): Interpretation of pathology specimens from the gastrointestinal tract. Japan Medical Center, 1999
25. Clark MA, et al: Lancet Oncol **5**: 149–157, 2004
26. Bilimoria KY, et al: Dis Colon Rectum **52**: 624–631, 2009
27. Hoots BE, et al: Int J Cancer **124**: 2375–2383, 2009
28. Masushita M, et al: Endoscopy **30**: 444–447, 1998
29. Yoshida T, et al: Gastroentest Endosc **59**: 288–295, 2004

Index

M. Muto et al. (eds.), *Atlas of Endoscopy with Narrow Band Imaging*,
DOI 10.1007/978-4-431-54243-8

The manufacturer's authorised representative in the EU is Springer
Nature Customer Service Centre GmbH, Europaplatz 3, 69115 Heidelberg,
Germany. If you have any concerns regarding our products, please
contact ProductSafety@springernature.com

Printed and bound by CPI Group (UK) Ltd, Croydon, CR0 4YY
22/09/2026
02220946-0012